SpringerWienNewYork

Acta Neurochirurgica
Supplements

Editor: H.-J. Steiger

New Trends of Surgery for Stroke and its
Perioperative Management

Edited by
Y. Yonekawa, Y. Sakurai, E. Keller, and T. Tsukahara

Acta Neurochirurgica
Supplement 94

SpringerWienNewYork

Prof. Dr. Yasuhiro Yonekawa
PD. Dr. Emanuela Keller
University Hospital, Zurich, Switzerland

Dr. Yoshiharu Sakurai
Department of Neurosurgery, Sendai National Hospital, Sendai, Japan

Dr. Tetsuya Tsukahara
Department of Neurosurgery, Kyoto National Hospital, Kyoto, Japan

© 2005 Springer-Verlag/Wien
Printed in Austria
SpringerWienNewYork is a part of Springer Science+Business Media
springeronline.com

Typesetting: Asco Typesetters, Hong Kong
Printing and Binding: Druckerei Theiss GmbH, 9431 St. Stefan, Austria, www.theiss.at

Printed on acid-free and chlorine-free bleached paper

SPIN: 11377313

Library of Congress Control Number: 2005924436

With partly coloured Figures

ISSN 0065-1419
ISBN-10 3-211-24338-0 SpringerWienNewYork
ISBN-13 978-3-211-24388-1 SpringerWienNewYork

Preface

In the last years progress has been made in stroke treatment. In July 2004 specialists in neurosurgery, neuroradiology, neurology and neurointensive care discussed recent trends at the 2nd Swiss Japanese Joint Conference on Cerebral Stroke Surgery held in Zurich, Switzerland. Prof. Dr. Y. Yonekawa, Zurich and Prof. D. Y. Sakurai, Sendai were the presidents of the conference. New concepts were worked out during the conference and are published in this volume. The book starts with the topic intracranial aneurysms, discussing microsurgical and endovascular treatment modalities, as well as new surgical approaches. Further chapters deal with the management of unruptured aneurysms and with subarachnoid hemorrhage. Practical guidelines for vasospasm treatment are given. Together with contributions about arteriovenous malformations and fistulas, cerebral revascularization techniques and surgery related to the intracranial venous system a comprehensive overview about stroke surgery is given with an interdisciplinary approach. The book should be of interest for all specialists involved in therapy of cerebrovascular disease. The editors extend their gratitude to the many contributors and to all those who participated in the conference. Publication of the proceedings is partially supported by Research Fund for Cardiovascular diseases from Japanese Ministry of Health, Labour and Welfare; Assessment of the quality of medical care in cardio- and cerebrovascular diseases and the principal national hospitals.

Y. Yonekawa, Y. Sakurai, E. Keller, and T. Tsukahara

Contents

Listed in Current Contents

Intracranial aneurysms

Acta Neurochir (2005) [Suppl] 94: 3–6
© Springer-Verlag 2005
Printed in Austria

Microsurgical clipping of cerebral aneurysms after the ISAT Study

M. Niemelä[1], **T. Koivisto**[2], **L. Kivipelto**[1], **K. Ishii**[1], **J. Rinne**[2], **A. Ronkainen**[2], **R. Kivisaari**[1], **H. Shen**[1], **A. Karatas**[1], **M. Lehecka**[1], **J. Frösen**[1], **A. Piippo**[1], **J. Jääskeläinen**[2], and **J. Hernesniemi**[1]

[1] Department of Neurosurgery, University Hospital Helsinki, Helsinki, Finland
[2] Department of Neurosurgery, University Hospital Kuopio, Kuopio, Finland

"The arduous work of countless researchers has already thrown much darkness on the subject, and if they continue, we shall soon know nothing at all about it"
Mark Twain

The ISAT Study nails low case load microsurgery of cerebral aneurysms

This landmark study [9] – somewhat Twainian at first glance – sets the stage for future microsurgery in cerebral aneurysms and SAH. *The ISAT Study does not nail microsurgery – it will nail microsurgery in low case load neurosurgical centers and in inexperienced hands.* In future neurovascular centers, exovascular and endovascular surgeons are forced to support each other by having the full responsibility over the population in a defined geographical area. Exosurgeons will become far more experienced – less in number but not the last Mohicans.

Population based treatment of cerebral aneurysms and SAH

In the national health ministries, it is wise to remember when deciding on the guidelines and facilities for endosurgery and exosurgery that aneurysmal SAH is a dismally deadly disease when treated with full population responsibility. One third of patients present with a large haematoma or severe hydrocephalus necessitating immediate surgery. Mortality and morbidity figures are unattractive when the treatment center functions as primary imaging center and accepts all patients at ultra early phase to prevent rebleeding. Selection and delayed aneurysm occlusion ensure low percentages of management morbidity and mortality – how about the patients who die of acute rebleeding [7] or haematoma and do not get a chance of decent recovery?

Kuopio and Helsinki Aneurysm Registries

Aneurysmal SAH is particularly frequent in Finland. There is a linkage to 19q13.3 in Finnish aneurysm families [17, 20] but the interplay of genetic and acquired risks [10] remains to be solved. The Kuopio and Helsinki Aneurysm Registries (a) support clinical trials [12, 13, 19], (b) collect basic clinical data [5, 6, 16], (c) characterize aneurysm families and collect blood samples [17, 20], and (d) collect aneurysm walls resected after clipping of the neck [4]. The first published prospective randomised study – well before ISAT – compared the outcome with acutely ruptured aneurysm after coiling or clipping at the Kuopio University Hospital in eastern Finland in 1995–1997 [11–13, 19, 21]. Of the 199 patients (≤ 75 years, ≤ 72 hours from bleeding), only 109 (55%) were randomizable either to endovascular occlusion or to exovascular occlusion – e.g., 37 patients were excluded because of haematoma or mass effect, and 33 because of aneurysm morphology unsuitable for endovascular occlusion [11].

Cellular and molecular biology of the cerebral aneurysm wall is poorly known

Saccular cerebral artery aneurysms are not just pressurized blebs that threaten to leak. *The cellular and molecular biology of the aneurysm wall is poorly under-*

stood because aneurysm sacs have not been resected for research purposes after clipping of the neck. A study of 24 unruptured and 42 ruptured aneurysm walls from the Helsinki Aneurysm Registry and Biomedicum Helsinki showed that the wall becomes unstable before rupture, showing proliferation, apoptosis, intimal hyperplasia, inflammatory cell infiltration, and thrombosis lining the lumen [4]. Consequently, non-invasive microneuroimaging methods are called for to identify aneurysms prone to leak because most aneurysm will not leak ever [8]. Gene expression profiling and proteome analysis of the wall will guide future development of both endovascular and exovascular occlusive techniques.

Successful endovascular occlusion is a wonder of nature – but is it permanent?

Exovascular occlusion of the aneurysm neck by clipping is hydrodynamically effective but it takes craniotomy and microneurovascular dissection to get the job done. Endovascular occlusion is hydrodynamically demanding. The occlusive material must stay in the lumen to induce and guide the fibrotizing wall reaction – with recruitment of circulating cells – to occlude the lumen and the entire base. Arteries adjacent to the aneurysm base must remain patent which further complicates the design of endovascular instrumentation. It is a wonder of nature that mechanical filling of the lumen with metal coils ever results in smooth re-arterialization over the occluded aneurysm orifice. Successful endovascular occlusion owes to the immense maintenance and healing capacity of the cerebral artery wall, the biology of which is incompletely understood. *Angiographically complete occlusion may fail in the long run which necessitates repeated angiographic follow up, a safety protocol that requires a lot of DSA and endosurgeon capacity at the moment.*

Exosurgery vs. endosurgery

In unselected aneurysm populations, e.g. in the total of 400 annual cases of Helsinki and Kuopio, in about 50% the aneurysm's anatomy or the patient's arteries will allow satisfactory endovascular occlusion. Exosurgery – in our opinion – is preferable at present in the following instances:

– large or giant aneurysm
– very small aneurysm

– wide base aneurysm
– large aneurysmal haematoma or severe hydrocephalus
– severely atherosclerotic or tortuous cerebral arteries

Endosurgery of very small, large, and wide base aneurysms will improve with technical development but not at all exclusive of exosurgery.

Restorative exosurgery after failed endosurgery is difficult

Failure in endovascular occlusion is more common than in clipping. Endovascular failure may call for restorative exosurgery in the acute phase (failed occlusion of aneurysm, rupture of aneurysm, occlusion of major artery), or in the long run (failed occlusion). Clipping of the aneurysm neck after failed coiling or stenting is difficult with the risk of parent artery damage and occlusion. Coils may project into the parent artery or into the brain tissue, e.g. into the brain stem from basilar tip or trunk aneurysms. Fibrotizing wall may engulf coils already within two weeks which supports early restorative surgery when coil material has to be removed. However, restorative exosurgery in acute SAH is particularly difficult because brain is swollen and affected by SAH. The overall situation may call for high-flow bypass surgery [18] – a further indication to keep exosurgery running. The stop of low-flow bypass surgery in the 1980's – inefficient in the EC/IC Bypass Study [3] but now under re-evaluation [15] – eroded neurovascular anastomosis skills that have to be acquired again.

Technical aspects of exovascular aneurysm occlusion

In experienced hands, most aneurysms can be ligated quickly and permanently [2] – in a bloodless field with gentle techniques, minimal or no brain retraction, intact vascular anatomy, and minimal or no skull base manipulation. The repertoire should include the following:

– careful opening and closure – preferably under the operating microscope from skin to skin
– slack brain achieved by opening the lamina terminalis or by frontal ventriculostomy
– avoidance of the use of brain retractors
– sharp dissection rather than blunt dissection
– removal of thrombotic tissue from large aneurysms

- speed of action to avoid ischaemic deficits when using temporary clips
- moulding of the aneurysm base with bipolar coagulation when necessary
- reconstruction of the parent arteries with clips when included in the base of aneurysm
- dissection and resection of the aneurysm sac to ensure perfect clip position after clipping
- intraoperative angiography in large and giant aneurysms
- arteriotomy and thrombectomy of major cerebral arteries
- both high-flow and low-flow bypass techniques

Exosurgery training

Comprehensive skills to clip most aneurysms and to perform intracranial arteriotomies and anastomoses are not easily acquired. Less neurosurgeons will take the track with the advent of endosurgery [14]. It takes a lot of passionate work and the learning curve is not short – in the senior author's (JH) hands, the operative time has dropped below one hour in most cases from two hours a decade ago. Taking digital high quality video clips and discussing them with others is extremely healthy – leading exosurgeons should produce comprehensive video libraries and make them widely available. Leading exosurgeons – like concert pianists – may trace back master-apprentice or senior-junior lineages, with professor Yasargil affecting them all [22]. Professor Yasargil emphasizes (a) profound knowledge of microneurosurgical anatomy acquired in cadaveric laboratories [1], and (b) gentle handling of cerebral arteries and veins acquired by performing microvascular anastomoses in rats – vessels of mice are particularly educative. Delicate endomicroscopes and instrumentations are already being developed, but exosurgeons are still married to the dinosauric exomicroscope. The practice of using a mouth-controlled microscope from skin to skin – freeing both hands to operative work – greatly helps to tame the beast.

CT angiography saves time and money

The use of DSA might have biased the ISAT result as the mean allocation-to-treatment interval was 1.1 days in the endovascular group as against unbelievable 1.7 days in the microsurgical group. In acute SAH, CT angiography as the first imaging method spares time and the patient. With ultrarapid CTA, aneurysm patients can be transferred within one hour after their SAH to the exosurgery room [4] or the endosurgery DSA room – or to the future exo-endo-surgery suite. *The problem of coil and clip artefacts in CTA has to be vigorously solved* – present titanium clips may still obscure postoperative CTA. Future refinement of CTA may allow detailed verification of (a) the immediate post clipping anatomy in the aneurysm region, and (b) the follow up for re-filling after endovascular occlusion.

Future neurovascular center

Competent exovascular and endovascular surgeons should form neurovascular teams to discuss and tailor an individual treatment for each patient, including aneurysm patients. One center with a team of five to six surgeons – exosurgeons and endosurgeons working together – could easily occlude all aneurysms diagnosed in Finland per year – some 600 patients. However, SAH patients require a lot treatment before and after the actual imaging and occlusion – taking few hours at most – of the aneurysms. One national center is not conceivable in Finland because of long transfer distances but could be practical in small densely populated nations.

Conclusions

1. Only specialized neurovascular exosurgeons should continue open aneurysm surgery.
2. Competent exovascular and endovascular surgeons should collaborate in population based neurovascular centers, discussing and tailoring an individual treatment for each patient, including aneurysm patients.
3. The cellular and molecular biology of the aneurysm wall as well as the interplay of genetic and environmental riks factors should be elucidated. Biological prevention – avoidance of smoking as a prime example – will improve management results far more than any endovascular or exovascular mechanical approach.

References

1. Aboud E, Al-Mefty O, Yasargil MG (2002) New laboratory model for neurosurgical training that simulates live surgery. J Neurosurg 97: 1367–1372
2. Drake CG, Peerless SJ, Hernesniemi JA (1996) Surgery of vertebrobasilar aneurysms. London, Ontario Experience on 1767 patients. Springer, Wien New York

3. Failure of extracranial-intracranial arterial bypass to reduce the risk of ischemic stroke. Results of an international randomized trial. The EC/IC Bypass Study Group (1985) N Engl J Med 313: 1191–1200

4. Frösen J, Piippo A, Paetau A, Kangasniemi M, Niemelä M, Pyy I, Hernesniemi J, Jääskeläinen J (2004) Remodeling of saccular cerebral artery aneurysm wall is associated with rupture. Histological analysis of 24 unruptured and 42 ruptured cases. Stroke 35: 2287–2293

5. Hernesniemi J, Vapalahti M, Niskanen M, Kari A, Luukkonen M (1992) Saccular aneurysms of the distal anterior cerebral artery and its branches. Neurosurgery 31: 994–999

6. Hernesniemi J, Vapalahti M, Niskanen M, Kari A, Luukkonen M, Puranen M, Saari T, Rajpar M (1993) One-year outcome in early aneurysm surgery: a 14 years experience. Acta Neurochir (Wien) 122: 1–10

7. Hillman J, Fridriksson S, Nilsson O, Yu Z, Saveland H, Jakobsson KE (2002) Immediate administration of tranexamic acid and reduced incidence of early rebleeding after aneurysmal subarachnoid hemorrhage: a prospective randomized study. J Neurosurg 97: 771–778

8. International Study of Unruptured Aneurysm Investigators (1998) Unruptured intracranial aneurysms – risk of rupture and risks of surgical intervention. N Engl J Med 3339: 1725–1733

9. International Subarachnoid Aneurysm Trial (ISAT) Collaborative Group (2002): International Subarachnoid Aneurysm Trial (ISAT) of neurosurgical clipping versus endovascular coiling in 2145 patients with ruptured intracranial aneurysms: a randomized trial. The Lancet 360: 1267–1274

10. Juvela S, Porras M, Poussa K (2000) Natural history of unruptured intracranial aneurysms: probability of and risk factors for aneurysm rupture. J Neurosurg 93: 379–387

11. Koivisto T (2002) Prospective outcome study of aneurysmal subarachnoid hemorrhage (PhD Thesis). Kuopio University Publications D Medical Sciences 284. 2002. 140p. ISBN 951-781-884-X, ISSN 1235-0303 (http://www.uku.fi/tutkimus/vaitokset/2002/isbn951-781-884-X.pdf)

12. Koivisto T, Vanninen R, Hurskainen H, Saari T, Hernesniemi J, Vapalahti M (2000) Outcomes of early endovascular versus surgical treatment of ruptured cerebral aneurysms: a prospective randomized study. Stroke 31: 2369–2377

13. Koivisto T, Vanninen E, Vanninen R, Kuikka J, Hernesniemi J, Vapalahti M (2002) Cerebral perfusion before and after endovascular or surgical treatment of acutely ruptured cerebral aneurysms: a 1-year prospective follow-up study. Neurosurgery 51: 312–325

14. Lindsay KW (2003) The impact of the International Subarachnoid Aneurysm Treatment Trial (ISAT) on neurosurgical practice. Acta Neurochir (Wien) 145: 97–99

15. Neff KW, Horn P, Dinter D, Vajkoczy P, Schmiedek P, Duber C. (2004) Extracranial-intracranial arterial bypass surgery improves total brain blood supply in selected symptomatic patients with unilateral internal carotid artery occlusion and insufficient collateralization. Neuroradiology Jul 29

16. Rinne J, Hernesniemi J (1993) De novo aneurysms: special multiple aneurysms. Neurosurgery 33: 981–985

17. Ronkainen A, Hernesniemi J, Puranen M, Niemitukia L, Vanninen R, Ryynanen M, Kuivaniemi H, Tromp G (1997) Familial intracranial aneurysms. Lancet 349: 380–384

18. Streefkerk HJ, van der Zwan A, Verdaasdonk RM, Beck HJ, Tulleken CA (2003) Cerebral revascularization (review). Adv Tech Stand Neurosurg 28: 145–225

19. Vanninen R, Koivisto T, Saari T, Hernesniemi J, Vapalahti M (1999) Ruptured intracranial aneurysms: acute endovascular treatment with electrolytically detachable coils – a prospective randomized study. Radiology 211: 325–336

20. van der Voet M, Olson J, Kuivaniemi H, Dudek D, Skunca M, Ronkainen A, Niemelä M, Jääskeläinen J, Hernesniemi J, Helin K, Leinonen E, Biswas M, Tromp G (2004) Intracranial aneurysms in Finnish families: confirmation of linkage and refinement of the interval to chromosome 19q13.3. Am J Human Genet 74: 564–571

21. Yaşargil MG (2002) Reflections on the Thesis "Prospective Outcome Study of Aneurysmal Subarachnoid Hemorrhage" of Dr Timo Koivisto. Kuopio University Publications D Medical Sciences 284B. 51 p. ISBN 951-780-338-9, ISSN 1235-0303 (http://www.uku.fi/tutkimus/vaitokset/2002/isbn951-780-338-9.pdf)

22. Yaşargil MG: Microneurosurgery, Volumes I–IV in 1982–1997

Correspondence: Juha Hernesniemi, Department of Neurosurgery, Helsinki University Central Hospital, Topeliuksenkatu 5, 00260 Helsinki, Finland. e-mail: juha.hernesniemi@hus.fi

Acta Neurochir (2005) [Suppl] 94: 7–9
© Springer-Verlag 2005
Printed in Austria

Endovascular treatment for elderly patients with ruptured aneurysm

K. Sugiu, K. Tokunaga, K. Watanabe, W. Sasahara, M. Tagawa, N. Tamesa, S. Ono, K. Onoda, and I. Date

Department of Neurological Surgery, Okayama University Medical School, Okayama, Japan

Summary

We report our results of endovascular treatment for elderly patients with ruptured aneurysm and discuss the indication for treatment. One hundred and thirty four consecutive patients with ruptured aneurysm treated in our institute during the last 4 years were retrospectively evaluated. Fifty eight patients were included in group A (over 70 years old), and 76 patients in group B (under 69 years old). In both groups, the outcome was strongly related to the preoperative Hunt & Kosnik grade. However, significant risk factors (i.e. pneumonia, rupture of extracranial aneurysm) which make prognosis poor were more common in group A. Group A showed poor outcome in grade III patients, although there were no outcome differences between the two groups in patients of other grades. Endovascular treatment for elderly patients with ruptured aneurysms seemed to be useful. Their outcome was strongly related to their preoperative condition. General risk factors should be evaluated before treatment, especially in elderly patients. Patients with low Hunt & Kosnik grade seem to be most suitable for endovascular treatment. On the other hand, outcome of patients with poor preoperative grade was worse despite the less invasive nature of endovascular treatment. An improvement of outcome in grade III patients is desirable.

Keywords: Cerebral aneurysm; rupture; subarachnoid hemorrhage; elderly patient; coil embolization; endovascular treatment.

Introduction

Surgical treatment of ruptured cerebral aneurysms in elderly patients is difficult, and their prognosis is worse as compared to younger patients [4]. Endovascular treatment using Guglielmi Detachable Coil (GDC) is an important alternative in the treatment of cerebral aneurysms [1, 3]. We report our results of endovascular treatment in elderly patients with ruptured aneurysm and discuss the indication for treatment.

Materials and methods

From January 2000 to March 2004, 182 consecutive patients with cerebral aneurysm, treated with endovascular embolization using GDC in our institute, were retrospectively evaluated. Of these 134 patients with ruptured aneurysm were treated at acute stage of subarachnoid hemorrhage. They were divided into two groups according to their age at onset. Group A included patients older than 70 years and group B included those who were younger than 69 years. Several factors such as preoperative condition (Hunt & Kosnik grade), complications, and outcome (Glasgow Outcome Scale: GOS) were retrospectively evaluated.

Results

Group A (>70 years) included 58 patients (Male : Female = 14:44), and group B (<69 years) included 76 patients (Male : Female = 34:42). Their mean age was 78.6 (range 70–99) years in group A, and 53.9 (range 23–68) years in group B. Location of aneurysms is shown in Fig. 1. The relationship between preoperative Hunt & Kosnik grade and GOS is demonstrated in Fig. 2. Patients' outcome was strongly related to their preoperative condition in the two groups. Group A showed poor outcome in grade III patients as compared to group B, but there were no outcome differences between both groups in other grade patients.

Poor outcome in group A patients was attributable to initial brain damage in 7 patients, pneumonia or respiratory failure in 3 patients, bleeding from extracranial aneurysm in 2 patients (abdominal aorta aneurysm and splenic aneurysm), rebleeding from embolized aneurysm in 2 patients, multiple organ failure in 1 patient, liver failure in 1 patient, and vasospasm in 1 patient. Poor outcome in group B patients was attributable to initial brain damage in 19 patients, rebleeding from embolized aneurysm in 2 patients, bleeding from another cerebral aneurysm in 1 patient, and vasospasm in 1 patient.

Both groups showed the same number of complications, which included rebleeding from embolized

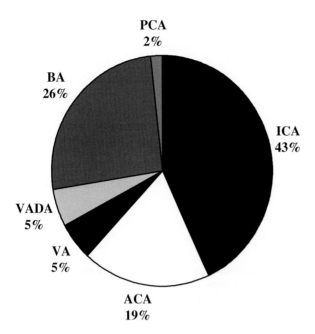

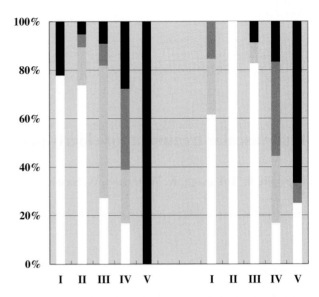

Fig. 2. Preoperative Hunt & Kosnik grade and outcome (Glasgow outcome scale) (left; group A, right; group B). ■ D; ▨ SD; ▨ MD; ☐ GR

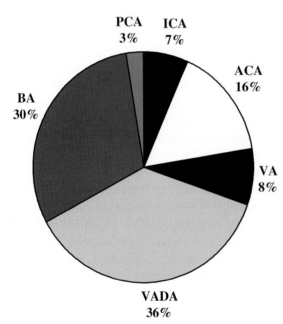

Fig. 1. Location of aneurysms (upper; group A, lower; group B)

aneurysm in two patients, cerebral infarction in two patients, and intra-procedural aneurysmal rupture in one patient in each group.

Discussion

Since the proportion of elderly in the population of developed countries is increasing, we are faced with a growing number of aged patients with ruptured cerebral aneurysms [4]. Surgical treatment of elderly patients is usually difficult, and their prognosis is generally not so good as in younger patients. Since the introduction of GDC, endovascular embolization of cerebral aneurysms has become an important alternative in the treatment of cerebral aneurysms [1, 3]. This technique can be very useful for elderly patients because of its less invasive nature. A recent randomized controlled study suggests that in patients with ruptured intracranial aneurysm, for which endovascular coiling and neurosurgical clipping are therapeutic options, a significantly better outcome in terms of survival free of disability at one year is achieved with endovascular coiling [2].

We have actively used this new technique in the past years for the treatment of ruptured cerebral aneurysms especially in the older age group. Our current indications for GDC embolization include vertebral artery dissecting aneurysm (VADA), high risk for general anesthesia, aged patients (over 70–75 years old), poor neurological grading (H & K grade IV–V), surgical difficulty (location), and vasospasm period. One limiting factor in this study is the different location of aneurysms between the two groups. In the younger patient group one third of patients had VADA, whereas a high frequency of internal carotid artery aneurysm occurred in the elderly patient group.

In this retrospective study, the overall outcome and complication rate in the older age group were similar to that of the younger patient group, which was in line with our expectations. However, significant general risk factors, such as pneumonia and rupture of extracranial aneurysms, made their prognosis poor and were more common in the elderly patient group. General risk factors should be checked before treatment of elderly patients. In addition, Hunt & Kosnik grade III patients in group A tended to have more neurological problems including muscle power weakness and cognitive dysfunction, which made their outcome moderately disabled (MD). This is another specific problem in older subjects as the majority of grade III patients in the younger patient group showed good outcome. Aged patients need to resume their preinsult activities as soon as possible after treatment to improve their chances for a good outcome. Early rehabilitation and meticulous general care should be provided to elderly patients. From this point of view, endovascular treatment might have an advantage over surgical treatment because of its less invasiveness. A comparison between endovascular and surgical treatment would be needed to prove this hypothesis, and we are pursuing such a study in the near future.

Conclusion

Endovascular treatment for elderly patients with ruptured aneurysm seems to be useful. Outcome is strongly related to their preoperative condition. General risk factors should be evaluated before treatment, especially in elderly patients. Good H & K grade patients are suitable for endovascular treatment, on the other hand, outcome of poor grade patients was worse despite the less invasive nature of endovascular treatment. An improvement of outcome in grade III patients is desirable.

References

1. Guglielmi G, Vinuela F, Dion J, Duckwiler G (1991) Electrothrombosis of saccular aneurysms via endovascular approach. Part 2: Preliminary clinical experience. J Neurosurg 75: 8–14
2. Molyneux A, Kerr R, Stratton I, Sandercock P, Clarke M, Shrimpton J, Holman R, International Subarachnoid Aneurysm Trial (ISAT) Collaborative Group (2002) International Subarachnoid Aneurysm Trial (ISAT) of neurosurgical clipping versus endovascular coiling in 2143 patients with ruptured intracranial aneurysms: a randomised trial. Lancet 360: 1267–1274
3. Raymond J, Roy D (1997) Safety and efficacy of endovascular treatment of acutely ruptured aneurysms. Neurosurgery 41: 1235–1246
4. Yano S, Hamada J, Kai Y, Todaka T, Hara T, Mizuno T, Morioka M, Ushio Y (2003) Surgical indications to maintain quality of life in elderly patients with ruptured intracranial aneurysms. Neurosurgery 52: 1010–1016

Correspondence: Kenji Sugiu, Department of Neurological Surgery, Okayama University Medical School 2-5-1 Shikata-cho, Okayama, 700-8558, Japan. e-mail: ksugiu@md.okayama-u.ac.jp

Acta Neurochir (2005) [Suppl] 94: 11–15
© Springer-Verlag 2005
Printed in Austria

Conventional microsurgical technique and endovascular method for the treatment of cerebral aneurysms: a comparative view

Y. Kaku

Department of Neurosurgery, Asahi University Murakami Memorial Hospital Gifu, Gifu, Japan

Summary

Endovascular embolization using Guglielmi Detachable Coils (GDCs) for complicated intracranial aneurysms has become widely accepted as an alternative to direct surgery. There is now a choice of therapeutic options for the management of cerebral aneurysms. The decision for treatment of an individual patient should be based on objective selection of the safest and most effective treatment. In addition, less invasive and cost effective treatment should be chosen. It is self-evident that the primary consideration in the selection process must be the immediate and long-term welfare of the individual patient, rather than the physician's preference for any specific treatment modality.

GDC embolization is a less invasive and safe treatment with low incidence of periprocedural morbidity, and has been successful in preventing acute subsequent bleeding, whereas follow-up results are less satisfactory in cases involving incompletely obliterated lesions. High incidence of recanalization was promoted in cases with neck remnant and/or body filling.

In contrast, the most important advantage of direct surgery is long-term durability, while conditions of patients and aneurysmal geometry limit the indication of direct surgery. In addition, direct surgery could be applied to complicated aneurysms with wide-neck or branching from the neck in combination with vascular reconstruction technique, such as EC-IC bypass.

With these limitations in mind, patients need to be very carefully chosen for GDC embolization or direct surgery.

Keywords: Cerebral aneurysm; direct surgery; endovascular treatment; GDC.

Introduction

Recent advancement in neurosurgery and interventional neuroradiology has brought us a new aspect to the treatment of cerebral aneurysms. There is now a choice of several therapeutic options for the management of cerebral aneurysms [1, 2, 9]. The selection of interventional neuroradiologic techniques with GDC, therefore, requires consideration of neurosurgical techniques, just as the selection of neurosurgical treatment requires an analysis of endovascular alternatives. Decision for the treatment of an individual patient should be based on objective selection of the safest and most effective treatment. It is self-evident that the primary consideration in the selection process must be the immediate and long-term welfare of the individual patient, rather than the physician's preference for any specific treatment modality.

Safety, efficacy and limitations of treatment

As for the safety of treatment, there is no significant difference between coil embolization and direct surgery regarding the periprocedural mortality and morbidity. Concerning the degree of invasion, GDC embolization is apparently less invasive and has been successful in preventing acute subsequent bleeding, whereas follow-up results are less satisfactory in cases involving incompletely obliterated lesions. High incidence of recanalization was promoted in such cases. From my personal experience, 64.9% of incompletely obliterated aneurysms displayed recanalization or regrowth on follow-up angiography, 13.5% of incompletely obliterated aneurysms exhibited progressive thrombosis, 21.6% remained unchanged. The most important advantage of direct surgery is long-term durability, while conditions of patients and aneurysmal geometry limit the indication of direct surgery. In contrast, the advantage of coil embolization is that patients' medical condition and aneurysmal geometry do not affect the indication of coil embolization. Figure 1 demonstrates a ruptured large fenestrated basilar artery aneurysm. Direct surgery for this aneurysm was considered to be extremely difficult, while complete occlusion of aneurysm could be achieved by coil embolization.

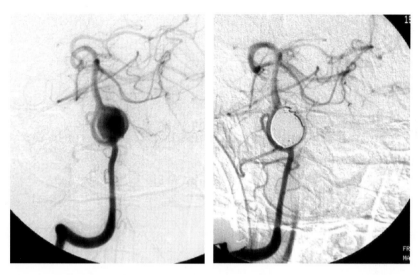

Fig. 1. *Left:* Right vertebral angiogram demonstrates a ruptured large fenestrated basilar artery aneurysm. *Right:* Angiogram obtained after coil embolization demonstrates complete occlusion of aneurysm

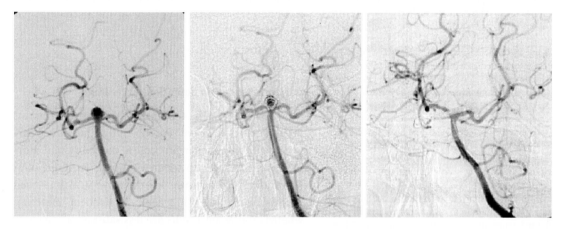

Fig. 2. *Left:* Left vertebral angiogram shows a small basilar tip aneurysm with relatively wide neck. *Center:* The first coil protruded to the basilar artery, so that the coil was retrieved to avoid thrombo-embolic complication. *Right:* Angiogram obtained after surgical neck clipping demonstrates complete obliteration of aneurysm

Aneurysms with ill-defined neck or branching from the neck or dome of aneurysm are not suitable for coil embolization. Figure 2 shows a small basilar tip aneurysm with relatively wide neck. Coil embolization was attempted once, but the first coil protruded to the basilar artery, so that the coil was retrieved to avoid thrombo-embolic complication. Surgical neck clipping was performed without any insults.

Aneurysms with mass effect may be a contraindication for coil embolization. Direct surgery is to be preferred for this lesion.

Limitation of access route, such as marked atherosclerosis, makes endovascular coiling difficult. Figure 3 shows a low positional basilar tip aneurysm with limitated access via endovascular route, left VA was occluded and right VA origin exhibited coiling. Direct surgical clipping was done with modern skull base surgical technique, thus low positional basilar tip aneurysms could be managed safely. Through the standard pterional approach, the operative view is quite restricted. Anterior clinoidectomy enhanced mobilization of IC and widened the operative field, so that the posterior clinoid process could be removed. Definitive clipping could be achieved with preservation of all performating branches.

Coil embolization could not be applied to compli-

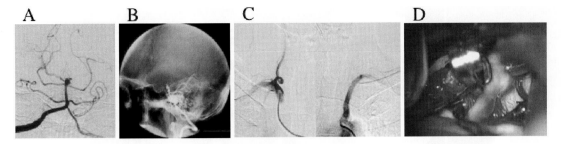

Fig. 3. (A) Left vertebral angiogram shows a small basilar tip aneurysm. (B) Lateral view of angiogram demonstrates that the neck of aneurysm was below the posterior clinoid process. (C) Angiograms demonstrate that a left VA was occluded and origin of right VA exhibited coiling. (D) Definitive clipping could be achieved with preservation of all the perforating branches

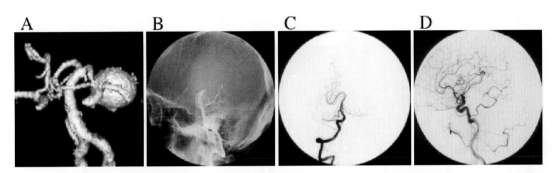

Fig. 4. (A) 3D CT angiogram shows a high positioned large left PCA (P2) aneurysm. (B) Lateral view of angiogram demonstrates that the aneurysm was 2 cm above the posterior clinoid process. (C) Angiogram obtained after surgical trapping demonstrates complete obliteration of aneurysm. (D) The post-operative left carotid angiogram demonstrates that the distal left PCA was perfused via STA-PCA anastomosis

cated aneurysms with occlusion intolerance, whereas such aneurysms could be managed by direct surgery in combination with vascular reconstruction technique, such as EC-IC bypass. Figure 4 shows a high positioned large left P2 aneurysm. Balloon occlusion test of left P1 indicated that the patient was intolerable for permanent PCA occlusion. Direct surgery is preferable for such complicated aneurysms with occlusion intolerance. STA-PCA anastomosis and trapping of aneurysm was performed. Proximal PCA was approached via supra IC bifurcation space, as aneurysm was high positional. Distal PCA was approached through partial corticotomy of entorhinal cortex. The post-operative angiogram demonstrated that the aneurysm was completely trapped and distal left PCA could be seen via STA-PCA anastomosis.

Collaboration between direct surgery and endovascular coiling

Collaboration between direct surgery and endovascular coiling has become an important factor. Not only when the procedure failed or to attempt another treatment modality, but also real collaboration, such as tentative coiling followed by definitive clipping or surgical vascular reconstruction followed by coil embolization, is useful in the treatment of complicated aneurysms. Figure 5 shows a case with ruptured right MCA aneurysm with ill-defined neck and mild vasospasm adjacent to the aneurysm. The patient consulted our clinic on day 7. In order to prevent rebleeding as well as deterioration of vasospasm, tentative coil embolization was performed with aneurysmal neck patent. It is one of the great advantages of coil embolization to occlude the aneurysm without manipulation of the brain parenchyma and the cerebral vasculatures. Two weeks later, definitive neck clipping was performed without any difficulty. Figure 6 shows large VA union aneurysm located midline, and left PICA was delivered from the dome of the aneurysm. OA-PICA anastomosis was made, and left PICA was clipped at its orifice. Coil embolization was followed by OA-PICA anastomosis.

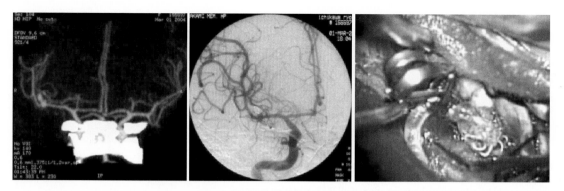

Fig. 5. *Left:* 3D CT angiogram shows a ruptured right MCA aneurysm with ill-defined neck and mild vasospasm adjacent to the aneurysm. *Center:* Right carotid angiogram obtained after tentative coil embolization demonstrates that the rupture site of aneurysm was occluded with aneurysmal neck patent. *Right:* Definitive neck clipping was performed without difficulty

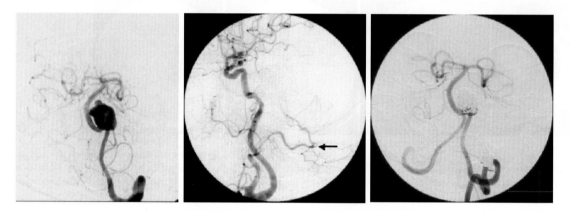

Fig. 6. *Left:* Left vertebral angiogram shows a large VA union aneurysm located midline, and the left PICA was delivered from the dome of the aneurysm. *Center:* Left carotid angiogram obtained after left OA-PICA anastomosis demonstrates that the left PICA was perfused via OA-PICA anastomosis (arrow). *Right:* Angiogram obtained after coil embolization demonstrates occlusion of aneurysm

Discussion

Endovascular embolization using GDCs for complicated intracranial aneurysms has become widely accepted as an alternative to direct surgery. Published reports of early clinical and angiographical results have been promising [1, 2, 9], but long-term efficacy of the GDC methods remains to be determined. International Subarachnoid Aneurysm Trial of neurosurgical clipping versus endovascular coiling (ISAT) suggested that in patients with a ruptured aneurysm, for which endovascular coiling and surgical clipping are therapeutic options, outcome is significantly more favorable with endovascular coiling [5]. The ISAT also suggests that the risk of rebleeding is higher and retreatment has to be performed somewhat more frequently with endovascular coiling. Longer term follow-up is vital to answer the question of durability of endovascular coiling. Endovascular coil embolization is a safe treatment with low incidence of periprocedural morbidity, and has been successful in preventing acute subsequent bleeding, whereas follow-up results are less satisfactory in cases involving incompletely obliterated lesions. High incidence of recanalization was promoted in such cases. 64.9% of incompletely obliterated aneurysms showed aneurysmal recanalization or regrowth in my series [7]. Incomplete endovascular occlusion of aneurysm leaves the patient at risk for future expansion and future subarachnoid hemorrhage [3, 4, 6, 8, 10]. Coil embolizations should not be chosen unless complete obliteration of aneurysms can be achieved. Surgical clipping can be applied to complicated aneurysms which have unsuitable configuration for coil embolization, such as ill-defined neck or branching from the neck, in combination with the vascular reconstruction technique. With this limitation in mind, patients need to be very carefully chosen for GDC.

Conclusions

The selection of interventional neuroradiologic techniques requires consideration of neurosurgical techniques, just as the selection of neurosurgical treatment requires an analysis of endovascular alternatives. The decision for treatment should be based on objective selection of the safest and most effective treatment. Further refinements of GDC technology are necessary to improve morphological and clinical outcomes.

References

1. Gruber DP, Zimmerman GA, Tomsick TA, van Loveren HR, Link MJ, Tew Jr JM (1999) A comparison between endovascular and surgical management of basilar artery apex aneurysms. J Neurosurg 90: 868–874
2. Guglielmi G, Viñuela F, Dion J, Duckwiler GR (1991) Electrothrombosis of saccular aneurysms via endovascular approach. Part 2: Preliminary clinical experience. J Neurosurg 75: 8–14
3. Hayakawa M, Murayama Y, Duckwiler GR, Gobin YP, Guglielmi G, Viñuela F (2000) Natural history of the neck remnant of a cerebral aneurysm treated with the Guglielmi detachable coil system. J Neurosurg 93: 561–568
4. Hodgson TJ, Carroll T, Jellinek DA (1998) Subarachnoid hemorrhage due to late recurrence of a previously unruptured aneurysm after complete endovascular occlusion. AJNR 19: 1939–1941
5. International Subarachnoid Aneurysm Trial (ISAT) Collaborative Group (2002) International Subarachnoid Aneurysm Trial (ISAT) of neurosurgical clipping versus endovascular coiling in 2143 patients with ruptured intracranial aneurysms: a randomised trial. Lancet 360: 1267–1274
6. Kaku Y, Yoshimura S, Hayashi K, Ueda T, Sakai N (1999) Follow-up study on intra-aneurysmal embolization for unruptured cerebral aneurysms. Interventional Neuroradiology 5 [Suppl] 1: 89–92
7. Kaku Y, Hayashi K, Sawada M, Sakai N (2001) Long-term angiographical follow-up of cerebral aneurysms after coil embolization. Interventional Neuroradiology 7 [Suppl] 1: 149–154
8. Kaku Y, Yoshimura S, Kokuzawa J, Sakai N (2003) Clinical and angiographic results of intra-aneurysmal embolization for cerebral aneurysms and histopathological findings in an aneurysm treated with GDC. Interventional Neuroradiology 9 [Suppl] 1: 35–40
9. Koivisto T, Vanninen R, Hurskainen H, Saari T, Hernesniemi J, Vapalahti M (2000) Outcomes of early endovascular versus surgical treatment of ruptured cerebral aneurysms A prospective randomized study. Stroke 31: 2369–2377
10. Mericle RA, Wakhloo AK, Lopes DK, Lanzino G, Guterman LR, Hopkins LN (1998) Delayed aneurysm regrowth and recanalization after Guglielmi detachable coil treatment. J Neurosurg 89: 142–145

Correspondence: Yasuhiko Kaku, Department of Neurosurgery, Asahi University Murakami Memorial Hospital, Gifu Hashimoto-cho 3-23, Gifu 500-8523, Japan. e-mail: kaku@murakami.asahi-u.ac.jp

Acta Neurochir (2005) [Suppl] 94: 17–21
© Springer-Verlag 2005
Printed in Austria

Lateral supraorbital approach as an alternative to the classical pterional approach

J. Hernesniemi[1], **K. Ishii**[1,2], **M. Niemelä**[1], **M. Smrcka**[3], **L. Kivipelto**[1], **M. Fujiki**[1,2], and **H. Shen**[1,4]

[1] Department of Neurosurgery, Helsinki University Central Hospital, Helsinki, Finland
[2] Department of Neurosurgery, Oita University Faculty of Medicine, Oita, Japan
[3] Department of Neurosurgery, Brno University Hospital, Brno, Czech Republic
[4] Department of Neurosurgery, Shenzhen Nanshan Hospital, Shenzhen, China

Summary

Objective. The standard pterional approach has been used to approach aneurysms of the anterior circulation and the basilar tip, suprasellar tumors, cavernous lesions. The senior author (JH) established a lateral supraorbital approach as an alternative to the pterional approach after continuous trial and error. We describe the techniques of this approach based on clinical experiences.

Methods. The lateral supraorbital approach is more subfrontal and anterior than the pterional approach. This approach has been regularly used by the senior author (JH) in the last decade in more than 2000 operations for mostly aneurysms of anterior circulation, but also for tumors of the anterior fossa and parasellar area as well as the sphenoid wing area.

Results. This approach can be used to operate on most cases, in which the classical pterional approach would be used. There are almost no craniotomy-related complications with this approach. This approach is not suitable in certain lesions which need to be exposed from a more temporal perspective.

Conclusion. This approach is simpler, faster, safer and less invasive than the classical pterional approach.

Keywords: Approach; supraorbital; pterional; cerebral aneurysm; intracranial aneurysm; subarachnoid hemorrhage; surgery.

Introduction

The standard pterional approach introduced and established by Yaşargil is widely recognized and has been a gold standard to approach lesions in the sellar and suprasellar region, Circle of Willis, Sylvian fissure and even the superior part of the clivus and basilar artery [7–9]. This approach has been proved of great benefit for safe microsurgery, and can be successfully used for both tumors and vascular pathologies. The senior author (JH) has established and developed a modified approach which is simpler and faster than the standard pterional approach [4]. We call this the lateral supraorbital approach which is different from the so-called "eye-brow incision" with a very small bone flap and more anterior location used in some institutions [1–3, 5, 6]. The lateral supraorbital approach is more subfrontal and located more anteriorly than the pterional approach. This approach is simple, less invasive and useful as an alternative to the classical pterional approach. This approach has been regularly used by the senior author (JH) in the last decade in more than 2000 operations, mainly in aneurysm surgery, but also in tumors of anterior fossa – parasellar – sphenoid wing area.

Operative procedure

The patient is positioned supine, the head elevated above the cardiac level to reduce bleeding. Head is fixed with three or four pins in the head frame (Mayfied or Sugita) and is rotated 15–45 degrees towards the opposite side and tilted slightly dependent on the precise location of the lesion. Hair shaving should be minimal still allowing a large enough oblique frontotemporal skin incision behind the hairline if possible. The skin incision is short and does not even go down in front of the ear to the level of zygomatic arch (Figs. 1, 2A). The line of skin incision is usually behind the hair line, but its medial part can be done in a skin wrinkle in bold or partially bold patients. The one layer skin-galea-muscle flap is dislocated after detachment from the bone by diathermy, thus avoiding any injury of the branches of facial nerve, and spring hooks are used to retract the flap anteriorly until the superior orbital rim and the anterior zygomatic arch are exposed (Fig. 2B). The temporal muscle is split only in its superior and anterior part. Only one burr hole is

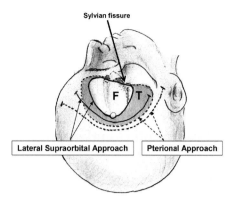

Fig. 1. A drawing illustrating the skin incision, the craniotomy margins, and the location of the Sylvian fissure in lateral supraorbital approach (a solid line) compared to pterional approach (a dotted line). *F* frontal lobe, *T* temporal lobe

placed posteriorly just below the insertion line of the temporal muscle (Fig. 2C). If necessary, depending on the size of the flap, thickness of the bone and adherence of the dura in elderly patients, another burr hole may be added over the pterion. The bone flap is detached mainly by side-cutting craniotome, but basal part is drilled off before lifting the flap (Fig. 2C). The bone flap is sized from 3 × 3 to 4 × 4 cm (Fig. 2E). The lateral sphenoid ridge and vertical bone on its both sides is drilled off until the bony exposure is along the skull base (Fig. 2D). Oozing from the bony surfaces is controlled by hot drilling (without saline irrigation) with diamond tipped drill. The dura mater is opened in a curvilinear incision pointing anterolaterally, and elevated with stitches (Fig. 2F). The operating microscope is brought in place. The Sylvian fissure is just on the temporal edge of the craniotomy and all the work to open the fissure is done from the frontal side (Fig. 1, 2G). After opening the Sylvian fissure minimally, it is filled with water injection technique and opened proceeding towards the aneurysm site. During these maneuvers, the Sylvian fissure is dissected with move towards midline of the opening. The use of retractors for brain dislocation is not necessary in most cases. In closure, the fixation of the bone flap with two Caniofix[O, R] is used (Fig. 2H).

Discussion

The gold standard pterional approach has been used for many years to access both tumors and vascular lesions, located in the sellar and suprasellar area as well as Circle of Willis, Sylvian fissure, the superior part of the clivus and basilar artery in many institutions [7–9]. However, this approach is quite extensive and includes a lot of drilling of the skull base especially in the temporal region, including the sphenoid wing. Removal of the anterior clinoid may have complications: the sphenoidal sinus can be entered quite frequently causing CSF leak leading often to an infection, and optic or oculomotor nerve lesions are possible. Epidural hematoma and an injury of the upper branch of the facial nerve may be caused by this approach. All these complications are not frequent but do occur even in the best hands. Also the cosmetic effect after the pterional craniotomy is not always satisfactory because of possible temporal muscle atrophy.

The lateral supraorbital approach has been developed and established as an alternative to this classical approach. The development of this approach was gradual just to make the procedure as simple and fast as possible and to reduce the craniotomy-related complications. Our approach is different from the "key-hole" supraorbital approach with an "eyebrow incision" and a very small frontal bone flap [1–3, 5, 6]. We do not use it except for some rare cases. Eyebrow incision is not accepted by our Finnish patients for cosmetic reasons because they have thin, blond eye brows. In elderly patients without specific cosmetic needs who have been operated on mainly for olfactory meningiomas or some aneurysms, the eye brow incision has been used without difficulties but also with no advantages as compared to lateral supraorbital approach. The anatomy is different, and the distance to the optic nerve is longer from the eyebrow, and the small craniotomy may be risky if some difficult hemorrhagic complications occur. It is noted during the years, that a difficult aneurysm is usually operated on through a larger flap than necessary. It is the fear and respect of the lesion that makes a large flap seem safer.

Fig. 2. The skin incision is placed just behind the hairline and does not go so far down in front of the ear as in the pterional approach (A). Pterion is still the central point of the craniotomy (A). The soft tissues are retracted as one layer flap and the anterior attachment of the zygomatic arch and the superior orbital rim have to be exposed (B). Only a small frontal part of the temporal muscle is split and detached from the temporal line (B). One burr hole is made approximately 4 cm above the pterion in the temporal line (C). Small craniotomy is then made extending 2–3 cm anteriorly from the burr hole and 2–3 cm posteriorly from it, ending at the sphenoid wing (C, D, E). Skull base at the superior orbital rim needs usually only a little drilling (D). The anterolateral part of the frontal lobe is disclosed after dural opening, and the Sylvian veins are hidden just below the posterior and basal edge of the craniotomy (G). The bone flap fixation using two Craniofix[O, R] is sufficient (H)

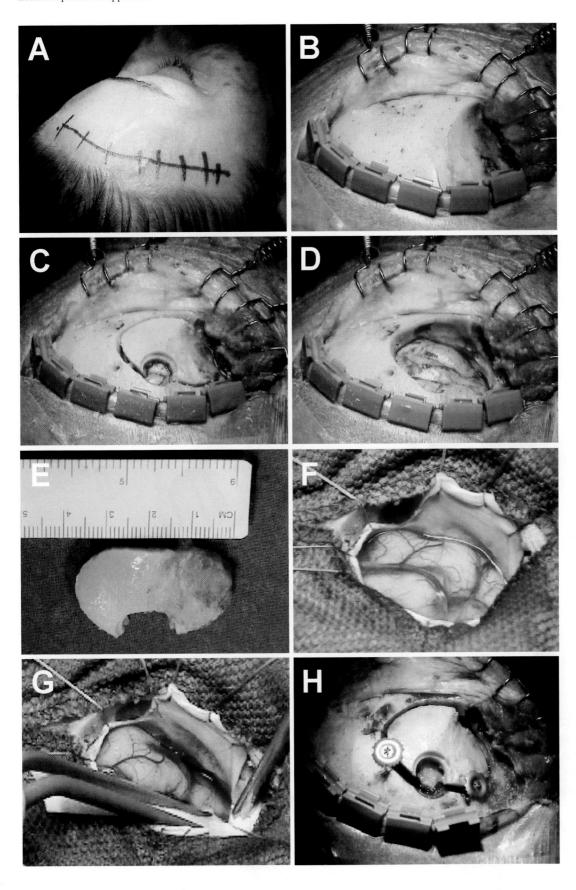

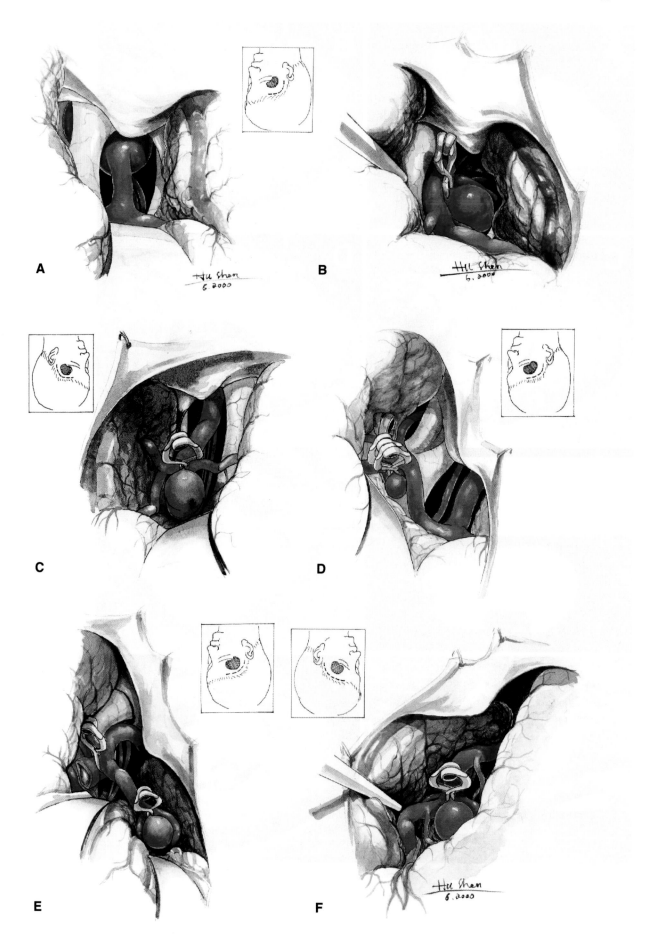

The advantage and disadvantage of the lateral supraorbital approach is as follows. The craniotomy is very fast, can be performed in 5–10 minutes which substantially shortens the overall operation times (shortest operation time from skin-to-skin 25 minutes in an MCA aneurysm). The short skin incision does not even go down in front of the ear to the level of zygomatic arch as in pterional approach causing less trauma to the temporal muscle. There is no risk to injure the upper branch of the facial nerve, because the use of a combined skin and muscle flap. The cosmetic result of this incision is good since it is usually behind the hair line. The medial part of the incision can be done in a skin wrinkle in bold or partially bold patients. Even here the wound is at first visible, but after healing the cosmetic result is excellent. The temporal muscle is split only in its superior and anterior part which decreases the postoperative problems with chewing, and as mentioned earlier, late muscle atrophy is practically not seen. One burr hole is usually sufficient for the craniotomy, but if the dura mater is tightly attached to the bone it may be torn, particularly in elderly patients. The bone flap can be quite small which decreases the risk of craniotomy-related complications, particularly CSF leak, postoperative epidural hematoma, and also infection. The size of the craniotomy is absolutely sufficient to reach the whole anterior part of the Circle of Willis, sellar, suprasellar legion and also anterior part of the basilar artery if it is located superiorly from the posterior clinoid process. This approach has certainly some limitations, and is not suitable and not used for some lesions; certain lesions need to be exposed from a more lateral (temporal) perspective: posterior communicating artery aneurysms pointing posteriorly, large and giant middle cerebral artery (MCA) aneurysms, particularly those pointing laterally against the sphenoid wing and lower positioned basilar tip artery aneurysms. In these situations, a pterional or subtemporal approach (even combined) is necessary. The other approaches by a more temporal craniotomy are also required in MCA aneurysms with a large temporo-parietal intracerebral hematoma.

Conclusion

The pterional craniotomy is the classic approach to lesions in the anterior part of the Circle of Willis, the sellar and suprasellar area, the Sylvian fissure, and also to the upper part of the clivus and basilar artery. As a simple alternative we present the lateral supraorbital approach, which is useful in most of the indications where the pterional approach would be used. The lateral supraorbital approach is fast, simple and rather atraumatic, which are advantages as compared to other approaches. Notably, there are almost no craniotomy-related complications with this approach. We still have a classic pterional approach in our armamentarium, since some of the pathologies cannot be removed by the described approach.

References

1. Brock M, Dietz H (1978) The small frontolateral approach for the microsurgical treatment of intracranial aneurysms. Neurochirurgia 21: 185–191
2. Menovsky T, Grotenhuis A, de Vries J, Bartels RHMA (1999) Endoscope-assisted supraorbital craniotomy for lesions of the interpeduncular fossa. Neurosurgery 44: 106–112
3. Reisch R, Perneczky A, Filippi R (2003) Surgical technique of the supraorbital key-hole craniotomy. Surg Neurol 59: 223–227
4. Rinne J, Shen H, Kivisaari R, Hernesniemi JA (2000) Surgical management of aneurysms of the middle cerebral artery. In: Schmidek HH (ed) Operative neurosurgical techniques: indications, methods, and results, 4th edn. WB Saunders Co., Philadelphia, pp 1159–1180
5. van Lindert E, Perneczky A, Fries G, Pierangeli E (1998) The supraorbital keyhole approach to supratentorial aneurysms: concept and technique. Surg Neurol 49: 481–490
6. Wilson DH: Limited exposure in cerebral neurosurgery (1971) Technical note. J Neurosurg: 102–106
7. Yaşargil MG, Fox JL, Ray MW (1975) The operative approach to aneurysms of the anterior communicating artery. Adv Tech Stand Neurosurg 2: 113–170
8. Yaşargil MG, Antic J, Laciga R, Jain KK, Hodosh RM, Smith RD (1976) Microsurgical pterional approach to aneurysms of the basilar bifurcation. Surg Neurol 6: 83–91
9. Yaşargil MG (1984) Vertebrobasilar aneurysms. In: Microneurosurgery, vol 2. Georg Thieme Verlag, Stuttgart, pp 232–295

Correspondence: Juha Hernesniemi, Department of Neurosurgery, Helsinki University Central Hospital, Topeliuksenkatu 5, 00260 Helsinki, Finland. e-mail: juha.hernesniemi@hus.fi

Fig. 3. Drawing illustrating the operative various views in lateral supraorbiral approach. An aneurysm located at right proximal internal carotid artery (A), right posterior communicating artery (B), left internal carotid artery bifurcation (C), anterior communication artery (D), anterior communication artery and right middle cerebral artery bifurcation (E), and left middle cerebral artery bifurcation (F)

Acta Neurochir (2005) [Suppl] 94: 23–29
© Springer-Verlag 2005
Printed in Austria

Conventional microsurgical treatment of paraclinoid aneurysms: state of the art with the use of the selective extradural anterior clinoidectomy SEAC

N. Khan[1], S. Yoshimura[1], P. Roth[1], E. Cesnulis[1], D. Koenue–Leblebicioglu[1], M. Curcic[2], H.-G. Imhof[1], and Y. Yonekawa[1]

[1] Department of Neurosurgery, University Hospital Zurich, Zurich, Switzerland
[2] Department of Anesthesiology, University Hospital Zurich, Zurich, Switzerland

Summary

Surgical treatment of paraclinoid aneurysms is considered to be difficult due to their complicated anatomical location in the vicinity of important neural, vascular and bony structures. We present our clinical experience of the past 10 years of conventional microsurgical treatment of 81 paraclinoid aneurysms in 75 patients with the use of selective extradural anterior clinoidectomy SEAC and discuss the method of therapy option by reviewing recent reports on results of endovascular coiling method and the combination of these with conventional microsurgical therapy. The favorable surgical results with the use of SEAC and no recurrence of the treated aneurysm after clipping procedure in our series indicate that direct surgery can still be a standard technique for paraclinoid aneurysms in view of the fact that the endovascular aneurysm coiling methods are still associated with a considerable percentage of incomplete occlusion and present the problem of coil packing.

Keywords: Paraclinoid aneurysm; clipping; SEAC; endovascular surgery; outcome; complication.

Introduction

Paraclinoid aneurysm is a term coined for aneurysms arising from the segment of the internal carotid artery as it exits from the cavernous sinus (CS) to the point of origin of the posterior communicating artery. The internal carotid artery ICA in this segment runs through the clinoid space and the subarachnoid space. Aneurysms of this paraclinoid segment remain to be one of the technically challenging topics for neurosurgeons [4, 18, 35, 39, 45]. Before the development of microsurgical cranial base techniques, direct access to these aneurysms was often hampered by the obstructing anterior clinoid process (ACP). Satisfactory clipping was also technically difficult in terms of preservation of patency of the ICA and its branches due to

existence of considerable number of giant or large aneurysms with or without partial thrombosis in this region [1, 24, 29]. In 1997, the technique of selective extradural anterior clinoidectomy SEAC was reported by our group. This technique facilitates both radical removal of tumors and radical neck clipping of aneurysms in the supra- and parasellar regions by providing a wide operative exposure and hence better illumination, and therefore making this method suitable for routine use in the treatment of these lesions [46].

On the other hand, endovascular aneurysm embolization with Guglielmi detachable coils (GDCs) has become an alternative treatment in the management of cerebral aneurysms [5, 17–19]. This endovascular method of treatment has many advantages not only for patients who are at a high risk for surgery, but also in cases of aneurysms where surgery is difficult due to their special location, size and form. However, the method of obliteration of aneurysms with this treatment is not the same as with surgery. Indeed, it has also been reported that embolized aneurysms often recanalize, i.e. the well known problem of coil packing or coil compaction, where remnants of aneurismal necks have been observed, especially in cases of large and giant aneurysms [13, 23, 26, 43], making the optimal treatment for these lesions still open to evaluation [25, 26], although treatment modality of combined surgical and endovascular approaches are also being tried and reported [1, 34, 42].

In this study was review our recent experience using a pure surgical approach to paraclinoid aneurysms using SEAC in order to assess the role of direct surgery for these aneurysms.

Table 1. *Patients and total number of aneurysms*

75 patients: 60 female (80%) vs 15 male (20%). Age: 50.9 $\pm$ 10.9 (mean $\pm$ SD)

Multiplicity	Number of patients	Number of aneurysms
1	43 (57.3%)	43
2	19 (25.3%)	38
3	7 (9.3%)	21
4	3 (4.0%)	12
5	3 (4.0%)	15
Total	75	129

Patients

From 1993 to March 2003, 81 aneurysms in the paraclinoid segment of the ICA in 75 patients were treated in the Department of Neurosurgery, University Hospital Zurich. Of these 75 patients, 53 patients presented with subarachnoid hemorrhage (SAH) and 22 were diagnosed as having paraclinoid aneurysms during routine neuroradiological examinations for various neurological symptoms and signs or other reasons. Fourty nine patients presenting with SAH were admitted to our hospital within 3 weeks after the ictus (average: 4.7 days), these were classified into the SAH group. Four patients with SAH were admitted at 2 months, 3 months, 5 months and 4 years after SAH, respectively, and were classified into the "non" SAH group together with 22 patients with non ruptured aneurysms. Glasgow Coma Scale (GCS) of the SAH patients on admission was 3–15 points (average: 12.3 points). Of the 26 patients from the non SAH group, all but five had no neurological deficits on admission; four patients presented with visual disturbance and one with a left hemiparesis due to thalamic hemorrhage.

Patients included 60 females (80%) and 15 males (20%) with mean age of 50.9 $\pm$ 10.9 years. Among the 75 patients, 32 patients (42.6%) had multiple aneurysms (Table 1).

The paraclinoid aneurysms were diagnosed as follows: (unruptured 37 (46%); SAH caused by their rupture 35 (43%); symptomatic i.e. visual disturbance 6 (7%) and incidental 3 (4%). Unruptured aneurysms were aneurysms associated with ruptured aneurysms at other sites and one with a ruptured arteriovenous malformation. Three incidental aneurysms (two at the time of headache work-up and one at the time of a hypertensive thalamic hemorrhage) were also found.

In 4 cases, coil embolization had been attempted by neuroradiologists. Two aneurysms were successfully embolized, but recanalized during follow-up period. In the other 2 cases, embolization was attempted but failed.

Methods

Classification of paraclinoid aneurysms

We defined paraclinoid aneurysms as those aneurysms arising from the segment of the internal carotid artery (ICA) that runs through the clinoid space and subarachnoid space between its point of exit from the the cavernous sinus (CS) with the landmark of proximal dural ring and the point of origin of the posterior communicating artery, corresponding with the C3 and C2 segments of the internal carotid artery after Fischer [14]. The lesions that originated in the CS and extended into the subdural space (so-called transitional aneurysms), and the lesions located completely within the CS were excluded. We used the anatomical land marks for classification of paraclinoid aneurysms based on the aneurysm's presumed origin on the ICA.

Clinoid aneurysms arise from the ICA segment between the proximal and distal dural rings, namely C3 segment. Carotid cave aneurysms arise at the pouch of the distal dural ring of the ICA including also the so called superior pituitary artery aneurysms. IC-ophthalmic aneurysms arise from the origin of the ophthalmic artery. Superior carotid wall aneurysms on the superior wall of the ICA distal to the dural ring and project superiorly. Inferior carotid wall aneurysms arise on the inferior wall of the ICA and project inferiorly.

The locations of the 81 paraclinoid aneurysms were grouped; clinoid 8 (10%), carotid cave 5 (6%), IC-ophthalmic 34 (42%), inferior wall 17 (21%) and superior wall 17 (21%) as is shown in Fig. 1. Of the 81 aneurysms, 16 (20%) were large (12–25 mm), and 3 (4%) were giant (>25 mm) aneurysms.

Surgical treatments

Most of cases were operated upon by the senior author Yonekawa [46, 47]. Direct neck clipping was attempted on all aneurysms and this could be done in 76 aneurysms (93%), wrapping was performed in one aneurysm with atheromatous and calcified wall and neck (1%) and the 4 remainig aneurysms were treated with trapping combined with extracranial-intracranial EC-IC arterial bypass (5%); three large clinoid aneurysms, in which two were partially thrombosed and one large IC-ophthalmic aneurysm of early case of this series. In patients with SAH, the ruptured aneurysm was initially clipped, followed by clipping of other aneurysms, when possible, through the original craniotomy and in the same session. The mean GCS just before operation was 12.3 $\pm$ 3.8 points in the SAH patients.

Our procedure of SEAC has been reported elsewhere previously [46]. This procedure enables exposure of the clinoid segment of the ICA (C3) and aneurysm dissection of this segment. So the proximal control at the clinoid segment becomes secure. Better mobilization of the optic nerve and of the ICA yields additional working space and better illumination.

Among 76 clipping procedures, one wrapping procedure and 4 trapping and EC-IC bypass procedures for 81 paraclinoid aneurysms, in 70 aneurysms (86.4%), the SEAC procedures were performed. Seven paraclinoid aneurysms (8.6%) were occluded from the contralateral side at the time of clipping of ruptured and/or larger aneurysms of ipsilateral side.

Results

Angiographic results

Follow-up cerebral angiography was performed routinely postoperatively around 1 week after sur-

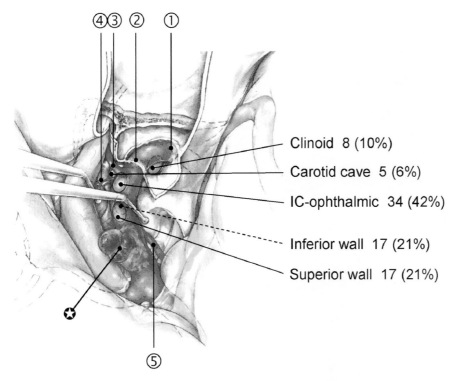

Fig. 1. Schematic drawing of aneurysm locations and their distribution in this study. Site of predilection of the blistering aneurysm "chimame aneuysm" is also indicated as star symbol, Also the proximal and distal dural rings ① and ②, the ophthalmic artery ③ and the superior hypophyseal artery ④ and posterior communicating artery ⑤ are also migrated respectively

gery in all patients but one, who rejected this examination.

Clipping condition assessed by postoperative angiography is as follows: Neck clipping was performed in 76 procedures, and complete clipping was confirmed in 73 (96%) cases. In the 2 patients whose aneurysms recanalized after previous embolization with coils, complete obliteration of the aneurysm was obtained by direct surgery. One of them had both recanalization of the aneurysm and migration of the placed coils from the aneurysm extending to the M2 segment. Neck clipping was successfully performed without removal of intraluminal coils in the MCA segment because of tight adhesion of the coils to the arterial wall (Fig. 2). Small neck remnant was demonstrated in 4 patients (5.1%) on postoperative angiography. One patient in which whole dome opacification was demonstrated due to the slipping out was reoperated for complete clipping. The other 3 patients received further clinical and angiographic follow-up, and no regrowth of the aneurysm was observed on repeated angiography usually at three months then a year later. In one patient, angiography could be performed 5 years after the op-

eration, showing no change in the size of this residual neck.

Clinical outcome

Patient outcomes were evaluated at three months and expressed as a score calculated according to the Glasgow Outcome Scale (GOS). A GOS score of 5 is an outcome of good recovery GR, 4 is moderately disabled MD, 3 severely disabied SD, 2 vegetative state VS, and 1 death D.

The clinical outcome was evaluated at 3 months after surgery and expressed by the GOS score. Among 29 patients of the non SAH group, clinical outcomes were: GR (GOS 5) in 23 (79.3%), and MD (GOS 4) in 4 (13.7%). In two patients (4.2%), whose outcome was GOS 3, the pre-exisiting neurological deficit did not change by the clipping procedure. There was no mortality. Surgery-related permanent morbidity was observed in 4 patients (13.7%); visual field defect in 2 patients, deterioration of visual acuity and oculomotor nerve palsy in another patients respectively. Among 46 patients of the SAH group, clinical out-

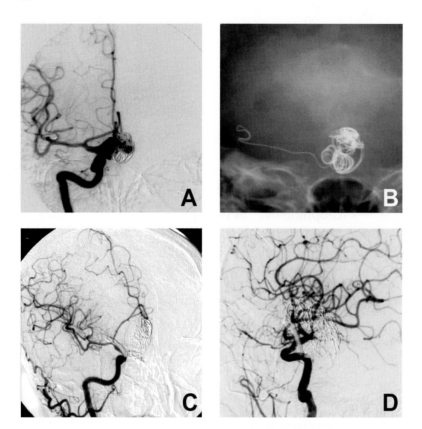

Fig. 2. A 66-year-old female. Preoperative right internal carotid angiogram (A) and skull X-ray (B) showing recanalization and regrowth of the aneurysm which was successfully embolized previously with Guglielmi detachable coils. Migration of the coil from the aneurysm lumen to the left M2 segment of the middle cerebral artery *(MCA)* can be seen. Postoperative A-P (C) and lateral (D) carotid angiograms showing complete clipping of the aneurysm, remaining migrated coil in the internal carotid artery to the MCA

comes were: GR (GOS 5) in 28 patients (60.8%), MD (GOS 4) in 10 (21.7%), SD (GOS 3) in 4 (8.6%), and death (GOS 1) in 4 (8.6%). Surgery-related permanent morbidity was observed in 6 patients (13.0%); ischemic stroke in 5 patients, including 2 patients with probable thorombus migrations from the aneurysms, and visual field defect in one patient. Surgery related mortality rate was 0%.

Furthermore, in the SAH group, 12 patients (25.6%) showed ischemic symptoms and signs due to severe cerebral vasospasm. 11 of those 12 patients were treated with intraarterial infusion of papaverine and balloon angioplasty, barbiturate coma and hypothermia therapy according to our structured vasospasm therapy protocol [47]. Ischemic neurological deficits persisted in 6 patients resulting in permanent morbidity in 4 patients and death in 2. One patient died of direct hemorrhagic injury. Another patient death resulted from rebleeding from a ruptured small aneurysm of the posterior cerebral artery, which could not be detected on the preoperative anigography, but was confirmed at

autopsy. Thus, overall morbidity was 12 (26.0%) and mortality was 4 (8.7%) in this group.

As far as the size of aneurysms is concerned, surgical outcomes of the large and giant aneurysm were analyzed. In the non-SAH group, complete clipping was performed in all 4 cases and trapping combined with EC-IC bypass in 3 cases. Ipsilateral visual disturbance complicated in a case of the former (25%) and a case in the latter (33%). In the SAH group, neck clipping was performed in 10 of 11 patients. In the remaining case, wrapping was performed due to severe calcification especially at the neck of the aneurysm. In one of the patients (9%) treated with neck clipping, a small infarction at the genu of the internal capsule causing a hemiparesis of mild degree was seen.

Discussion

Paraclinoid aneurysms were historically treated by Hunterian ligation of proximal occlusion of the ICA or the common carotid artery and recently endovascu-

Table 2. *Recent comparable treatment series*

	Cases	Treated aneurysms	SAH	Clip	Wrap	Coil	Occl.	Morbidity	Mortality
Day 1990	80	54	35%					7%	6%
Batjer 1994	89	89	44%				4	12%	1%
De Jesus 1999	28	35	24%				3	18%	4%
Roy 1997	26	28	30%			25		4%	0%
Thornton 2000	71	61	18%			49	12	3%	2%
Hoh 2000	216	238	25%	180		57	1	6%	0.4%
Park 2001	70	73	11%	3		84		8.3%	0%
Iihara 2003	112	111	0%	35		77		5.4%	0%
Present series	*75*	*81*	*61%*	*76*	*1*		*4*	*12%*	*0%*

larly [7, 10, 15, 30, 33, 41], also in use with combination with EC-IC bypass, especially for large and giant aneurysms of this location in cases where clipping is unfeasible [2, 16, 27, 38, 39]. However, this method does not always prevent ischemic complications [21]. Also late occurrence of hemodynamically induced aneurysms after the carotid ligation have been reported experimentally and clinically [10, 22]. Therefore, neck clipping of the aneurysm with preservation of patency of the ICA is the most appropriate treatment, although this has been considered and reported to be technically difficult.

Complete neck clipping with partial clinoidectomy [3, 35] and use of specially formed clips [40] have been the subsequent technical development in combination with microsurgery followed by the extensive clinoidectomy to be credited to Dolenc [9].

In this study, we reviewed our recent experience of surgical treatment for patients with paraclinoid aneurysms with or without SAH separately. Our surgical treatment provided favorable results in both groups. One possible reason to explain this good result is that we have routinely performed the SEAC for confirming aneurysmal shape, location and relationship between aneurysm and surrounding bone, neural and vascular structures. The SEAC gives a wider surgical working space hence also better illumination for careful observation and manipulation of the aneurysm and of the ICA branches and enables secure proximal control, leading to a better outcome. Sometimes the space gained by the SEAC procedure proved to be the only possible room available in which aneurysms could be managed in view of the swollen or angry brain in the SAH group. The SEAC procedure is less time-consuming (usually within 20 min.) and less extensive as compared with the method described by Dolenc [9] and Kattner [29]. This procedure, enables use of the trapping and "puncture and collapse" method of aneurysms obviating complicated and time consuming combined methods of endovascular temporary occlusion of the ICA and aspiration of blood-contents of large or giant aneurysms through an indwelling catheter [1, 34, 42]. In our series, the SAH group had more frequent complications as compared with the non SAH group. This can be well understood from the pathophysiological difference of the presenting disease back ground; combination or non combination of SAH. The former was complicated with perforating artery infarctions, bleeding from an untreated (preoperatively undetected) aneurysm in the acute stage and with devastating vasospasm in spite of our structured therapy. Postoperative persistent visual deterioration was observed in four cases (5%) so that the careful manipulation of the optic nerve at the time of drilling procedures of SEAC and of aneurysm clipping procedure can not be overemphasized in the presence already impaired optic nerve function or anatomical derangement [12, 31].

We reviewed recent comparable reports regarding treatment of paraclinoid aneurysms and have summarized them in Table 2. Day [6], Batjer [3], De Jesus [8] and Park [36] reported surgical results of paraclinoid aneurysm. On the other hand, endovascular embolization with GDC is gaining a considerable position as an alternative method in the treatment of aneurysms [17, 19]. As shown in Table 2, Thornton [43] reported their experience with endovascular treatment for paraclinoid aneurysms. Morbidity-mortality was impressively low (5.5%) in their series. 10 of 71 paraclinoid aneurysms (14.1%) showed regrowth of the aneurysms after embolization on repeat angiography. Roy [37] also reported low morbidity (4%) as compared to previous surgical series with complete occlusion in 14 of 28 aneurysms (50%). Ho [25] and

Iihara [28] have reported overall good results by selecting cases of high risk in the former or by selecting cases according to aneurysm projection in the latter for coil embolization. The rate of regrowth/coil compaction was 26% after successful embolization and 5 of their patients required retreatment, whereas no recurrence was observed in the surgical group [25].

These facts suggest that interventional risk is generally lower in coil embolization than in surgical clipping. However, aneurysms harboring broad neck have been reported to be difficult to have sufficient anatomical occlusion with embolization with GDC embolization. Paraclinoid aneurysms often present with large or giant aneurysms with broad neck, posing difficulties in complete obliteration by currently available coiling methods [44]. Acceptable coiling of aneurysms tends to be complicated with recanalization (coild packing or coil compaction and anreurysm regrowth. These facts suggest that current coil embolization technique is applicable principally only for narrow-necked (less than 4 mm) aneurysms even when neck plasty method with a balloon catheter is available [13]. This limitation may partially be overcome by development of new stent-assisted system in the near future [32], although additional interventional procedure can be a new source of further complication. Given the apparent difference between clipping and embolization in terms of recurrence of the treated aneurysms, underlying mechanisms for recanalization or regrowth of aneurysms should be further investigated to overcome this problem.

Therefore, one would consider the combination of coiling and clipping modalities in order to mutually compensate their disadvantages [20]. However, adhesion or incorporation of coils within the aneurysm wall and protrusion of coils into the vicinity of aneurysm neck would make future neck clipping more difficult, as was shown in our case of Fig. 2. Accordingly, especially in aneurysms with broad-neck, primary direct surgery is considered to be better as a first treatment.

Conclusion

Paraclinoid aneurysms are known to demand special therapeutic considerations due to their special location of close vicinity to bony structures and important neural and vascular structures. Most appropriate treatment is to occlude aneurysms without compromizing patency of the internal carotid artery and with-

out causing any new neurological sequelae. The SEAC procedure enables appropriate surgical management of the aneurysms. Our results indicate that microsurgical aneurysm clipping in combination with this procedures can still be a standard treatment inspite of recent development of endovascular coiling procedures. In light of the contemporary evidence available, endovascular treatment does frequently present with incomplete occlusion and coil compaction for aneurysms of this location.

References

1. Arnautovic KI, Al-Mefty O, Angtuaco E (1998) A combined microsurgical skull-base and endovascular approach to giant and large paraclinoid aneurysms. Surg Neurol 50: 504–520
2. Barnett DW, Barrow DL, Joseph GJ (1994) Combined extracranial-intracranial bypass and intraoperative balloon occlusion for the treatment of intracavernous and proximal carotid artery aneurysms. Neurosurgery 35: 92–98
3. Batjer HH, Kopitnik TA, Giller CA, Samson DS (1994) Surgery for paraclinoidal carotid artery aneurysms. J Neurosurg 80: 650–658
4. Benedetti A, Curri D (1977) Direct attack on carotid ophthalmic and large internal carotid aneurysms. Surg Neurol 8: 49–54
5. Brilstra EH, Rinkel GJ, van der Graaf Y, van Rooij WJ, Algra A (1999) Treatment of intracranial aneurysms by embolization with coils: a systematic review. Stroke 30: 470–476
6. Day AL (1990) Aneurysm of the ophthalmic segment. A clinical and anatomical analysis. J Neurosurg 72: 677–691
7. Debrun G, Fox A, Drake C, Peerless S, Girvin J, Ferguson G (1981) Giant unclippable aneurysms: treatment with detachable balloons. AJNR Am J Neuroradiol 2: 167–173
8. De Jesus O, Sekhar LN, Riedel CJ (1999) Clinoid and paraclinoid aneurysms: surgical anatomy, operative techniques, and outcome. Surg Neurol 51: 477–488
9. Dolenc VV (1985) A combined epi- and subdural direct approach to carotid-ophthalmic artery aneurysms. J Neurosurg 62: 667–672
10. Drake CG, Peerless SJ, Ferguson GG (1994) Hunterian proximal arterial occlusion for giant aneurysms of the carotid circulation. J Neurosurg 81: 656–665
11. Dyste GN, Beck DW (1989) De novo aneurysm formation following carotid ligation: case report and review of the literature. Neurosurgery 24: 88–92
12. Ferguson GG, Drake CG (1981) Carotid-ophthalmic aneurysms: visual abnormalities in 32 patients and the results of treatment. Surg Neurol 16: 1–8
13. Fernandez Zubillaga A, Guglielmi G, Vinuela F, Duckwiler GR (1994) Endovascular occlusion of intracranial aneurysms with electrically detachable coils: correlation of aneurysm neck size and treatment results. AJNR (abbreviation of Am J Neuroradiol) 15: 815–820
14. Fischer E (1938) Die Lageabweichungen der vorderen Hirnarterie im Gefässbild. Zbl Neurochir 3: 300–313
15. Fox JL, Vinuela F, Pelz DM, Peerrless SJ, Ferguson GG, Drage CG, Debrun G (1987) Use of detachable balloons for proximal artery occlusion in the treatment of unclippable cerebral aneurysms. J Neurosurg 66: 40–46
16. Gelber BR, Sundt TM Jr (1980) Treatment of intracavernous

and giant carotid aneurysms by combined internal carotid ligation and extra- to intracranial bypass. J Neurosrug 52: 1–10

17. Guglielmi G, Vinuela F, Dion J, Duckwiler G (1991) Electrothrombosis of saccular aneurysms via endovascular approach. Part 2: preliminary clinical experience. J Neurosurg 75: 8–14

18. Guidetti B, La Torre E (1979) Carotid-ophthalmic aneurysms. A series of 16 cases treated by direct approach. Acta Neurochir (Wien) 22: 289–304

19. Gurian JH, Vinuela F, Guglielmi G, Gobin YP, Duckwiler GR (1996) Endovascular embolization of superior hypophyseal artery aneurysms. Neurosurgery 39: 1150–1156

20. Hacein-Bey L, Connolly ES Jr, Mayer SA, Young WL, Pil-Spellman J, Solomon RA (1998) Complex intracranial aneurysms: combined operative and endovascular approaches (review). Neurosurgery 43: 1304–1313

21. Hashi K, Nin K (1985) Complications following carotid ligation combined with EC-IC bypass. Neurosurgeons 4: 359–366 [Jpn]

22. Hashimoto N, Handa H, Hazama F (1978) Experimentally induced cerebral aneurysms in rats. Surg Neurol 10: 3–8

23. Hayakawa M, Murayama Y, Duckwiler GR, Gobin YP, Guglielmi G, Vinuela F (2000) Natural history of the neck remnant of a cerebral aneurysm treated with the Guglielmi detachable coil system. J Neurosurg 93: 561–568

24. Heros RC, Nelson PB, Ojemann RG, Crowell RM, DeBrun G (1983) Large and giant paraclinoid aneurysms: surgical techniques, complications, and results. Neurosurgery 12: 153–163

25. Hoh BL, Carter BS, Budzik RF, Putman CM, Ogilvy CS (2001) Results after surgical and endovascular treatment of paraclinoid aneurysms by a combined neurovascular team. Neurosurgery 48: 78–90

26. Hope JK, Byrne JV, Molyneux AJ (1999) Factors influencing successful angiographic occlusion of aneurysms treated by coil embolization. AJNR (abbreviation of Am J Neuroradiol) 20: 391–399

27. Hopkins LN, Grand W (1979) Extracranial-intracranial arterial bypass in the treatment of aneurysms of the carotid and middle cerebral arteries. Neurosurgery 5: 21–31

28. Iihara K, Murao K, Sakai N, Shindo A, Sakai H, Higashi T, Kogure S, Takahashi JC, Hayashi K, Ishibashi T, Nagata I (2003) Unruptured paraclinoid aneurysms: a management strategy. J Neurosurg 99: 241–247

29. Kattner KA, Bailes J, Fukushima T (1998) Direct surgical management of large bulbous and giant aneurysms involving the paraclinoid segment of the internal carotid artery: report of 29 cases (review). Surg Neurol 49: 471–480

30. Kothandaram P, Dawson BH, Kruyt RC (1971) Carotid-ophthalmic aneurysms. A study of 19 patients. J Neurosurg 34: 544–548

31. Kumon Y, Sakaki S, Kohno K, Ohue S, Oka Y (1997) Asymptomatic, unruptured carotid-ophthalmic artery aneurysms: angiographical differentiation of each type, operative results, and indications. Surg Neurol 48: 465–472

32. Lanzino G, Wakhloo AK, Fessler RD, Hartney ML, Guterman LR, Hopkins LN (1999) Efficacy and current limitations of intravascular stents for intracranial internal carotid, vertebral, and basilar artery aneurysms. J Neurosurg 1: 538–546

33. Larson JJ, Tew JM Jr, Tomsick TA, van Loveren HR (1995) Treatment of aneurysms of the internal carotid artery by intravascular balloon occlusion: long-term follow-up of 58 patients. Neurosurgery 36: 23–30

34. Mizoi K, Takahashi A, Yoshimoto T, Fujiwara S, Koshu K (1993) Combined endovascular and neurosurgical approach for paraclinoid internal carotid artery aneurysms. Neurosurgery 33: 986–992

35. Morgan F (1972) Removal of antertior clinoid process in the surgery of carotid aneurysm, with some notes on recurrent subarachnoid haemorrhage during craniotomy. Schweiz Arch Neurol Neurochir Psychiatr 111: 363–368

36. Park HK, Horowitz M, Jungreis C, Kassam A, Koebbe C, Genevro J, Dutton K, Purdy P (2003) Endovascular treatment of paraclinoid aneurysms: experience with 73 patients. Neurosurgery 53: 14–24

37. Roy D, Raymond J, Bouthillier A, Bojanowski MW, Moumdjian R, L'Esperance G (1997) Endovascular treatment of ophthalmic segment aneurysms with Guglielmi detachable coils. AJNR (abbreviation of Am J Neuroradiol) 18: 1207–1215

38. Serbinenko FA, Filatov JM, Spallone A, Tchurilov MV, Lazarev VA (1990) Management of giant intracranial ICA aneurysms with combined extracranial-intracranial anastomosis and endovascular occlusion. J Neurosurg 73: 57–63

39. Spetzler RF, Selman W, Carter LP (1984) Elective EC-IC bypass for unclippable intracranial aneurysms. Neurol Res 6: 64–68

40. Sugita K, Kobayashi S, Kyoshima K, Nakagawa F (1982) Fenestrated clips for unusual aneurysms of the carotid artery. J Neurosurg 57: 240–246

41. Swearingen B, Heros RC (1987) Common carotid occlusion for unclippable carotid aneurysms: an old but still effective operation. Neurosurgery 21: 288–295

42. Tamaki N, Kim S, Ehara K, Asada M, Fujita K, Taomoto K, Matsumoto S (1991) Giant carotid-ophthalmic artery aneurysms: direct clipping utilizing the "trapping-evacuation" technique. J Neurosurg 74: 567–572

43. Thornton J, Aletich VA, Debrun GM, Alazzaz A, Misra M, Charbel F, Ausman JI (2000) Endovascular treatment of paraclinoid aneurysms. Surg Neurol 54: 288–299

44. Vinuela F, Duckwiler G, Mawad M (1997) Guglielmi detachable coil embolization of acute intracranial aneurysm: perioperative anatomical and clinical outcome in 403 patients. J Neurosurg 86: 475–482

45. Yasargil MG, Gasser JC, Hodosh RM, Rankin TV (1977) Carotid-ophthalmic aneurysms: direct microsurgical approach. Surg Neurol 8: 155–165

46. Yonekawa Y, Ogata N, Imhof HG, Olivecrona M, Strommer K, Kwak TE, Roth P, Groscurth P (1997) Selective extradural anterior clinoidectomy for supra- and parasellar processes. Technical note. J Neurosurg 87: 636–642

47. Yonekawa Y, Khan N, Roth P (2002) Strategies for surgical management of cerebral aneurysms of special location, size and form – approach, technique and monitoring. Acta Neurochir (Wien) [Suppl] 82: 105–118

Correspondence: Yasuhiro Yonekawa, Neurochirurgische Universitätsklinik Zurich, Frauenklinikstrasse 10, 8091 Zurich, Switzerland. e-mail: yasuhiro.yonekawa@usz.ch

Acta Neurochir (2005) [Suppl] 94: 31–38
© Springer-Verlag 2005
Printed in Austria

Subtemporal approach to basilar bifurcation aneurysms: advanced technique and clinical experience

J. Hernesniemi[1], **K. Ishii**[1,2], **M. Niemelä**[1], **L. Kivipelto**[1], **M. Fujiki**[1,2], and **H. Shen**[1,3]

[1] Department of Neurosurgery, Helsinki University Central Hospital, Helsinki, Finland
[2] Department of Neurosurgery, Oita University Faculty of Medicine, Oita, Japan
[3] Department of Neurosurgery, Shenzhen Nanshan Hospital, Shenzhen, China

Summary

Objective. The surgical treatment of basilar bifurcation aneurysms is challenging, and many of these aneurysms are currently treated by endovascular means. However, the complete closure of the aneurysm by surgical clipping still remains the best and most permanent cure for the aneurysm. The "gold standard", subtemporal approach was established and introduced by Drake and it has been adapted by the senior author Hernesniemi. We describe our present modified technique of this approach based on clinical experience.

Methods. The subtemporal approach to basilar bifurcation aneurysms has been regularly used by the senior author Hernesniemi in recent 15 years in over 200 operations in Kuopio and Helsinki, Finland.

Results. This approach is suitable in most basilar bifurcation aneurysms except for those high above the posterior clinoid process. To avoid temporal lobe damage, cerebrospinal fluid drainage is necessary. Benefits of subtemporal approach are short operative and retraction times, and no need for skull base resection.

Conclusion. The subtemporal approach is simple and safe in experienced hands, and should be considered the standard method to approach most basilar bifurcation aneurysms.

Keywords: Approach; subtemporal; pterional; cerebral aneurysm; intracranial aneurysm; basilar bifurcation aneurysm; surgery.

Introduction

The surgical treatment of basilar bifurcation aneurysms (BBAs) remains one of the most difficult tasks in neurosurgery because of the anatomical and technical difficulties. Recently, many of these rare aneurysms located in a narrow space in front of the brain stem have been treated by endovascular procedures in many institutions. However, closure of the base of the aneurysm by clipping still remains the most effective cure for the aneurysm [12, 20]. Several surgical approaches, such as subtemporal approach, pterional approach, supraorbital approach, orbitozygomatic approach, transpetrosal approach and combined approaches are currently used for the treatment of BBAs [1–6, 8–11, 13–19]. The subtemporal approach is the oldest one, which was widely used by Drake and Peerless in more than 1000 patients [2–4]. The senior author Hernesniemi adopted the use the subtemporal approach in the 80's after studying chapters written by Drake and Peerless in different text books. This experience was later refined by coworking with these authors [4, 7]. We describe our recently modified operative technique of the subtemporal approach.

Operative procedure
Craniotomy, approach to tentorial edge and basilar bifurcation

The patient is positioned in the park bench position. A small subtemporal craniotomy through a linear incision is done. Ordinarily, the non-dominant, right side is used, unless the projection or complexity of the aneurysm, scarring from earlier operations, severe anatomical rotation of the basilar bifurcation, left oculomotor palsy, left sided blindness or right hemiparesis, makes an approach from the dominant side necessary.

The subtemporal approach can be converted into a pterional or posterior temporal bone flap, which, however, is rarely needed. The skin incision is at right angle to the zygoma about 1 cm in front of the ear and is carried down to the level of the zygomatic arch (Fig. 1A). Here, care must be taken not to injure the upper branch of the facial nerve, and it is advisable to retract the lower part of the incision downwards with a "fish hooks" (Fig. 1A, C). After incising the fascia and temporal muscle along its fibers to the arch, it is important

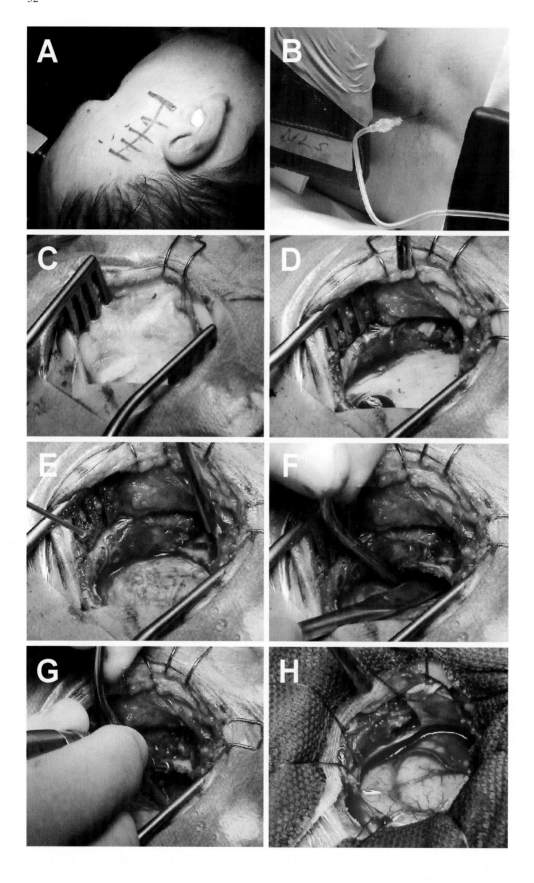

to detach the muscle with its fascia posteriorly from the temporal root of the zygoma (Fig. 1D). Anteriorly, both leaves of the temporal fascia are separated from the arch one centimeter's distance with blunt dissection, not to injure the nerve (Fig. 1D). This allows wider spreading of the temporal muscle with a curved retractor and fishhooks (Fig. 1D). A small bone flap sized 3 × 3 cm is done with one burr hole and craniotome taking care not to injure the dura which may be heavily attached to the skull at the most based part of the craniotomy (Fig. 1D, E). Resection of a part of the zygomatic arch can be done with a diamond drill, but is not often necessary or very helpful (Fig. 1F, G).

The trick of the proper use of the subtemporal approach lies in getting in quickly, without heavy compression of the temporal lobe, and with just enough space to reach the tentorial edge. Lumbar drainage installed by the neurosurgeon before surgery, is the key to successful surgery (Fig. 1B). Modern neuro-anesthesia with Mannitol may be helpful to accelerate slack brain, but without CSF drainage we would not be recommend to start a subtemporal approach. In the presence of hydrocephalus a frontal ventricular drainage has been applied, and when widening the opening into a pterional approach lamina terminalis can also be opened.

With spinal drainage of 50–100 ml of CSF, the brain will be slack when the dura is opened, even in early surgery for ruptured aneurysms in good grade patients (Fig. 1B, H). After opening the dura in V-shaped form, base downwards, and after very careful fixation of the dura with stitches to the surrounding muscles or draping, the microscope should be brought into position (Fig. 1H). Fibrin glue has proved to be extremely useful in stopping possible epidural bleedings. Absolute hemostasis is done before proceeding deeper; otherwise blood may be poured on the operation field at the most critical moments of deep surgery. The retraction of the temporal lobe should be slowly increased. The brain is covered with oxidized cellulose and large wet cottonoids. The line of retraction goes first slightly downwards, then across the floor of the middle fossa and after that upwards to the tentorial

edge. The course of creating the operative route is like taking the temporal lobe in your retracting hand and pulling upwards to see the tentorial edge. A broad Aesculap ^{o,R} retractor is used, very gently, and another may assist to hold the temporal pole anteriorly.

The angle of the subtemporal approach ordinarily is nearly perpendicular to the sagittal plane, but even through a small craniotomy the angle can be changed. An opposite P1 hidden behind a large sac with its perforators can usually be seen by angling the retractor forward a few degrees under the temporal pole, changing the angle of the operating microscope and then displacing the waist of the sac posteriorly. This maneuver is particularly appropriate when a larger bone flap has been used. Associated ipsilateral intact carotid aneurysms are easily exposed for clipping by moving the retractor tip forward a few centimeters under the temporal pole.

One or two temporal lobe bridging veins crossing to the floor of the middle fossa in the line of approach must be divided, but usually other veins on either side can be spared. The adjacent bridging veins are under stretch but they may be dissected a few millimeters from arachnoid to get more freedom for retraction. The junction of the vein of Labbé with the lateral sinus is further away posteriorly located and not in jeopardy in this approach. It is critical that this vein is not injured, to avoid major temporal lobe hemorrhagic infarction.

As the edge of the tentorium comes slowly into view, having the temporal lobe in your "hand", the uncus will leave its position inside the edge of the tentorium. The uncus is the landmark for this retraction, as its elevation by the retractor tip exposes the opening into the interpeduncular cistern. A medial temporal vein may be divided before the final retractor placement on the temporal lobe mesially at the base or under the tip of the uncus.

As the uncus is raised with the tip of the retractor, the third nerve is elevated with it, without placing disturbing angular tension on it. It is usually possible to work below the third nerve to clip the aneurysm except for the case of a higher basilar bifurcation or a giant

◄ ───

Fig. 1. (A) Skin incision. The skin incision is at right angle to the zygoma about 1 cm in front of the ear and is carried to the level of the zygomatic arch. (B) Setting of lumbar spinal drainage. (C) Retraction. Care must be taken not to injure the upper branch of the facial nerve, and it is better to retract the lower part of the incision downwards with a fish hook. A curved retractor and fish hooks allow wider spreading of the temporal muscle. (D) Location of the burr hole. (E) Craniotomy. A small bone flap sized 3 × 3 cm is done with one burrhole. (F) Detaching the heavily attached dura at the lowest part of the craniotomy. (G) Removal of lowest part of the skull by drilling. (H) Dural opening. Dura was opened in a V-shaped form, base downwards, and fixed very carefully with stiches to the surrounding muscles or draping sac, when it may be necessary to separate the third nerve from the uncus. The third nerve may be relaxed by dividing the arachnoid bands holding it. The third nerve tolerance to manipulation varies greatly: an oculomotor palsy may follow a most delicate dissection, and sometimes no palsy is seen even after a relatively strong, long lasting manipulation.

Even with the uncal retraction of the third nerve, the opening into the interpeduncular cistern is narrow. It can be widened significantly by the original simple maneuver of placing a suture in the edge of the tent just in front of, but free of, the insertion and intradural course of the fourth nerve. This suturing is awkward in the deep small gap, and it has been replaced by the use of a small Aesculap [o, R] clip reflecting the edge of the tentorium by about 1 cm towards the surgeon to the floor of the middle fossa. The bleeding is stopped by the use of fibrin glue. The fourth nerve is freed from its arachnoid adhesions, and can be tucked below a cottonoid under the tentorial edge for safety. If necessary, the tentorium is divided and fixed also with a small Aesculap clip(s) to get better access for temporary clipping of the basilar artery. In the case of a low lying basilar bifurcation, tentorium division remains absolutely necessary, and a more posterior approach with a larger flap is planned from the beginning of the operation.

All the arachnoid is widely opened beginning just above the fourth nerve and the superior cerebellar artery below the third nerve on the side of the midbrain, going forward anterior to the third nerve freeing also carotid and posterior communicating arteries. A small space exists between the peduncle and the dorsum sellae laterally. The brain stem can be compressed against the clivus, hiding the interpeduncular fossa. With careful preparation of the arachnoid and further removal of CSF, the peduncle is retracted with the dissecting instruments and cottonoids to see the basilar artery and the base of the aneurysm. The posterior clinoid is not removed as the working field in this position is lateral (posterior) to it.

Depending on the extent of the patient's hemorrhage and the interval between the bleeding and surgery, the interpeduncular fossa may be either filled with clear CSF, packed with fresh or disintegrating clot, or, occasionally in long delayed cases, obliterated with dense arachnoiditis. To avoid heavier retractor pressure in order to see the PCA above the third nerve, it is convenient to follow the superior cerebellar artery back under the third nerve to the BA, sucking away clot to expose its origin just below that of P1. The

lower aspect of P1 will disappear underneath the third nerve. Even though still covered by a clot, the position of the lateral aspect of the neck and waist of the aneurysm is just medial to P1 and usually partially covered laterally and posteriorly by the P1 perforators. The PCoA should be carefully preserved in case some injury to P1 occurs or if it becomes necessary to include P1 in the clip. Furthermore, the PCoA gives rise to important diencephalic branches (anterior thalamoperforating arteries) the integrity of which may be compromised by its occlusion.

Intraoperative hypotension and temporary clipping

Tension in the aneurysm wall is related in an almost linear fashion to systemic blood pressure. Induced hypotension by various means has contributed to the safety of aneurysm surgery with minimal risk of ischemia. Systemic hypotension, down to mean arterial pressure (MAP) of 40–50 mmHg has been widely recognized to reduce the tension and fragility of the aneurysm wall. Recently, local or regional hypotension induced by temporary occlusion of the parent artery has replaced systemic hypotension.

Temporary clipping of BA, which requires most demanding, difficult dissection and a lot of work, has been recently replaced by balloon occlusion. P1 is always above the third nerve and the PCoA joins it; the SCA is always below. A segment of the BA below the SCA and free of perforators for 2 or 3 millimeters should be always exposed for placement of a temporary clip. Our experience indicates that nearly none of these aneurysms should be treated without the use of temporary occlusion of BA.

Temporary clipping is safe and useful when very low tension in the aneurysm is deemed essential for dissection, coagulation or clipping. For difficult aneurysms, especially large ones at the basilar bifurcation, and when one or both PCoAs are large, temporary trapping has been used by occluding one or both PCoAs during the BA occlusion. The opposite PCoA is usually seen unless the aneurysm fills the space. It is more convenient to leave the temporary basilar clip in place while removing and replacing the clip on a large PCoA to provide the intervals for reflow.

Dissection of the aneurysm base

There is a big difference if the BBA is projected forward (rare; may be attached to clivus when low),

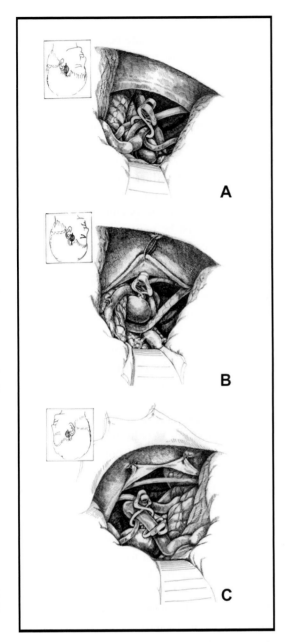

Fig. 2. (A) Schematic drawing shows the skin incision and a small left sided tic craniotomy, and the operative sketch after total occlusion of a basilar bifurcation aneurysm failed to be occluded by earlier coiling and pterional right sided approach. A short ring clip leaves P1–P2 and posterior communicating artery and third nerve inside the ring. (B) Schematic drawing shows the skin incision and small left sided tic craniotomy, and the operative sketch after total occlusion of a BA-SCA aneurysm with a curved microclip before opening and coagulating the aneurysm. The tenting suture has nowadays been replaced by a short straight microclip. (C) Schematic drawing shows the skin incision and small right sided tic craniotomy, and the operative sketch after total occlusion of a large basilar bifurcation aneurysm with two ring clips leaving P1–P2 and posterior communicating artery inside the rings. The tenting sutures have nowadays been replaced by short straight microclips

upwards (most common) or backwards (most difficult due to vicinity of the perforators). The front of the BA is cleared of clot gently upward across the ipsilateral P1 origin where the bulging of the anterior aspect of the neck of the aneurysm is first seen. If the clot can be sucked or teased away easily, the whole of the front of the neck and waist of the aneurysm can be exposed quickly. Occasionally, the clot is tough and adherent to a thin neck; then, only enough neck is cleared to accept the width of the clip blade. Depending on the bulge of the neck and the projection of the aneurysm, the opposite P1 can usually be seen by displacing the waist of the sac posteriorly with a dissector. This will confirm the angle the clip blades must take during application, and further, will often help to visualize the perforators arising from the opposite P1, as well as the opposite third nerve. Sometimes, it will be necessary to clear arachnoid with blunt or sharp dissection on the other side of the neck to see the opposite P1 origin clearly with its perforators.

The major difficulties with this aneurysm lie behind the sac. Rarely, it will stand free in the interpeduncular space; usually, it will be half buried in the interpeduncular fossa. Clearing the base of P1 behind will prepare the way for the important task of finding and separating the perforators. Gentle retraction of the crus is well tolerated and will expose the posterolateral aspect of the neck and waist of the sac, sucking or teasing away old clot if needed. Most of the perforators arise from P1 near its origin and course obliquely upward and backward on the side and back of the base and waist of the sac. They are often free or only lightly adherent to small sacs, but are usually adherent, sometimes densely, to large aneurysms. Not infrequently, one or more perforators arising from the upper BA course upward on the back of the neck. Getting behind the neck usually requires gentle retraction forward of the waist of the sac with the sucker tip, while using a small curved dissector to clear and separate any perforators clinging to the back of the neck. Usually, the perforators can be teased off, but occasionally one or more can be quite adherent to a thin-walled neck. More forceful dissection to free them is made less dangerous by temporary occlusion of BA. Ordinarily, the neck can be displaced forward far enough to see across the interpeduncular fossa to the opposite peduncle, the origin of the opposite P1 and the root of the opposite third nerve. Adherent perforators must be separated upward far enough so that the posterior clip blade can slip inside them without kinking or tearing their origin.

Clipping

The neck of an aneurysm is most completely obliterated when the clip blades fall across the neck in parallel with the parent bifurcation; then there is less risk of kinking P1, particularly with large necks. This ideal placement is more likely to occur with the subtemporal exposure, and is identical to the principles used to treat the much more common middle cerebral artery bifurcation aneurysms. Clips placed more perpendicular to this crotch often leave tags of neck in front and behind ("dog ears"), as the sides of the neck are approximated and the bifurcation crimped. "Dog ears" of residual neck can grow into new aneurysms in our "and others" experience.

The upward curve of P1 only stands free beside small aneurysms, but is usually adherent to larger sacs, often tightly. With the design of the fenestrated clip in 1969 by Drake, P1 can be left adherent to the sac, but open in the aperture while the blades fall across the neck of the aneurysm. Some perforators or the third nerve, too, may be included safely in the aperture. To obscure vision least during clip application, a very low profile clip applier should be used. The fenestrated ring beyond the applier tips tends to obscure vision in the narrow confines, especially behind the aneurysm. The clip blades must be no longer than the flattened, occluded neck or else the P1 origin(s) and its perforators may be stenosed or occluded. Exact measurement of the base in anterior-posterior projection of the aneurysm in CT angiography has proved very useful. A flattened neck is about 1.5 times the width of an open, circular neck (for example a 6 mm aneurysm base needs a clip with 9 mm blades for complete occlusion). Placing the clip too far out on the neck leave a part of the aneurysm base unsecured. The origin of the SCA may not be mistaken for P1, as inadvertent occlusion of the basilar bifurcation will occur. Not uncommonly a bit of the neck is left open in the aperture just medial to the P1 root. This is usually the cause of an aneurysm that still pulsates or bleeds on needling, although it must be certain that the clip tips cross to the far side of the neck. Repositioning of the clip a little higher or addition of a straight tandem clip may suffice to occlude the remaining neck. As the posterior blade is passed behind the neck, one must be certain that it is inside the perforators while using temporary basilar occlusion to soften a dangerously thin neck. As the blades are allowed to close and narrow the neck, the opposite P1 will come into view so that

final alignment, flush with the neck at the upper origins of P1 on each side, can be made before final closure. The posterior blade must not be put too far across, for the root of the opposite third nerve courses up just behind the opposite P1 and can be brushed or actually injured by this blade. As for any aneurysm, immediate inspection is done in front of and behind the neck to determine whether each P1 is open and no perforators are caught or kinked by the blades. Rotating the clip handle forward usually exposes the posterior blade and looking just above the blade will determine whether or not any perforators emerge from underneath it. The clip must be removed and reapplied as many times as necessary for perfect placement. Not infrequently with the first placement, the blades will be too high or too low on the opposite side and it is sobering how often, when surely all the perforators have been seen and separated, one or more are still found caught under the blade.

If single fenestrated clip blades cannot be positioned perfectly without concern for the P1 origins or perforators, then shorter, fenestrated blades should be placed so as to occlude accurately the far two-thirds of the neck, leaving the near neck and P1 and perforators open in the fenestration. Usually then it is simple to separate this open but narrowed portion of the neck from P1 and the perforators, and occlude it by adding a tandem straight clip. This short clip may be applied in front of or behind P1 and the perforators while being certain that it crosses all the neck remaining open in the aperture of the first clip. Instead of using short blades for the tandem clip just to occlude the remaining neck in the fenestration, longer straight blades are used and worked across the whole of the neck, just beyond the fenestrated clip, which then can be removed. The straight clip blades then can be repositioned lower on the neck if necessary. This is of particular value if the fenestrated clip has slid down to obliterate the P1(s) or if the fenestrated blades cannot be positioned so as to occlude both sides of the neck. Provided they do not kink P1, straight blades are more satisfactory; there is no worry about any open near neck and without the obscuration of the fenestrated rings, the tips can be positioned very accurately on the far side of the neck. If the aneurysm base is thick, it may keep the blades of a long clip open on the far side to allow continued filling of the aneurysms. A tandem, fenestrated clip will close the far side of the neck. Because of the small gap and the clip handles, it may be difficult to needle and collapse the sac to prove completed clipping, but it should be done. When coming subtemporally, bipolar coagulation is occasionally useful to shrink and firm up bulbous or otherwise awkward necks of aneurysms, but the fear for occlusion of nearby or hidden perforators always remain. In clipping of SCA and proximal PCA aneurysms, the perforators are usually not of so much concern, but the height and direction of the aneurysm besides its size deserve careful preoperative planning.

Local papaverine is applied after clipping of the aneurysm. The wound is closed to the last stitch under microscope in several layers extremely carefully without leaving any drains.

Discussion

In 1958, the approaches to various segments of the basilar artery were worked out by Drake in the post-mortem room [2–4]. The anterior subtemporal approach across the floor of the middle fossa and tentorial edge into the mouth of the incisura in front of the midbrain seemed to provide the most direct and widest exposure of the interpeduncular region. Consequently, the subtemporal approach was used by Drake and Peerless in 1250 cases in their never-to-repeated series of 1767 patients with vertebrobasilar artery aneurysms (VBAAs) in 1959–1992. Eighty percent (80%) of the 1234 patients with basilar tip aneurysms were treated by subtemporal approach. The main reason for the use of frontotemporal approach for Drake and Peerless was the multiplicity with other aneurysms on the anterior circulation. Much of the merit of this approach is a matter of continued use and familiarity with the anatomy. There is an awkward far side of the operative field with its related difficulties by every approach [1–6, 8–11, 13–19]. The major difficulties with the basilar bifurcation aneurysm lie behind the sac. The advances of the subtemporal approach are that basilar tip aneurysms, especially their backside can be visualized simply and quickly regardless of their size, height, direction or multilocularity. The inner third of the tent can be divided for very low necks and placement of a temporary basilar artery clip, and there is no necessity to open the cavernous sinus, to remove the posterior clinoid or inner petrous apex. This approach has been used by the senior author also for posterior projecting ruptured carotid aneurysms. For associated middle cerebral, carotid bifurcation and anterior communicating aneurysms, the subtemporal exposure usually has been abandoned for the transsylvian approach. However, optic tract and trajectory above it are well seen during subtemporal approach, and it seems possible that at least some of the anterior communicating aneurysms could be clipped through this approach. On the other hand, the transmastoid-transpetrosal presigmoid approach, through a completely divided tentorium, has been used for difficult, large, low placed necks, as well for basilar trunk aneurysms.

In regard to temporary occlusion of basilar artery, the safe time for temporary basilar clipping in normothermia is unknown. Our experience indicates that three to four minute intervals are safe for any artery, and much dissection can be done in that time. The highly variable collateral circulation will be a major factor in the time element for each artery. Under barbiturates and Mannitol protection (1–2 gm/kg), up to ten minutes of single total occlusion times seems to be safe; between 10 to 15 minutes in small and large basilar bifurcation aneurysms the mortality and morbidity rised implying technically more difficult aneurysms.

Conclusion

The advantages of the subtemporal approach to the basilar tip aneurysms (especially their backside) are its simplicity and quickness regardless of the aneurysm size, height, direction or multilocularity. In addition, it is not necessary to open the cavernous sinus and remove the posterior clinoid or inner petrous apex. This classical approach is still most useful for the surgical treatment of basilar bifurcation aneurysms.

References

1. Al-Mefty O (1987) Supraorbital-pterional approach to skull base lesions. Neurosurgery 21: 474–477
2. Drake CG (1961) Bleeding aneurysms of the basilar artery: Direct surgical management in four cases. J Neurosurg 18: 230–238
3. Drake CG (1965) Surgical treatment of ruptured aneurysms of the basilar artery: Experience with 14 cases. J Neurosurg 23: 457–473
4. Drake CG, Peerless SJ, Hernesniemi JA (1996) Surgery of vertebrobasilar aneurysms. London, Ontario Experience on 1767 Patients. Springer, Wien New York
5. Fujitsu K, Kuwabara T (1985) Zygomatic approach for lesions in the interpeduncular cistern. J Neurosurg 62: 340–343
6. Hakuba A, Liu S, Nishimura S (1986) The orbitozygomatic infratemporal approach: a new surgical technique. Surg Neurol 26: 271–276
7. Hernesniemi J, Vapalahti M, Niskanen M, Kari A (1992) Management outcome for vertebrobasilar artery aneurysms by early surgery. Neurosurgery 31: 857–862

8. Heros RC, Lee SH (1993) The combined pterional/anterior temporal approach for aneurysms of the upper basilar complex: technical report. Neurosurgery 33: 244–251

9. Ikeda K, Yamashita J, Hashimoto M, Futami K (1991) Orbito-zygomatic temporopolar approach for a high basilar tip aneurysm associated with a short intracranial internal carotid artery: a new surgical approach. Neurosurgery 28: 105–110

10. Jane JA, Park TS, Pobereskin LH, Winn HR, Butler AB (1982) The supraorbital approach: technical note. Neurosurgery 11: 537–542

11. Kawase T, Toya S, Shiobara R, Mine T (1985) Transpetrosal approach for aneurysms of the lower basilar artery. J Neurosurg 63: 857–861

12. Koivisto T (2002) Prospective outcome study of aneurysmal subarachnoid hemorrhage. Kuopio University Publications, Medical Sciences 284B, pp 140

13. Lawton MT, Vates GE, Spetzler RF (2004) Surgical approaches for posterior circulation aneurysms. In: Winn HR (ed) Youmans neurological surgery: hemorrhagic vascular disease: aneurysms, 4 Vol, 5th edn. Saunders, Philadelphia, pp 1971–2005

14. Le Roux PD, Winn HR (2004) Surgical treatment of basilar bifurcation aneurysms. In: Le Roux PD, Winn HR, Newell DW (eds) Management of cerebral aneurysms: surgical techniques of aneurysm occlusion. Saunders, Philadelphia, pp 809–827

15. Pitelli SD, Almeida GG, Nakagawa EJ, Marchese AJ, Cabral ND (1986) Basilar aneurysm surgery: the subtemporal approach with section of the zygomatic arch. Neurosurgery 18: 125–128

16. Sano K (1980) Temporopolar approach to aneurysms of the basilar artery at and around the distal bifurcation. Technical note. Neurol Res 2: 361–367

17. Yaşargil MG, Fox JL, Ray MW (1975) The operative approach to aneurysms of the anterior communicating artery. Adv Tech Stand Neurosurg 2: 113–170

18. Yaşargil MG, Antic J, Laciga R, Jain KK, Hodosh RM, Smith RD (1976) Microsurgical pterional approach to aneurysms of the basilar bifurcation. Surg Neurol 6: 83–91

19. Yaşargil MG (1984) Vertebrobasilar aneurysms. In: Rand RW (ed) Microneurosurgery, vol 2. Thieme, Stuttgart, pp 232–295

20. Yaşargil MG (2002) Reflections on the thesis "Prospective outcome study of aneurysmal subarachnoid hemorrhage" of Dr Timo Koivisto. Kuopio University Publications, Medical Sciences 284B, pp 51

Correspondence: Juha Hernesniemi, Department of Neurosurgery, Helsinki University Central Hospital, Topeliuksenkatu 5, 00260 Helsinki, Finland. e-mail: juha.hernesniemi@hus.fi

Acta Neurochir (2005) [Suppl] 94: 39–44
© Springer-Verlag 2005
Printed in Austria

Basilar bifurcation aneurysms. Lessons learnt from 40 consecutive cases

Y. Yonekawa, N. Khan, H.-G. Imhof, and P. Roth

Department of Neurosurgery, University Hospital Zurich, Zurich, Switzerland

Summary

Basilar bifurcation aneurysms are lately treated frequently with endovascular technique. Microsurgical clipping occlusion technique has, however, still its solid position because of its completeness. This standard technique is required often due to unfeasibility and/or incompleteness at the time of application of the endovascular technique for aneurysms of this location. The authors suggest following strategies and tactics for safe and secure occlusion of aneurysms of this location: pterional approach, selective extradural anterior clinoidectomy SEAC, no transection of the posterior communicating artery, isolation of perforating arteries at the time of neck clipping with oxycellulose and combination of the use of fenestrated clip and conventional clip (especially for aneurysms projected posteriorly), controlled hypotension (systolic pressure of around 100 mmHg), temporary clipping (trapping) procedures of usually less than 15 min.

All these are aimed for prevention of intraoperative premature rupture, and of injury of perforating arteries and for complete occlusion of aneurysms in the narrow depth of the operative field.

Keywords: Basilar bifurcation aneurysm; selective extradural anterior clinoidectomy SEAC; perforating artery injury; microsurgical neck clipping; endovascular coiling.

Introduction

Treatment of basilar bifucation aneurysms has always been a challenging topic even since the introduction of microsurgery. In patients with relatively good risk, mortality of less than 10% (ranged 2–8%) and good outcome between 70–80% have been reported by neurosurgeons of extreme expertise [3, 9, 10, 12, 13, 16]. Perforating artery injuries rendering unfavourable results have been reported between 7–10% [3, 9, 12]. Introduction of the endovascular coiling method and its application to basilar bifurcation aneurysms has become another modality of treatment [6, 13, 15]. The immediate results have been reported as good or even better as compared to direct clipping methods. Incomplete occlusion of more than 10%, coil compaction of around 25% and impossible to perform coiling procedures of around 5% [13, 15] have been often enumerated to be the common drawbacks of coiling procedures. So the microsurgical treatment is still considered to be the standard method also superior to the endovascular treatment as a result of its completeness.

The purpose of this communication is to describe our recent strategies and tactics at the time of the microsurgical management learnt from our experience of more than 40 consecutive cases of aneurysms of this location.

Patients and results

From 1993 through October 2003, 42 cases (female 31 vs male 11) of basilar bifurcation aneurysm were surgically treated in our department. The age ranged from 28 to 81 years old with median of 50.2 years old. Ruptured aneurysms amounted to 31 cases (74%), unruptured 2 cases (5%), incidental 7 (17%) and symptomatic 1 (2%). Postoperative outcome at 3 months were as follows (Fig. 1): Good recovery GR 29 (69%), Moderately disabled MD 6 (14%), Severely disabled SD 1 (2%), Vegetative state VS 4 (10%), Dead 2 (5%). Complete neck clipping was possible in 88% of cases. The observed surgical complications were: perforator injuries 4 (9.5%), residual neck 2 (4%) and rupture 1 (2%) which took place four months later at the site where a complete neck clipping could be initially performed.

Discussion

Preoperative evaluation of angiography

Beside size, form, neck width, direction of aneurysms and their geographical relation to both P1 origins, height of aneurysm neck has been considered to be of cardinal importance to evaluate technical difficulties beforehand and to select the suitable approaches [19].

Height of aneurysm neck on angiography (lateral view) in most of the cases was within the range of 1.5 cm above the posterior clinoid process PCP. In five

WFNS Grade	GR	MD	SD	VS	D
Ruptured aneurysms — I	●ˣ●ˣ●ˣ●°●°● ●●●●●				●ᵃ
II	●●●●●●	●			
III	●●◑	●●	◑		
IV	●●●●	●▲		●ᵇ●	●ᵇ
V				●ˣ●	
	23	**4**	**1**	**4**	**2**
Incidental aneurysms	OˣO°O O O O	O⊗			
	6	**2**			

Fig. 1. Outcome of microsurgical treatment of basilar bifurcation aneurysms. Outcome at three months: *GR* good recovery, *MD* moderately disabled, *SD* severely disabled, *VS* vegetative state, *D* death. ˣ: coiled after failed clipping procedure, °: clipped after failed coiling procedure, ▲: coating, (a): giant aneurysm, (b): severe vasospasm, ⊗: symptomatic aneurysm, ◑: unruptured aneurysm

cases of this series (10%), necks were positioned lower than the level of the PCP: two of them (7 mm and 10 mm) were managed with subtemporal approach and the rest could be managed with pterional approach combined with selective extradural anterior clinoidectomy SEAC [20]. Need of further combination of posterior clinoidectomy depended on the distance between the PCP and the basilar artery trunk. The smaller this distance is, the more difficult is the placement of a permanent clip to the aneurysm neck or of a temporary clip to the basilar artery without additional use of posterior clinoidectomy. So the distance of more than 5 mm between the PCP and the basilar artery signifies some technical ease of this procedure also in cases with low positioned aneurysms.

Craniotomy with SEAC

There is no doubt that the subtemporal approach pioneered by Drake *et al.* is one of the standards approach for the basilar bifurcation aneurysm [2, 3]. Especially this has been reported to be effective in preservation of the perforating arteries running at the posterior surface of the aneurysm of this location even of those aneurysms that are posteriorly projected. One of the main drawbacks of this approach lies in the use of it in aneurysm cases where there is accompanying brain swelling at the acute stage of bleeding. We applied subtemporal approach only in three cases with low positioned aneurysms. In one of these cases presenting at the subacute stage of bleeding and with the height of the aneurysm neck 3 mm below the PCP, surgery through this approach was interrupted because of swollen brain and therefore the patient was operated upon later with the classical pterional approach with additional SEAC.

Pterional approach developed by Yasargil *et al.* [17] was applied for all cases except for cases mentioned above and SEAC was combined (except for four cases in the early series) in 90% of cases. One of the great advantages of pterional approach is considered to be applicability also for surgery in the acute stage, especially in combination with SEAC and with opening of the lamina terminalis for cerebrospinal fluid CSF drainage [19]. The SEAC procedure adds several advantages to surgery: a wider working space hence also better illumination and better mobility of the internal carotid artery and the optic nerve, this being of cardinal importance [20]. Posterior clinoidectomy [16] and/or transcavernous approach [4] to the aneurysm can be performed with more ease (Fig. 2). SEAC procedure has been reported to enlarge the carotid-oculomotor space and the opticocarotid triangle OCT to more than double [5, 22] so that the space gained can be

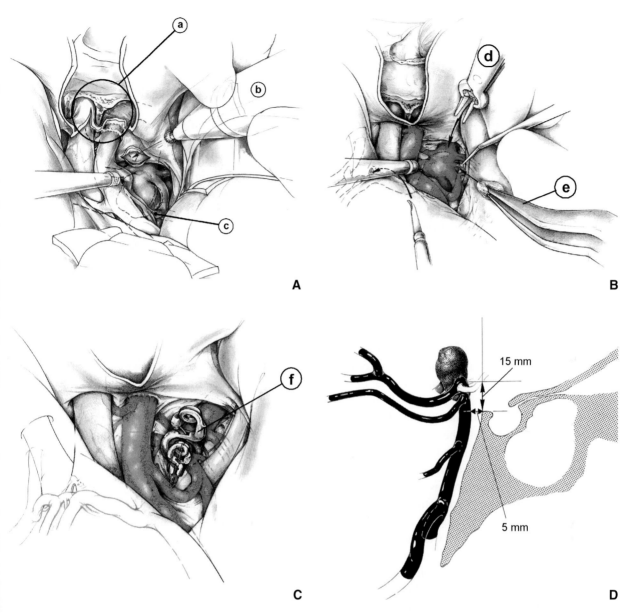

Fig. 2. Artists drawing of our procedure in the microsurgical treatment of basilar bifurcation aneurysms by pterional approach. (A) *a* SEAC, *b* Posterior clinoidectomy, *c* O – no transection of the Pcom A. (B) *d* Temporary clipping. *e* Oxycellulose insertion. (C) *f* Combined clipping procedure with the use of a fenestrated clip and a straight clip in which P1 and a part of the aneurysm neck incorporated to the P1 is preserved at the fenestration of the former clip. The distal part of the incompletely occluded aneurysm is closed with a straight clip. (D) PCP-basilar artery distance: if the distance is more than 5 mm, clipping procedures can be performed with more ease even if the aneurysm necks are 3 mm below the level of PCP

used more effectively for placement of a temporary clip even to the opposite P1 and for placement of a permanent clip to aneurysms of relatively high position.

Transection of the posterior communicating artery

This technique has been recommended to be a helpful and harmless procedure for the access to aneurysms of special location [17]. However, the occurrence of tuberothalamic infarction due to ischemia of the anterior thalamoperforating arteries territorial supply especially after transection of the posterior communicating artery PcomA [1, 11] is becoming increasingly evident. This transection was performed in 15 of cases of our early series: 11 cases were without any neurological and neuroradiological sequellae, 3 cases presented with initial slight hemiparesis followed by complete recovery as a consequence of tuberothalamic infarction on CT scan, and 1 case presented with persistent hemiparesis along with the infarction extending to the posterior limb of the internal capsule. The complication of persistent hemiparesis was considered to be due to an individual variation of the perfusion territory pattern of the sacrificed anterior thalamoperforating arteries arising from the PcomA. After this complication of persistent hemiparesis, our strategy of the use of PcomA transection as a routine procedure has been abandoned. Additionally the introduction of SEAC has also made this procedure unnecessary. However also to mention is that this type of infarction was also observed in a further two cases of this series with subarachnoid hemorrhage SAH without a PcomA transection.

Temporary clipping and trapping

Temporary clipping method (including temporary trapping method in about half of the cases) to obtain secure aneurysm dissection and appropriate placement of permanent clip was used in all but one case. In 75% of the cases the duration was of less than 15 min. The rest ranged between 15 min and 30 min. The longest duration was 40 min. During the aneurysm dissection the blood pressure was controlled and maintained at 100 mmHg of systolic pressure, under which local cortical bood flow lCBF measured with thermal clearlance probe did nit change from the orginal lCBF values. As additional neuroprotective measures Mannitol, barbiturate and heparine were used in accordance to our protocol prior to and during the temporary clipping procedure [18]. Damaging sequellae due to temporary clipping procedure could not be detected in our series except for in one case presenting with bilateral thalamic infarction presumably due to timing of surgery being carried out at the very stage of vasospasm.

Posteriorly projected aneurysms

Beside height and size of aneurysms, their projection have been considered to be one of the factors which make clipping procedures difficult especially at the time of pterional approach, as the running course of perforating arteries is behind aneurysms and therefore hidden in this projection. Subtemporal approach has been reported to be superior to the former for the management of such aneurysms at the time of dissection of perforating arteries from aneurysms and hence their

preservation [3]. But even with subtemporal approach this dissection procedure in the depth is troublesome especially in the presence of swollen brain at the acute stage of SAH.

In this series five cases of which recently three were treated successfully with the method of insertion of oxycellulose between the back side of the aneurysm and perforating artery for isolation [7, 14] followed by occlusion of aneurysms by combination of a fenestrated clip and a conventional clip have been reported elsewhere [21].

Others

For extremely high positioned aneurysms, some special approaches have been reported: transorbital transzygomatic approach and transthird ventricular approach followed by subfrontal interhemispheric approach [8]. Although we did not encounter the need of these approaches in our series, as none of the aneurysms were of such extremely high position, one might take into consideration the approach of transrostrum corporis callosi-lamina terminalis. This approach has been developed for craniopharyngiomas or hypothalamic tumors extending into the third ventricle and into the intercrural and prepontine cistern [18]. This approach offers an unexpextedly wide view of the upper part of the basilar artery after opening the lamina terminalis and the floor of the third ventricle by a one sided (non dominant side) craniotomy without compromising either the olfactory nerve or the frontal sinus. Preservation of hypothalamic branches running on the lamina terminalis and the wall of the third ventricle is considered to be mandatory to prevent postoperative deterioration of cognitive function.

This series includes five cases that required an additional endovascular coiling procedure due to incompleteness or impossibility of neck clipping and four cases of neck clipping procedures; two cases of posteriorly projected aneurysms, a case of residual neck of one large aneurysm, a case of large aneurysm with calcificed neck and a case of a de novo aneurysm after neck clipping of basilar – superior cerebellar artery aneurysm 12 years ago in which neck clipping procedure was hampered by previously placed clips. This series includes, on the other hand, three cases after coiling procedures; one case of coil compaction (Fig. 3) and two cases of unfeasibility of the coiling procedure due to small size of the ruptured aneurysm and due to tortuousness of vessels.

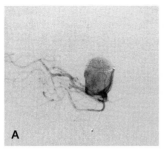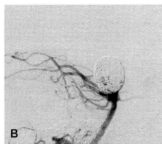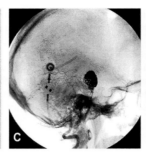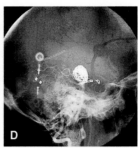

Fig. 3. A case of coil packing followed by clip occlusion. (a) Before coiling. (b) Directly after coiling. (c) 3 months later. (d) Follow-up angiography after the clipping.

Conclusion

Microsurgical occlusion of basilar bifurcation aneurysms should be the standard treatment of use in the face of the presently developing endovascular techniques due to the completeness of aneurysm occlusion acquired through this procedure. After having experienced more than 40 consecutive cases of basilar bifurcation aneurysms, the authors describe their strategies and tactics in the surgical management of basilar bifurcation aneurysms along with the surgical outcome. The safe and effective use of SEAC procedure along with pterional approach, no use of the technique of PcomA transection, clips-combination technique along with use of oxycellulose insertion for posteriorly projected aneurysms and possible application of transrostrum corporis callosi-lamina terminalis approach for extremely high positioned aneurysms have been emphasized.

References

1. Bogousslavsky J, Regli F, Assal G (1986) The syndrome of unilateral tuberothalamic artery terrtory infarction. Stroke 17: 434–441
2. Drake CG (1961) Bleeding aneurysms of the basilar artery. Direct surgical management in four cases. J Neurosurg 18: 230–238
3. Drake CG, Peerless SJ (1996) Small aneurysms at the bifurcation of the basilar artery 493 patients. Chapter 3. In: Drake CG, Peerless SJ, Hernesniemi JA (eds) Surgery of vertebrobasilar aneurysms: London, Ontario Experience on 1,767 Patients. Springer, Wien New York, pp 17–41
4. Dolenc VV, Skrap M, Sustersic J, Skrbec M, Morina A (1987) A transcavernous-transsellar approach to the basilar tip aneurysms. Br J Neurosurg 1: 251–259
5. Evans JJ, Hwang YS, Lee JH (2000) Pre- versus post-anterior clinoidectomy measurements of the optic nerve, internal carotid artery and opticocarotid triangle: a cadaveric morphometric study. Neurosurgery 46: 1018–1023
6. Gruber DP, Zimmerman GA, Tomsick TA, van Loveren HR, Link MJ, Tew JM Jr (1999) A comparison between endovascular and surgical management of basilar artery apex aneurysms. J Neurosurg 90: 868–874
7. Kodama N, Matsumoto M, Sasaki T (1995) Preservation of the arteries around an aneurysm: practical use of oxycellulose. Technical note. J Neurosurg 83: 748–749
8. Kodama N, Sasaki T, Sakurai Y (1995) Transthird ventricular approach for a high basilar bifurcation aneurysms. Report of three cases. J Neurosurg 82: 664–668
9. Lozier AP, Kim GH, Sciacca RR, Connolly ES Jr, Solomon RA (2004) Microsurgical treatment of basilar apex aneurysms: perioperative and long-term clinical outcome. Neurosrgery 54: 286–299
10. Nagashima H, Kobayashi S, Tanaka Y, Hongo K (2004) Endovascular therapy versus surgical clipping for basilar artery bifurcation aneurysm: retrospective analysis of 117 cases. J Clin Neurosci 11: 475–479
11. Regli L, de Tribolet (1991) Tuberothalamic infarct after division of a hypoplastic posterior communicating artery for clipping of a basilar tip aneurysm. Case report. Neurosurgery 28: 456–469
12. Samson D, Batjer HH, Kopitnik TA Jr (1999) Current results of the surgical management of aneurysms of basilar apex. Neurosurgery 44: 697–704
13. Sluzewski M, Bosch JA, van Rooij WJ, Nijssen PC, Wijnalda D (2001) Rupture of intracranial aneurysms during treatment with Guglielmi detachable coils: incidence, outcome, and risk factors. J Neurosurg 94: 238–240
14. Sundt TM (1990) Surgical techniques for saccular and giant intracranial aneurysms. Williams & Wilkins, Baltimore, pp 238–239
15. Tateshima S, Marayama Y, Gobin YP, Duckwiler GR, Guglielmi G, Vinuela F (2000) Endovascular treatment of basilar tip aneurysms using Guglielmi detachable coils: anatomic and clinical outcomes in 73 patients from a single institution. Neurosurgery 47: 1332–1342
16. Yasargil MG (1984) Vertebrobasilar aneurysm, Chapter 5. In: Yasargil MG (ed) Microneurosurgery, vol II. Thieme, Stuttgart, pp 232–295
17. Yasargil MG, Antic J, Laciga R, Jain KK, Hodosh RM, Smith RD (1976) Microsurgical pterional approach to aneurysms of the basilar bifurcation. Surg Neurol 6: 83–91
18. Yonekawa Y (2003) Radical removal of craniopharyngiomas – Consideration on approaches and their consequences. 13th Meeting of Japan Society for Hypothalamic and Pituitary Tumors. Matsue, Japan, February 5. 2002
19. Yonekawa Y, Khan N, Roth P (2002) Strategies for surgical management of cerebral aneurysms of special location, size and form – approach, technique and monitoring. Acta Neurochir (Wien) [Suppl] 82: 105–118

20. Yonekawa Y, Ogata N, Imhof HG, Olivecrona M, Strommer K, Kwak TE, Roth P, Groscurth P (1997) Selective extradural anterior clinoidectomy for supra- and parasellar processes. Technical note. J Neurosurg 87: 636–642

21. Yonekawa Y, Roth P, Khan N (2005) Backwards projecting ruptured basilar bifurcation aneurysm combined with hypoplasia of the internal carotid artery. In: Kobayashi S (ed) Complex tumors and vascular lesions: approaches. Thieme, New York (in press)

22. Youssef AS, Abdel Aziz KM, Kim EY, Keller JT, Zuccarello M, van Loveren HR (2004) The carotid-oculomotor window in exposure of upper basilar artery aneurysms: a cadaveric morphometric study. Neurosurgery 54: 1181–1189

Correspondence: Yasuhiro Yonekawa, Neurochirurgische Universitätsklinik Zurich, Frauenklinikstrasse 10, 8091 Zurich, Switzerland. e-mail: yasuhiro.yonekawa@usz.ch

Perioperative management

Acta Neurochir (2005) [Suppl] 94: 47–51
© Springer-Verlag 2005
Printed in Austria

Endovascular treatment of cerebral vasospasm following aneurysmal subarachnoid hemorrhage

B. Schuknecht

Institute of Neuroradiology, University Hospital of Zurich, Zurich Switzerland

Summary

Endovascular treatment by balloon angioplasty or intra-arterial papaverine infusion has been established as a valuable treatment option in patients with cerebral vasospasm refractory to maximal medical therapy. A summary of the indications, applications and limitations is provided for microcatheter guided selective papaverine infusion and transluminal balloon angioplasty in patients who sustain cerebral vasospasm following subarachnoid haemorrhage. Structured neuro-intensive and endovascular treatment of imminent vasospasm integrate papaverine administration and balloon angioplasty as complimentary rather than alternative techniques.

Keywords: Transluminal balloon angioplasty; microcatheter guided papaverine infusion; endovascular treatment; cerebral vasospasm; subarachnoid haemorrhage.

Introduction

Cerebral vasospasm remains a leading cause of morbidity and mortality following aneurysmal subarachnoid hemorrhage [9]. Preventive measures include surgical, medical and endovascular treatment. Surgical measures are performed in conjunction with clipping of the aneurysm and consist of flushing of the subarachnoid space and opening of the lamina terminalis. In case of endovascular treatment of the ruptured aneurysm, angiographic vasospasm may be treated within the same session following occlusion of the aneurysm. Endovascular means therefore are only rarely preventive but are usually aimed at targeted treatment of symptomatic and/or angiographic vasospasm. Medical preventive treatment is always instituted consisting of calcium antagonist therapy in a first step and hypertensive, hypervolemic therapy and hemodilution (triple H therapy) when rising flow velocities in basal cerebral arteries indicate impeding vasospasm.

The discrepancy between a high incidence of angiographic vasospasm or high flow velocity recordings by transcranial colour Doppler sonography (TCD) between day 7 and 15 and a significantly lower incidence of symptomatic vasospasm is explained by several factors. The high sensitivity of angiography and TCD to detect and localize vasospasm, the individuals potential to compensate vasospasm by way of collaterals, and last but not least the ability to judge a patients clinical condition and its deterioration depending on the Hunt and Hess grade.

Indication and methods

Cerebral vasospasm that is refractory to maximal medical management is an indication for endovascular therapy. In patients being well amenable to clinical assessment progressive vasospasm is indicated by confusion, deterioration in the level of consciousness and/or development of a new focal neurologic deficit. In patients with Hunt and Hess grade IV and V and in patients being intubated and ventilated recognition of vasospasm is dependent on indirect means only. Several techniques (bulbus oximetry, internal jugular vein lactic acid differences) have been investigated to substantiate the presence and location of cerebral vasospasm. TCD recordings have proven to be efficient and sensitive but not specific for cerebral vasospasm. TCD performed on a regular basis provides support to non-invasive recognition of vasospasm when time averaged maximal flow velocities exceed 140–160 cm/s within the anterior, or middle cerebral artery and intracranial internal carotid artery. A sudden rise of 50 cm/s is indicative of moderate to severe vasospasm as well. Prior to the decision to perform endovascular treatment a cranial CT is performed. The objective is to exclude hydrocephalus, haemorrhage, infarction or infection as causes of clinical deterioration or rising intracranial pressure values.

A new technique that is progressively being integrated into the diagnostic regimen is perfusion CT. Cerebral infarction either evident on noncontrast CT or on blood volume parameter maps is a contraindication to perform endovascular therapy. However, significant differences in territorial or hemispheric transit times not only substantiate the need to perform endovascular therapy but may help to direct treatment to the vascular territory most severely affected.

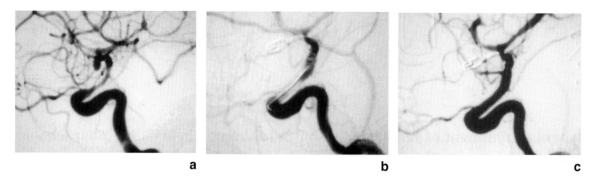

a   b   c

Fig. 1. 58 year old female with ruptured middle cerebral artery bifurcation aneurysm. Progressive right sided hemiparesis on day 8 following subarachnoid haemorrhage. The lateral projection of the left carotid angiography (a) reveals marked vasospasm of the supraclinoid internal carotid artery. Transluminal balloon angioplasty (b) due to circumscribed proximal location of vasospasm. Left lateral projection of carotid angiography following angioplasty (c) depicts elimination of vasospasm with restoration of normal vessel calibre

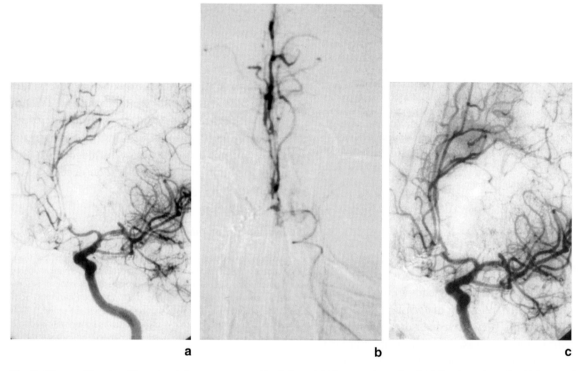

a   b   c

Fig. 2. 65 year old male with ruptured Acom aneurysm. Confusion, right leg paresis on day 11 following subarachnoid haemorrhage. The antero-oblique projection of the left carotid angiography (a) demonstrates marked vasospasm of both pericallosal arteries which are supplied via a moderately narrowed left A1 segment. The A1 on the right side was hypoplastic. Ap projection after contrast injection via the selectively positioned microcatheter with the tip within the distal left A1 segment (b). Antero-oblique projection of left carotid angiography following administration of 300 mg papaverine (c) shows marked vasodilatation within both A2 segments. The anterior cerebral artery and the proximal middle cerebral artery have increased in calibre as well

The presence, location and degree of vasospasm are confirmed by digital subtraction angiography (DSA). DSA as an invasive diagnostic procedure is performed only with the intent to perform endovascular treatment.

Endovascular treatment

The objective of endovascular treatment of cerebral arterial vasospasm is to restore adequate blood flow and to prevent cerebral ischemia and infarction. Cerebral arterial vasospasm consists of an active and passive component. The active constituent is caused by actin-myosin cross linking, while the passive component is due to a fixed contractile apparatus within the tunica media of the vessel wall. Endovascular treatment is aimed at reversal of both components. Two different techniques are applied: mechanical or pharmacological vessel dilatation. Mechanical vasodilatation is achieved by means of transluminal balloon angioplasty and is directed towards a circumscribed proximal vessel segment. Balloon angioplasty was first introduced in 1984 in the setting of clinical vasospasm [18]. Balloon angioplasty reverses both active and passive components of vasospasm.

Pharmacological endovascular dilatation is based on continuous intraarterial infusion of papaverine via a microcatheter positioned within the proximal intracranial vessel territory affected by vasospasm. Papaverine treatment is effective within the entire vessel territory primarily treated and recirculation exerts an effect within other vascular territories as well. Its action is predominantly directed towards the active component of arterial vasospasm.

Treatment by balloon angioplasty is targeted to proximal intracranial arterial vasospasm. Proximal vasospasm affects the supraclinoid internal carotid artery, the middle cerebral artery mainstem, the proximal middle cerebral artery branches (M 2 segments) and the A1 segment of the anterior cerebral artery [3, 16]. The arteries of the vertebro-basilar system including the proximal posterior cerebral arteries (P1) are accessible to balloon angioplasty as well, but only rarely exhibit vasospasm. Vasospasm occurring distal to the aforementioned vessel segments is not accessible to endovascular balloon treatment due to small vessel size. Balloon angioplasty is performed with compliable balloon systems with a diameter of 1.5 and 2.0 to 3.0 mm. Even though angioplasty is directed to and effective on a morphological basis in circumscribed proximal vessel segments only, the rational is to improve blood flow, oxygenation and metabolism within the distal arterial territory as well [1, 5].

In order to achieve sufficient dilatation within a longer proximal vessel segment or in multiple vessels, repeated balloon inflations may be required in different positions. In patients with maximum degree proximal vasospasm pre-treatment with intraarterial papaverine injection is at times the only means to achieve sufficient predilation to allow a balloon to be placed without obstructing blood flow. Additional balloon angioplasty on the other hand remains an option in patients with proximal vasospasm refractory to papaverine treatment [11].

Balloon angioplasty mechanically reverses the active and passive component of vasospasm. By distension of the internal elastic lamina and tunica media, smooth muscle constriction and fixation of the con-

tractile filaments and muscle fibres are thus eliminated. Balloon angioplasty therefore bears the risk of vessel rupture in case of overdistension of the vessel.

Vasospasm following angioplasty is not prone to recurrence. The dilating effect of transluminal balloon angioplasty was found to persist in 99% [3] and 100% [16] of vessel segments treated.

Limitations of balloon angioplasty include the segmental nature of dilatation and the inaccessibility of distal vessel segments. A contraindication to balloon angioplasty is a vasospastic vessel segment harbouring a clipped or coil treated side wall aneurysm and an unsecured aneurysm at or distal to the vessel segment affected by vasospasm. Manifest cerebral ischemia proven by CT or diffusion MR is a contraindication for any endovascular intervention as well. In patients with symptomatic or severe vasospasm at the time of initial angiography after subarachnoid hemorrhage a combined treatment approach may be performed starting with obliteration of the aneurysm followed by initiation of spasmolytic therapy. In 12 patients with severe vasospasm on admission combined GDC occlusion of the aneurysm and balloon angioplasty was performed in 6 patients, papaverine infusion in two cases or both treatment modalities in 4 patients in a single session. In all patients angiographic improvement of vasospasm was obtained [12].

Microcatheter guided intraarterial papaverine infusion is an alternative or supplementary treatment to balloon angioplasty in patients affected by vasospasm. First introduced in 1992 Kaku and Yonekawa [7] established superselective application of papaverine via a microcatheter. The authors were the first to report administration of papaverine in conjunction with PTA. Superselective papaverine application via a microcatheter which is placed within the proximal vessel segment has since evolved as a standard technique. Kassell and coworkers [8] established 300 mg papaverine as a standard dose dissolved within 100 ml of saline. Heparine should not be added in order to prevent crystal formation. Infusion is performed over a minimum of 30 minutes. Papaverine may also be administered as an adjunct following proximal angioplasty in order to reverse additional distal vasospasm. The long term effects of intraarterial papaverine treatment as the sole therapy has been questioned in view of its short pharmacologic half life of 8.5 minutes. After papaverine infusion a beneficial effect was found to be limited to the first three hours only by continuous long term thermal diffusion rCBF measurements [17].

Recurrence of vasospasm following papaverine treatment is not uncommon. Repeated infusions due to recurrence of vasospasm have been reported in 23.3% [16] and even in 37.5% of patients [13]. The incidence of a second recurrence following standard dose papaverine treatment is low [6.7%] and tends to affect different vessels than the ones previously treated [16]. In case of multi-territorial vasospasm or recurrence, the papaverine dose may be increased up to 600 mg [13, 16]. Recurrence of vasospasm accounts for the major limitation of papaverine treatment. However, repetitive papaverine administrations may be performed based on symptoms, TCD recordings or angiographic findings. Even though the efficacy of papaverine has been questioned within a later stage of vasospasm, a maintained effect corresponding to initial treatments has been shown. In 17 patients with recurrent vasospasm papaverine administration reversed prolonged circulation time in 90 of 91 (99%) vessels treated. Repeated infusions were as successful as the primary treatment [10]. In case of symptomatic vasospasm treatment should be instituted as early as possible. A two hour window was found to exist for restoration of blood flow by endovascular treatment [15].

Preventive treatment without clinical or angiographic evidence of vasospasm is not indicated in view of the following limitations and side effects. Limitations of papaverine treatment are raised intracranial pressure, and systemic hypotension. Side effects consist of respiratory depression and brainstem dysfunction in vertebral artery infusions [5], systemic hypotension and propensity to seizures in supratentorial arterial infusions [2].

Both papaverine and combined angioplasty and papaverine treatment are conducted under general anaesthesia. Elevated intracranial pressure is strongly associated with poor outcome and death in a series of 62 patients treated by balloon angioplasty and papaverine at the University of Cincinatti [1]. Papaverine was most effective as a single dose treatment in distal monoarterial vasospasm, if balloon angioplasty was impossible or not considered safe. Balloon angioplasty was indicated as an early treatment in multi-territorial proximal vasospasm. In another study the efficacy of balloon angioplasty was assessed in comparison to papaverine therapy and to combined angioplasty and papaverine spasmolytic treatment [14]. While the effect on proximal flow velocities was most pronounced in 12 patients treated with balloon angioplasty, the effect on cerebral blood flow and increase in vessel diameter was

more prominent in 20 patients following papaverine application. Combined treatment by papaverine and angioplasty in 13 patients proved most effective with respect to increase in cerebral blood flow and arterial diameter.

Despite aggressive instantaneous and repetitive treatment attempts by endovascular interventions the overall benefit with respect to patients outcome is difficult to assess. Early clinical improvement following endovascular treatment is strongly associated with favourable outcome [4]. In a review of 38 patients enrolled as part of the American trial of tirilazad the authors state the effectiveness of transluminal balloon angioplasty but conclude that the superiority to medical management is questionable [5]. In a series of 30 patients treated with papaverine infusion and angioplasty permanent clinical improvement was achieved in 73.3% of patients [16]. These results compare favourably with a rate of 69% permanent improvement in a series of 24 patients with papaverine as the sole treatment [13] and are identical to a series of 101 PTA treated vessels with maintained clinical improvement in 74% of patients [3].

Conclusion

The complexity of vasospasm with respect to mono- or multiterritorial location, proximal or distal vessel territory involvement and different degrees of severity render correlation of angiographic improvement with clinical improvement difficult [5, 16]. This is not surprising in view of the fact that endovascular treatment is only one constituent of the challenging neuro-intensive management of patients after subarachnoid hemorrhage.

References

1. Andaluz N, Tomsick TA, Tew JM Jr, van Loveren HR, Yeh HS, Zuccarello M (2002) Indications for endovascular therapy for refractory vasospasm after aneurysmal subarachnoid hemorrhage. Experience at the University of Cincinatti. Surg Neurol 58: 131–138
2. Carhuapoma JR, Qureshi AI, Tamargo RJ, Mathis JM, Hanley DF (2001) Intra-arterial papaverine-induced seizures: case report and review of the literature. Surg Neurol 56: 159–163
3. Elliott JP, Newell DW, Lam DJ, Eskridge JM, Douville CM, Le Roux PD, Lewis DH, Mayberg MR, Grady MS, Winn HR (1998) Comparison of balloon angioplasty and papaverine infusion for the treatement of vasospasm following aneurysmal subarachnoid hemorrhage. J Neurosurg 88: 277–284
4. Fandino J, Schuknecht B, Yuksel C, Wieser HG, Valavanis A, Yonekawa Y (1999) Clinical, angiographic, and sonographic

findings after structured treatment of cerebral vasospasm and their relation to final outcomes. Acta Neurochir (Wien) 141: 677–690

5. Firlik KS, Kaufmann AM, Firlik AD, Jungreis CA, Yonas H (1999) Intra-arterial papaverine for the treatment of cerebral vasospasm following aneurysmal subarachnoid hemorrahge. Surg Neurol 51: 66–74

6. Hoelper B, Hofmann E, Sporleder R, Soldner F, Behr R (2003) Transluminal balloon angioplasty improves brain tissue oxygenation and metabolism in severe vasospasm after aneurysmal subaarchnoid hemorrahge: case report. Neurosurgery 52: 970–976

7. Kaku Y, Yonekawa Y, Tsukahara T, Kazekawa K (1992) Superselective intra-arterial infusion of papaverine for the treatment of cerebral vasospasm after subarachnoid hemorrhage. J Neurosurg 77: 842–847

8. Kassell NF, Helm G, Simmons N, Phillips CD, Cail WS (1992) Treatment of cerebral vasospasm with intra-arterial papaverine. J Neurosurg 77: 848–852

9. Kassell NF, Torner JC, Haley EC Jr, Jane JA, Adams HP, Kongable GL (1990) The international cooperative study on the timing of aneurysm surgery. Part 1: overall management results. J Neurosurg 73: 18–36

10. Liu JK, Tenner MS, Gottfried ON, Stevens EA, Rosenow JM, Madan N, MacDonald JD, Kestle JR, Couldwell WT (2004) Efficacy of multiple intraarterial papaverine infusions for improvement in cerebral circulation time in patients with recurrent cerebral vasospasm. J Neurosurg 100: 414–421

11. Morgan MK, Jonker B, Finfer S, Harrington T, Dorsch NW (2000) Aggressive management of aneurysmal subarachnoid haemorrhage based on a papaverine angioplasty protocol. J Clin Neurosci 7: 305–308

12. Murayama Y, Song JK, Uda K, Gobin YP, Duckwiler GR, Tateshima S, Patel AB, Martin NA, Vinuela F (2003) Combined endovascular treatment for both intracranial aneurysm and symptomatic vasospasm. AJNR Am J Neuroradiol 24: 133–139

13. Numaguchi Y, Zoarski GH, Clouston JE, Zagardo MT, Simard JM, Aldrich EF, Sloan MA, Maurer PK, Okawara SH (1997) Repeat intra-arterial papaverine for recurrent cerebral vasospasm after subarachnoid haemorrhage. Neuroradiology 39: 751–759

14. Oskouian RJ, Martin NA, Lee JH, Glenn TC, Guthrie D, Gonzalez NR, Afrari A, Vinuela F (2002) Multimodal quantitation of the effects of endovascular therapy for vasospasm on cerebral blood flow, transcranial doppler ultrasonographic velocities, and cerebral artery diameters. Neurosurgery 51: 30–43

15. Rosenwasser RH, Armonda RA, Thomas JE, Benitez RP, Gannon PM, Harrop J (1999) Therapeutic modalities for the management of cerebral vasospasm: timing of endovascular options. Neurosurgery 44: 975–980

16. Schuknecht B, Fandino J, Yuksel C, Yonekawa Y, Valavanis A (1999) Endovascular treatment of cerebral vasospasm: assessment of treatment effect by cerebral angiography and transcranial Doppler sonography. Neuroradiology 41: 453–462

17. Vajkoczy P, Horn P, Bauhuf C, Munch E, Hubner U, Ing D, Thome C, Poeckler-Schoeninger C, Roth H, Schmiedek P (2001) Effect of intra-arterial papaverine on regional cerebral blood flow in hemodynamically relevant cerebral vasospasm. Stroke 32: 498–505

18. Zubkov YN, Nikiforov BM, Shustin VA (1984) Balloon catheter technique for dilatation of constricted cerebral arteries after aneurismal SAH. Acta Neurochir (Wien) 70: 65–79

Correspondence: Bernhard Schuknecht, MRI Medizinisch Radiologisches Institut an der Privatklinik Bethanien, Toblerstr. 51, 8044 Zurich, Schweiz. e-mail: Schuknecht@mri-roentgen.ch

Acta Neurochir (2005) [Suppl] 94: 53–58
© Springer-Verlag 2005
Printed in Austria

The intracranial B-waves' amplitude as prognostication criterion of neurological complications in neuroendovascular interventions

V. B. Semenyutin, V. A. Aliev, P. I. Nikitin, and **A. V. Kozlov**

Russian Polenov Neurosurgical Institute, Saint-Petersburg, Russia

Summary

The purpose of this study was to evaluate dynamics of B-waves' amplitudes (BWA) of blood flow velocity (BFV) in patients with cerebrovascular diseases during endovascular operations. We examined 12 patients with neurovascular pathology during neuroendovascular interventions. Patients were divided into two groups: 1st group (6 cases) – without intraoperative neurological complications, 2nd group (6 cases) – with complications. Bilateral monitoring of BFV in middle cerebral arteries was carried out applying Multi Dop X. To estimate BWA Fourier analysis was used. In the 1st group preoperative BWA on the affected side was 3.9 ± 0.6 cm/s. Intraoperative (during an access to pathologic formation and its embolisation) BWA increased up to 7.7 ± 1.1 cm/s ($p < 0.05$). Postoperative BWA decreased to 4.2 ± 0.8 cm/s. In the 2nd group the preoperative BWA on the affected side was 9.6 ± 1.1 cm/s ($p < 0.05$), thus higher than in the 1st group. Intraoperatively we observed further increase of BWA up to 12.1 ± 2.6 cm/s, accompanied by occurrence or increase of neurological symptoms. Postoperative BWA decreased to 10.4 ± 2.9 cm/s, whereas we didn't observe regression of neurological symptoms.

Keywords: Cerebral blood flow; cerebral autoregulation; transcranial Doppler; spectral analysis; intracranial B-waves; neuroendovascular intervention.

Introduction

Efficient treatment of neurovascular disorders is strongly dependent on the state of cerebral circulation during endovascular intervention [3, 4, 10, 13]. Quick and timely estimation of mechanisms regulating cerebral blood flow (CBF) would allow to reveal impaired function of cerebral circulation system at a stage that precedes development of neurological complications, and, thus, prevent them by taking necessary treatment-and-prophylaxis measures.

Existing methods of regulation assessment are based on use of transcranial Doppler to monitor the linear blood flow velocity (BFV) in basilar arteries at different stages of treatment of neurosurgical cases [3, 4, 10].

Special attention is paid to studying cerebral blood flow autoregulation (CA) as one of the main properties of a system of cerebral circulation supporting constancy of CBF in case of changes of cerebral perfusion pressure (CPP) within certain limits [1, 4, 19].

From the 90ies on, conventional methods to study CA (in time domain) [1, 4, 6] were supplemented by applying spectral analysis (in frequency domain) [2, 5, 7, 9, 12, 16, 22]. Estimation of BFV and CPP in time domain enabled obtaining information on static (by changing CPP by pharmacological means) and dynamic (by using cuff or compression tests, as well as Valsava's maneuver) CA in case of normocapnia, hypocapnia and hypercapnia [1, 11, 15, 17, 20]. Studying CA on the basis of spectral analysis resulted in forming a concept according to which CA was a complex multi-component mechanism ensuring constancy of CBF not only in quick changes of CPP, but also in its slow spontaneous oscillations within MF (middle frequency) (0.1 Hz) and LF (low frequency) (0.02–0.07 Hz) ranges without any considerable effect on systemic and cerebral hemodynamics as a whole [2, 6, 9, 12]. From this point of view CA can be regarded as a high-pass filter transmitting HF oscillations of BFV (>0.2 Hz) which are characterized by high coherence and a smaller phase shift in comparison with analogous oscillations of the systemic blood pressure (BP). At the same time, this high-pass filter damps down MF and LF oscillations of BFV (Mayer's waves, etc.). It manifests itself in low coherence and a bigger phase shift between BFV and BP within the above mentioned range. These data demonstrate that CA depends on frequency and is more effective within MF and LF ranges, as compared to HF range. Disorders of CA lead to an increase of the filter's transmitting capacity and, as a result, to higher coherence and a smaller phase shift between BP and BFV within MF and LF ranges of spontaneous oscillations.

Spectral analysis is an informative, simple and absolutely safe method of CA estimation. Thanks to this fact, it is used in clinical practice for diagnosis of CA disorders in cases with intracranial aneurysms, arteriovenous malformations and occluding lesions of major cervical vessels [6, 9, 15, 18]. However, its wider use is limited by the – technically often not feasible – necessity of continuous recording of BP.

Though acknowledging that CA is a frequency-dependent phenomenon, many researchers pay more attention to studying the spontaneous oscillations within the range of Mayer's systemic waves and respiratory waves instead of focusing on the B-waves (0.008–0.03 Hz). For the first time these waves were detected in the spectrum of intracranial pressure [8] its rise causing an increase of B-waves' amplitude. Later on it was discovered that they originated within the spectrum of BFV [14]. However, the exact cause for their appearance is not entirely clear [14, 22]. B-waves are likely to reflect a state of regulatory mechanisms of CBF mediated via smooth-muscle cells of cerebral vessels or stem pace-makers which change CBF within certain periodicity by effecting the activity of vasomotor neurons.

Our investigation is based on a supposition, according to which disorders of CA not only cause changes of coherence and a phase shift between BFV and BP within the MF range, but also changes of B-waves' parameters. The purpose of the study is to evaluate an amplitude of intracranial B-waves of BFV and its dynamics in endovascular interventions performed in cases with neurovascular pathology.

Materials and methods

Description of patients

There were 12 cases (7 males and 5 females, aged 25–60) with different neurovascular pathology, including malformations (7), aneurysms (4) and carotid-cavernous fistula (1). Supratentorial and subtentorial localization of malformations were observed in 6 and 1 patients respectively; all aneurysms were localized in the region of the internal carotid artery.

Malformations and aneurysms manifested themselves in a single episode of subarachnoid hemorrhage or a seizure; carotid-cavernous fistula developed after head injury of moderate severity.

Accompanying somatic diseases were represented by coronary heart disease, observed in elderly patients (50–60 years old); though there was no need to prescribe additional cardiac drugs during the period of treatment.

The patients were admitted to a hospital a month after disease onset. As for admission, subsequent examination and intervention, they were characterized either by absence of any neurological symptoms or presence of oculomotor or minor motor disorders.

Interventions

Due to localization of malformations in eloquent cerebral areas, big and giant aneurysms or their localization at the level of an ophthalmic segment of the internal carotid artery, endovascular operation was considered to be preferable to open surgical intervention.

Operations were executed according to a standard method with an approach through the right femoral artery and use of catheters for endovascular interventions (Balt). Superselective embolization of malformations was performed through afferent vessels, using histoacryl as an embolizing substance; aneurysms and carotid-cavernous fistula were occluded with mechanically detachable coils and latex balloon. Anesthesiologic support consisted in sedation-analgesia (a standard-dose combination of propofol and fentanyl).

Monitoring

Perioperative bilateral monitoring of BFV in the middle cerebral artery was carried out applying Multi Dop X (DWL). BP was monitored invasively through the 20–22 GA catheter, introduced into the radial artery; the M-34 mingograph (Siemens) was used. Recorded indices were monitored every 5 min during operation; a patient was in a horizontal position with his head elevated up to 30°; monitoring was carried out at rest against a background of preserved spontaneous breathing.

A protocol of perioperative monitoring during neuroendovascular interventions was approved of by the Ethic Committee of the Polenov Neurosurgical Institute. Monitoring started after receiving the patient's written consent.

Data analysis

Spectral analysis of B-waves of BFV in the middle cerebral artery was carried out according to a standard algorithm with the help of Statistica 6.0 for Windows (Time Series/Forecasting module). A time series within an interval of 240–300 sec was chosen based on the Kotelnikov-Shannon's theorem stating the estimation of the spectrum of LF oscillations requires analysis of a time series for a period, which is at least twice as long as a maximum period of LF oscillations (120 sec for B-waves). To ensure stability of this series, spectral analysis was preceded by subtraction of the mean from values of a time series. Smoothing of values, characteristic of one period, was performed with the purpose of incidental noise suppression, reducing dispersion of a time series and revealing frequencies with high spectral densities, which contributed significantly to a periodic behavior of the whole time series. Smoothing was achieved by transformation of the running weighted mean in Hemming's window. Then the spectral density of all oscillations in a chosen time interval, including the range of intracranial B-waves (0.0083–0.033 Hz), was calculated. Calculation of B-waves' amplitude (BWA) was carried out in accordance with the following formula:

$$BWA = \sqrt{SD \times F} \ (cm/s)$$

(SD – spectral density, $(cm/s)^2/Hz$; F – frequency, Hz)

Statistics

Statistical processing of data was carried out with the help of standard methods (Statistica 6.0 for Windows). Criteria used were parametric (Student's t-criterion) and non-parametric (Kholmogorov-Smirnov's criterion, Pirson's χ^2 criterion). Difference was considered to be statistically reliable with $p < 0.05$.

Results

BWA was estimated in succession at three stages of intravascular intervention. The first stage preceded with the introduction of a catheter guide into major cervical vessels. The second stage corresponded to the period of microcatheter's delivery to the pathologic formation and the actual surgical intervention. The third stage corresponded to completion of the operation and removal of catheters.

The patients were subdivided into two groups, depending on the course of the intraoperative period. The 1st group included cases (6) without neurological complications during intraoperative period; the 2nd group (6) comprised patients with development of intraoperative neurological complications (headache, suppressed consciousness, nausea, vomiting, gross motor and speech disturbances). The causes of complications were as follows: thrombosis of the internal carotid artery – 2 cases with aneurysm and 1 case with carotid-cavernous fistula; cerebral vasospasm and intracranial hypertension – 1 female patient with aneurysm and 1 male patient with malformation; parenchymal-subarachnoid hemorrhage into cerebellar hemispheres – 1 female patient with malformation of subtentorial localization. As for the last female, development of marked bulbar symptoms resulted in a fatal outcome during the first postoperative day.

Patients without intraoperative complications

Mean values of BP, BFV and BWA, recorded on the side of operation and on the opposite side in patients of the 1st group at different stages of intravascular intervention, are given in Table 1.

Due to anesthesiologic support (sedation-analgesia) causing no considerable suppression of breathing and BP reduction and transnasal insufflation of an oxygen-air mixture, spontaneous breathing of patients corresponded to normoventilation conditions. It was confirmed by capnography data and measurements of pCO_2 in arterial blood. At the main stage of operation there was a reliable increase of BWA ($p < 0.05$) (Table 1) on the side of intervention and on the opposite side. On both sides no considerable changes of BP and BFV were observed during intervention (Table 1).

Table 1. *BP, BFV and BWA of patients of the first group at different stages of endovascular intervention*

Stages of operation	BP [mm Hg]	BF parameters [cm/s]			
		On the side of operation		On the opposite side	
		BFV	BWA	BFV	BWA
Preoperative	79 ± 9	77 ± 11	3.9 ± 0.6	82 ± 12	3.8 ± 0.7
Intraoperative	84 ± 10	85 ± 12	7.7 ± 1.1	75 ± 12	7.5 ± 1.3
Postoperative	84 ± 11	87 ± 14	4.2 ± 0.8	83 ± 15	4.0 ± 0.6

Figure 1 demonstrates monitoring of BFV and BWA on the side of operation at different stages of intravascular intervention performed in a 25 years old patient with giant aneurysm of the left internal carotid artery. Complete exclusion of the aneurysm from blood circulation was achieved by means of its occlusion by a latex balloon. There were no intraoperative and early postoperative neurological complications.

Patients with intraoperative complications

Mean values of BP, BFV and BWA, recorded on the side of operation and on the opposite side in patients of the 2nd group at different stages of intravascular intervention, are given in Table 2.

Perioperative changes of BFV and BP in patients of the 2nd group, as well as in cases of the 1st group, were insignificant. Their breathing was spontaneous and corresponded to normoventilation parameters. BWA was considerably higher already before operation ($p < 0.05$), i.e. before performing manipulations on major vessels (a change of an angiographic catheter for a catheter guide, introduction of a microcatheter into intracranial vessels), as compared to patients without complications (Table 2). However, there were no objective signs of augmentation of neurological symptoms. Further increase of BWA, observed on the side of operation and opposite side at the main stage of intervention, was accompanied by occurrence or increase of neurological symptoms (appearance of headache, nausea, vomiting, motor and speech disorders, sharp suppression of consciousness up to deep stupor, sopor). Reduction of BWA after operation (detachment of a spiral, balloon, injection of a glue composition, removal of catheters) was insignificant. There was no regression of neurological symptoms.

Figure 2 demonstrates monitoring of BFV and BWA on an operated side in a 42 years old female

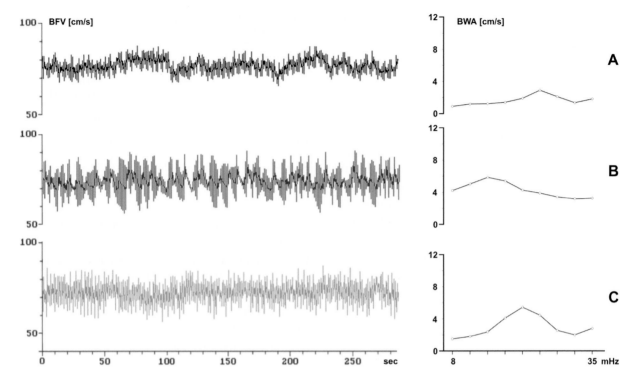

Fig. 1. Monitoring of BFV and BWA on the side of operation before (A), during (B) and after (C) the operation, performed in 25 years old patient with giant aneurysm of an ophthalmic segment of the left internal carotid artery

patient with a large saccular aneurysm of the supra-clinoid segment of the left internal carotid artery.

Before operation BWA on the side of the aneurysm was considerably higher than in patients without complications; it was watched against a background of relatively normal parameters of BFV in the left middle cerebral artery. The patient developed nausea, vomiting, psychomotor excitement, dysphasic disorders at the stage of an approach to aneurysm (introduction of a coil into aneurysm and its subsequent detachment). Monitoring of BFV, carried out just

before the described aggravation, did not reveal its considerable changes, though there was a further increase of BWA. After a coil detachment and catheters removal BWA reduced but did not reach the initial means before the operation. After operation the female patient was admitted to the Intensive Care Unit, where she spent a day and was subjected to intensive infusion therapy. Neurological symptoms regressed during a week.

Discussion

Volby *et al.*, in 1982 found in patients with acute subarachnoid hemorrhage, that correlation of B-waves amplitude increase during recording of intracranial pressure (ICP) with the severity of the bleeding according to the Hunt and Hess scale, as well as with the severity of intracranial hypertension and cerebral vasospasm [21]. Carrying out spectral analysis of BFV and ICP in patients with severe craniocerebral trauma, Newell *et al.* [14] concluded that B-waves of ICP were derivatives of B-waves of BFV, which, most likely, characterized a state of myogenic or neurogenic mechanisms of CBF regulation. In our opinion, intracranial

Table 2. *BP, BFV and BWA of patients of the second group at different stages of endovascular intervention*

Stages of operation	BP [mm Hg]	BF parameters [cm/s]			
		On the side of operation		On the opposite side	
		BFV	BWA	BFV	BWA
Preoperative	85 ± 11	71 ± 13	9.6 ± 1.1	79 ± 15	8.4 ± 1.4
Intraoperative	96 ± 9	89 ± 18	12.1 ± 2.6	83 ± 12	9.9 ± 2.3
Postoperative	90 ± 7	66 ± 12	10.4 ± 2.9	64 ± 13	7.9 ± 2.9

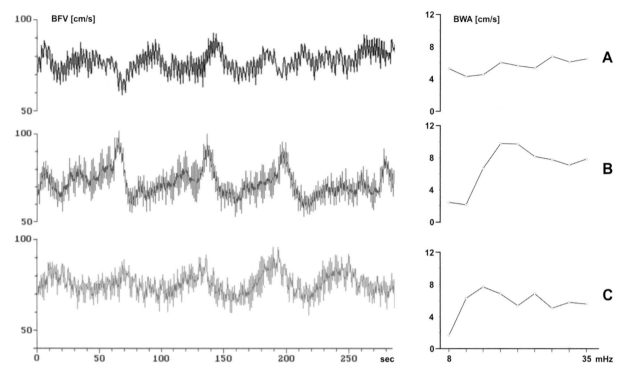

Fig. 2. Monitoring of BFV and BWA on the side of operation before (A), during (B) and after (C) the operation, performed in 42 years old patient with large aneurysm of a supraclinoid segment of the left internal carotid artery

B-waves reflect a state of regulatory mechanisms of CBF as a whole. It appears, that different pathologic states (intracranial hypertension, cerebral vasospasm, hemorrhage, brain compression) are accompanied by dysfunction of stem pace-makers, which control CBF, analogous with a effect of the brain stem on respiration rate, heart rate and other physiologic parameters. At the same time, these very states, causing changes of CPP, result in impairment of vasodilatation and vaso-constriction processes in cerebral vessels, which is re-vealed with a cuff test, cross-spectral analysis within the range of MF waves. One cannot answer exactly whether a neurogenic or myogenic mechanism is the first to be affected; thus, this problem requires further examination.

It is known, that low coherence and a big phase shift between BP and BFV within the range of MF waves, observed in healthy individuals with normal CA, are combined with a low BWA [4, 22]. Our examination of neurosurgical patients with preserved CA and a compensated function of the high-pass filter showed BWA indices close to normal values. As for cases with impaired CA and a decompensated function of the high-pass filter, BWA indices were far from nor-mal. Determining limits of normal values of BWA is a subject for further research.

Mean values of BWA were compared with mean indices of a phase shift within the range of MF waves. This was done in both groups of patients at rest and before intervention. As for the 1st group, the preoper-ative mean values of a phase shift between BFV and BP within the range of MF waves were 79.8 ± 11.4 on the side of operation and 83.4 ± 13.4 – on the op-posite side. In the 2nd group mean values of phase shift within the same range were much smaller: 17.2 ± 8.5 and 24.6 ± 8.5 respectively ($p < 0.05$). These data are similar to the ones previously presented by other au-thors [5, 6, 16].

The data obtained demonstrate possible use of BWA of BFV to estimate the state of a cerebral circu-lation system and prognosticating intra- and postoper-ative neurological complications in endovascular interventions performed in neurosurgical patients.

It is doubtless that simultaneous recording of BFV and other functionally important parameters (BP, ICP) gives more extensive information about the state of regulatory mechanisms of cerebral circulation sys-tem than studying BFV only. However, prolonged non-invasive recording of BP for some 4–5 minutes, carried out with the help of the Finapress apparatus, is accompanied by transient disorders of microcirculation in a finger and, often causes measurement errors and necessity to discontinue investigation and to place a cuff on another finger. Using this simple (and available) method – that does not demand additional continuous measurement of BP and ICP – to estimate BWA of BFV, would permit to reduce time and volume of intraoperative investigation without effecting diagnostic and prognostic significance of the obtained results which is extremely important as to ensure choosing an adequate algorithm of therapeutic and preventive measures.

References

1. Aaslid R, Lindegaard K, Sorteberg W, Nornes H (1989) Cerebral autoregulation dynamics in humans. Stroke 20: 45–52
2. Birch AA, Dirnhuber MJ, Hartley-Davies R, Iannotti F, Neil-Dwyer G (1995) Assessment of autoregulation by means of periodic changes in blood pressure. Stroke 26: 834–837
3. Chioffi F, Pasqualin A, Beltramello A, Da Pian R (1992) Hemodynamic effects of preoperative embolization in cerebral arteriovenous malformations: evaluation with transcranial Doppler sonography. Neurosurgery 31: 877–885
4. Diehl RR, Henkes H, Nahser HC, Kuhne D, Berlit P (1994) Blood flow velocity and vasomotor reactivity in patients with arteriovenous malformations. A transcranial Doppler study. Stroke 25: 1574–1580
5. Diehl RR, Linden D, Lucke D, Berlit P (1995) Phase relationship between cerebral blood flow velocity and blood pressure. A clinical test of autoregulation. Stroke 26: 1801–1804
6. Diehl RR (2002) Cerebral autoregulation studies in clinical practice. Review. Eur J Ultrasound 16: 31–36
7. Giller CA (1990) The frequency-dependent behavior of cerebral autoregulation. Neurosurgery 27: 362–368
8. Kjaellquist Ä, Lundberg N, Pont'en U (1964) Respiratory and cardiovascular changes during rapid spontaneous variations of ventricular fluid pressure in patients with intracranial hypertension. Acta Neurol Scand 40: 291–317
9. Kuo TB, Chern CM, Sheng WY, Wong WJ, Hu HH (1998) Frequency domain analysis of cerebral blood flow velocity and its correlation with arterial blood pressure. J Cereb Blood Flow Metab 18: 311–318
10. Lagalla G, Ceravolo MG, Provinciali L, Recchioni MA, Ducati A, Pasquini U, Piana C, Salvolini U (1998) Transcranial Doppler sonographic monitoring during cerebral aneurysm embolization: a preliminary report. AJNR Am J Neuroradiol 19: 1549–1553
11. Lam JM, Smielewski P, Czosnyka M, Pickard JD, Kirkpatrick PJ (2000) Predicting delayed ischemic deficits after aneurysmal subarachnoid hemorrhage using a transient hyperemic response test of cerebral autoregulation. Neurosurgery 47: 819–826
12. Lang EW, Diehl RR, Mehdorn HM (2001) Cerebral autoregulation testing after aneurysmal subarachnoid hemorrhage: the phase relationship between arterial blood pressure and cerebral blood flow velocity. Crit Care Med 29: 158–163
13. Laumer R, Steinmeier R, Gonner F, Vogtmann T, Priem R, Fahlbusch R (1993) Cerebral hemodynamics in subarachnoid hemorrhage evaluated by transcranial Doppler sonography: Part 1. Reliability of flow velocities in clinical management. Neurosurgery 33: 1–9
14. Newell DW, Aaslid R, Stooss R, Reulen HJ (1992) The relationship of blood flow velocity fluctuations to intracranial pressure B waves. J Neurosurg 76: 415–421
15. Newell DW, Weber JP, Watson R, Aaslid R, Winn HR (1996) Effect of transient moderate hyperventilation on dynamic cerebral autoregulation after severe head injury. Neurosurgery 39: 35–44
16. Panerai RB, Rennie JM, Kelsall AW, Evans DH (1998) Frequency-domain analysis of cerebral autoregulation from spontaneous fluctuations in arterial blood pressure. Med Biol Eng Comput 36: 315–322
17. Ratsep T, Asser T (2001) Cerebral hemodynamic impairment after aneurysmal subarachnoid hemorrhage as evaluated using transcranial Doppler ultrasonography: relationship to delayed cerebral ischemia and clinical outcome. J Neurosurg 95: 393–401
18. Reinhard M, Roth M, Müller T, Czosnyka M, Timmer J, Hetzel A (2003) Cerebral autoregulation in carotid artery occlusive disease assessed from spontaneous blood pressure fluctuations by the correlation coefficient index. Stroke 34: 2138–2144
19. Strandgaard S, Paulson OB (1984) Cerebral autoregulation. Review. Stroke 15: 413–416
20. Tiecks FP, Douville C, Byrd S, Lam AM, Newell DW (1996) Evaluation of impaired cerebral autoregulation by the Valsalva maneuver. Stroke 27: 1177–1182
21. Voldby B, Enevoldsen EM (1982) Intracranial pressure changes following aneurysm rupture. Part 1: clinical and angiographic correlations. J Neurosurg 56: 186–196
22. Zhang R, Zuckerman JH, Giller CA, Levine BD (1998) Transfer function analysis of dynamic cerebral autoregulation in humans. Am J Physiol 274: H233–H241

Correspondence: Semenyutin Vladimir Borisovich, Russian Polenov Neurosurgical Institute, 12 Mayakovsky St., 191104 Saint-Petersburg, Russia. e-mail: lbcp@rnsi.hop.stu.neva.ru

Acta Neurochir (2005) [Suppl] 94: 59–63
© Springer-Verlag 2005
Printed in Austria

Management of severe subarachnoid hemorrhage; significance of assessment of both neurological and systemic insults at acute stage

A. Satoh[1], **H. Nakamura**[2], **S. Kobayashi**[2], **A. Miyata**[2], and **M. Matsutani**[1]

[1] Department of Neurosurgery, Saitama Medical School, Saitama, Japan
[2] Department of Neurosurgery, Chiba Emergency Medical Center, Chiba, Japan

Summary

In order to elucidate mutual interrelationship between neurological and systemic dysfunctions in patients with subarachnoid hemorrhage (SAH) at acute stage, neurological condition, systemic complications and plasma catecholamine (CA) level were studied in 1431 consecutive cases admitted within 72 hours after the onset. Five hundred and twenty-four cases with Glasgow Coma Scale (GCS) score 8 or less were assigned to the group of severely ill cases (G-ill), 907 cases with GCS score 9 or more to that of the less ill group (G-well). Plasma CA level was extremely high at super-acute stage within an hour after bleeding and lowered fairly quickly within 24 hours to the normal range. Assuming the value obtained from a formula of [blood sugar level (mg/dl)/serum potassium concentration (mEq/L)] as stress index (SI), SI correlates well (r = 0.4~0.6) with serum catecholamine level at acute stage. Thus, sympathetic hyperactivity after SAH can be grossly estimated with SI. SI over 40 means that patients might have considerable neurological insults as well as systemic ones. For patients in G-well, SI over 50 means that there may be risks for systemic complications even in cases with good neurological condition.

Keywords: Subarachnoid hemorrhage; systemic complication; neurological grade; sympathetic storm.

Introduction

It is well known that patients with severe SAH are in severely ill condition not only by neurological but also by systemic insults. Systemic dysfunctions accompanying acute SAH are thought to be caused mainly by sympathetic hyperactivity which occurs at the onset of hemorrhage. Massive release of catecholamines (CA) by this abnormal sympathotonia often brings about life-threatening cardiopulmonary and systemic complications like varying types of arrhythmia, cardiac failure, neurogenic pulmonary edema (NPE) and/or extreme hypokalemia [1–8]. Clinical manifestation of neurological insults and that of systemic dysfunctions in patients with poor grade SAH have been studied well but separately so far. Thus, a precise relationship between these two clinical aspects of acute SAH have not yet been elucidated sufficiently [8]. In this paper, we describe the results of a study about relationship between these two conditions that are seemingly independent but actually connected well to each other.

Patients and methods

The cohort which was studied in this report comprised 1431 consecutive SAH patients admitted within 72 hours after the onset. Five hundred and twenty-four patients with Glasgow Coma Scale (GCS) score 8 or less on admission were studied as a severely ill group (G-ill), and 907 patients with GCS 9 or more were used as non-severely ill control (G-well). Blood sample for serum level of CA, potassium (K^+) or glucose (BS) was obtained at the emergency room immediately after patient's admission. Cases who had history of laboring renal insufficiency or diabetus mellitus and who underwent resuscitation for cardiopulmonary arrest caused by SAH were omitted from the cohort in order to exclude influences of these conditions on serum K^+ or BS level. Statistical analyses were made by Fisher's t-test, χ-square test or Kruskal-Wallis test. Regarding demographic background of the two groups, male to female ratio is 0.76 in G-ill and 0.64 in G-well that are not significantly different, while the average age is higher in the former group than in the latter (56.8 ± 13.1 vs 54.3 ± 12.0; P < 0.01).

Results

Serum CA level

Serum epinephrine level on admission in acute SAH patients is extremely elevated nearly up to the level of 800 pg/ml (almost 8–10 times higher than normal) immediately after the hemorrhage and then gradually falls down to the normal range within 24 hours. The spiky rising and rapid dropping of temporal profile

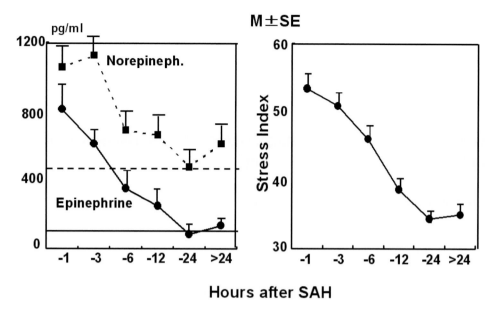

Fig. 1. *Left:* Time course of plasma CA after SAH. Dotted lines represent noradrenaline, and solid ones adrenaline. Horizontal lines are the upper normal limits. *Right:* Time course of SI. Note the identical pattern of CA level and SI

is almost the same as with serum norepinephrine levelin of which the initial peak value is around 1000–1200 pg/ml (3–4 times higher than normal) (Fig. 1, graph on the left).

Blood sugar, serum potassium level and stress index

An elevation of BS and reduction of K^+ are phenomena well-known to physicians treating patients suffering acute SAH. Serum level of these two substances correlate well to the neurological grade on admission with statistical significance ($P < 0.01$), that is mean BS level is higher and K^+ level is lower in the group of poorer grading. Consequently, providing a value calculated from BS level divided by serum potassium level ($BS^{mg/dl}/K^{+mEq/l}$) as Stress Index (SI), SI significantly correlates ($P < 0.01$) with clinical grade. Plotting a temporal profile of mean SI values at each time stage after SAH, time course of SI is almost identical with that of plasma CA (Fig. 1, graph on the right). A correlation coefficient between SI and catecholamines at each time interval from the onset of SAH is 0.5 to 0.6 with statistically significant probability ($P < 0.05$) at least up to 12 to 24 hours. Thus, one can roughly estimate the extent of sympathetic tone of patients with acute SAH in emergency rooms by using SI, which can easily be computed in ordinary clinical setting from serum BS and potassium level.

Comparing the composition of neurological grades in groups of every 5 SI scores, a significant difference is present between the groups with SI below and above 40 (Fig. 2, graph on the top). This means that groups with SI higher than 40 are significantly worse regarding neurological state than those with SI below 40 ($P < 0.01$).

Cardiopulmonary complications and SI

As manifestation of serious cardiopulmonary complications, neurogenic pulmonary edema (NPE) was observed in 14.6% of overall cases, apnea attack in 10.9%, cardiac failure in 2.6% and ventricular tachycardia or fibrillation (VT/VF) in 1.8%. Furthermore, ischemic ST/T changes on ECG were identified in 33.6%. These complications are more frequently observed in patients with higher SI, incidence of which is significantly different ($P < 0.05$) between the groups with SI below and above 40, and that with SI below or above 50 (Fig. 2, graph at bottom). Incidence of complications is 35.6% in G-ill and 12.5% in G-well with a significant difference ($P < 0.01$). Mean SI of G-ill is 58.0 ± 21.3 and that of G-well is 44.2 ± 16.4, which is significantly different ($P < 0.01$: Fig. 3, left columns). In G-ill, mean SI is 57.2 in cases with complications and 59.8 in those without (Fig. 3, columns in the mid), while in G-well, mean SI is significantly different ($P < 0.01$) in those with complications (SI = 52.5) and those without (SI = 41.9) (Fig. 3, right columns).

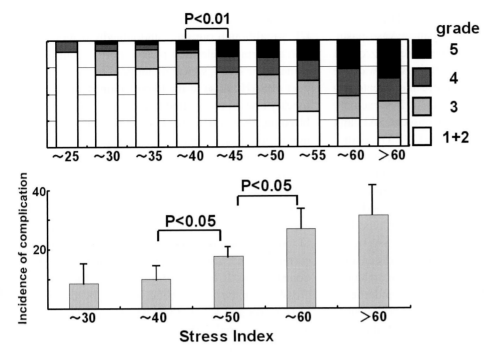

Fig. 2. *Top:* Relationship between neurological grade on admission and SI. Proportion of poor grade patients increases in higher SI group, and statistically significant difference is present between groups with SI above and below 40. *Bottom:* Relationship between incidence of systemic complications and SI. There are two significantly different points at SI 40 and 50. These SI scores may well be used as indices of high risk for systemic complications despite patient's neurological condition

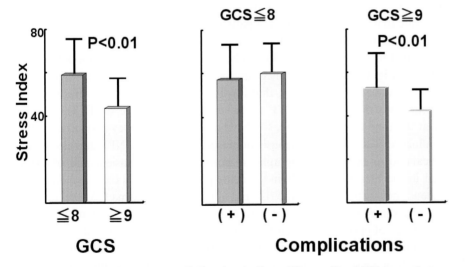

Fig. 3. *Left:* Mean SI of G-ill and G-well. There is a significant difference (P < 0.01) between the two groups (57.2 ± 21.3 vs 44.2 ± 16.4). *Mid:* Mean SI of G-ill with or without complications. No significant difference is present between the two groups (56.4 ± 17.1 vs 59.9 ± 19.1, respectively). *Right:* Mean SI of G-well with or without complications. The former is significantly higher (P < 0.01) than the latter (52.7 ± 18.2 vs 44.2 ± 16.4, respectively)

Discussion

Although management of patients suffering SAH at acute stage has been improved steadily in recent years, mortality still exceeds more than one third of overall patients and only less than a quarter of patients with SAH can make a complete recovery [4]. The major cause of mortality and morbidity from SAH can be attributed to direct brain damages by SAH per se, rebleeding from the ruptured aneurysm or vasospasm. However, in recent studies it has been recognized that nearly a quarter of overall deaths from SAH was due to systemic complications [9]. These life-threatening complications are caused by sympathetic hyperactivity which occurs immediately after the onset of SAH and brings about excess discharge of CA [1–8]. The pathophysiological mechanism of this drastic activation of the sympathetic system concurring with SAH is assumed to be due to damages to the tissue around the anterior hypothalamus [1, 6, 8]. Neil-Dwyer and Doshi [6] reported that histological changes of the hypothalamus in patients who had died following SAH consisted of small perivascular hemorrhages, distensions of perforated vessels with small ball hemorrhages, oedema or the vessel walls involving the endothelial cells with perivascular cuffing of polymorpholeucocytes and microinfarction. Even complete infarction of the hypothalamus was observed in some cases. These hypothalamic lesions are supposed to be induced by ischemic insults due to spasm of the small vessels which supply the region [5, 6]. Although in the literature there are numbers of reports describing that an elevation of CA is sustained throughout the acute phase for more than a week after SAH [2–6], data which are shown here clearly demonstrate that plasma CA rose up once to an extremely high level immediately after the bleeding, and then returned to normal range fairly quickly within 12 to 24 hours (Fig. 1). Discrepancies between the results of the literature and the presented data can be explained by our study method using blood samples obtained only at the time of patients' arrival, in order to avoid the influence of stresses on patients caused by surgical, medical and/or examination procedures, while those used in the literature were obtained on and after admission when patients may have been exposed to stressful procedures. Consequently, as we did not examine the change of plasma CA level after admission, our data can only delineate the features of CA surge at initial or super-acute stage after SAH. Moreover, it seems quite feasible that many patients with SAH might suffer from prolonged sympathetic hyperactivity, or more generally speaking, dysfunction of the autonomic nervous system for a certain period of time, because they have actual tissue damages in the hypothalamus as shown histopathologically in the literature [1, 6]. Some authors mentioned the acceleration of vagal as well as of sympathetic activity at 4–5 days after onset of SAH, which

might well be explained by these parenchymal lesions [2]. So, although our data undoubtedly demonstrates that abnormally elevated plasma norepinephrine and epinephrine levels, which are induced by the initial impact of SAH per se to the hypothalamus, are lowered quickly toward the normal range within 24 hours after bleeding, there might be a secondary effect of autonomic derangement which possibly is prolonged and may well influence, at least to some extent, the evolution of vasospasm [5].

In ordinary clinical setting, it is not easy to evaluate accurately the extent of sympathetic activity. However, judging from similarity of the time course of SI to that of plasma CA (Fig. 1) and a good statistical correlation between these two parameters as mentioned above, it is not arbitrary to say that one can grossly estimate sympathetic activity by calculating SI from BS and K^+, both of which can be easily and quickly measured in the emergency room [7, 8]. By using SI as an indicator of plasma CA level, we can demonstrate a relationship between neurological state and sympathetic activity at acute stage. The group of patients with SI over 40 comprises significantly larger numbers of neurologically ill patients than the group with SI less than 40 does (Fig. 2, top). Namely, SI over 40 means that the patients are quite ill due to systemic sympathetic hyperactivity and at the same time because of their neurological condition.

In this study, we adopted 5 typical cardiopulmonary dysfunctions as systemic complications caused by SAH, that involve NPE, apnea, cardiac insufficiency, VT/VF or ischemic ST/T change on ECG. Among those, NPE and cardiac insufficiency may occur simultaneously or in isolation [4]. Both NPE and electrocardiographic abnormalities are transient and observed only in the acute phase [4], that is corresponding well to the rise and fall pattern of plasma CA level demonstrated here (Fig. 1). A study as to relationship between SI and incidence of complications demonstrated that significant difference is observed between the groups with SI below and above 40, and also between those below and above 50 (Fig. 2, bottom). The presence of these 2 inflexion points of SI is compatible with a difference in G-well with or without complication, of which mean SI is 52.5 and 41.9, respectively (Fig. 3, right columns). Mean SI is significantly higher in G-ill than G-well (Fig. 3, left columns). Restricting to G-ill, however, average SI is not different between the cases with or without complications (Fig. 3, columns in the mid). On the other hand in G-well, mean SI is significantly higher in those with complications than without (Fig. 3, right columns). From these data, we can conclude that physicians treating patients with SAH at acute stage should pay much attention to possible cardiopulmonary complications in those who show high SI above 50 though their neurological condition can be assessed in G-well as well as in G-ill. Actually, a precise analysis restricted to the patients who belong to grade 1 or 2 revealed that mortality of 157 patients with SI over 40 was 10.8% and that of 64 patients with SI over 50 was 14.1%, and those figures were significantly worse ($P < 0.05$ and $P < 0.01$, respectively) than mortality of 5.0% in 278 patients of grade 1 or 2 with SI lower than 40.

Conclusion

Sympathetic hyperactivity at acute stage of SAH can be grossly estimated with SI, which is easily computed from serum BS and K^+. SI over 40 may well be used as an index showing the borderline between patients suffering considerable neurological insults as well as systemic ones and those not. Regarding patients in G-well, SI over 50 suggests that there may be a formidable risk for systemic complications even in cases with good neurological condition.

References

1. Dilraj A, Botha JH, Rambiritch V, Miller R, van Dellen JR (1992) Levels of catecholamine in plasma and cerebrospinal fluid in aneurysmal subarachnoid hemorrhage. Neurosurgery 31: 42–51
2. Kawahara E, Ikeda S, Miyahara Y, Kohno S (2003) Role of autonomic nervous dysfunction in electrocardiographic abnormalities and cardiac injury in patients with acute subarachnoid hemorrhage. Circ J 67: 753–756
3. Lambert G, Naredi S, Edén E, Rydenhag B, Friberg P (2002) Sympathetic nervous activation following subarachnoid hemorrhage: influence of intravenous clonidine. Acta Anesthesiol Scand 46: 160–165
4. Macmillan CS, Grant IS, Andrews PJD (2002) Pulmonary and cardiac sequelae of subarachnoid hemorrhage: time for active management? Intensive Care Med 28: 1012–1023
5. Naredi S, Lambert G, Edén E, Zäll S, Runnerstam M, Rydenhag B, Friberg P (2000) Increased sympathetic nervous activity in patients with nontraumatic subarachnoid hemorrhage. Stroke 31: 901–906
6. Neil-Dwyer G, Cruickshank JM, Doshi R (1990) The stress response in subarachnoid hemorrhage and head injury. Acta Neurochir, [Suppl] 47: 102–110
7. Satoh A (1998) Clinicopathological features and treatment of severely ill patients with subarachnoid hemorrhage. Jpn J Neurosurg 7: 24–31
8. Satoh A, Nakamura H, Kobayashi S, Miyata A, Wada M, Tsuru K (2004) Significance of assessment of both intracranial and systemic insults in treatment of severely ill patients with acute subarachnoid hemorrhage. Surg Cereb Stroke 32: 97–102
9. Solenski NJ, Haley ECJ, Kassell NF, Kongable G, Germanson T, Truskowski L, Torner JC (1995) Medical complications of aneurysmal subarachnoid hemorrhage: a report of the multicenter, cooperative aneurysmal study. Participants of the Multicenter Cooperative Aneurysmal Study. Crit Care Med 23: 1007–1017

Correspondence: Akira Satoh, Department of Neurosurgery, Saitama Medical School, Morohongo 38, Moroyama, Irumagun, Saitama, 350-0495 Japan. e-mail: satohak@saitama-med.ac.jp

Acta Neurochir (2005) [Suppl] 94: 65–73
© Springer-Verlag 2005
Printed in Austria

Cerebral vasospasm: results of a structured multimodal treatment

E. Keller, N. Krayenbühl, M. Bjeljac, and **Y. Yonekawa**

Department of Neurosurgery, University Hospital Zurich, Zurich, Switzerland

Summary

Symptomatic cerebral vasospasm (CVS) with delayed ischemic neurologic deficits affects about one third of the patients after aneurysmal subarachnoid hemorrhage (SAH). In spite of the lack of definite evidence of large clinical trials, the devastating outcome of the natural history of symptomatic CVS demands an aggressive CVS treatment in a practically oriented, structured multimodal treatment regimen. With our treatment protocol good functional outcome could be reached in 66% of the patients with symptomatic CVS. This policy requires close and fast multidisciplinary collaboration between neurosurgeons, neuroradiologists, competent in endovascular interventions, and specialists for neurointensive care. We report on our experience with 79 cases with symptomatic CVS and delayed ischemic neurologic deficit (DIND) after aneurysmal SAH. The different treatment options with CVS are reviewed and practical guidelines for a step by step treatment are given.

Keywords: Cerebral vasospasm; triple h therapy; ischemia; spasmolysis; hypothermia; barbiturate coma.

Introduction

With early aneurysm clipping delayed ischemic neurologic deficit (DIND) due to cerebral vasospasm (CVS) became the most common cause of death and disability due to aneurysmal subarachnoid hemorrhage (SAH) [30]. Symptomatic CVS with DIND affects about one third of the patients and, without specific treatment, the outcome of DIND is devastating, causing death (30%) and permanent disability (34%) [14, 16].

We report on our experience with 79 cases with symptomatic CVS after aneurysmal SAH. The different treatment options with CVS are reviewed and practical guidelines for a structured step by step multimodal treatment protocol are given.

Materials and methods

Patient population

The study was approved as a part of the project E-015/99 by the Ethics Committee of the University of Zurich. Between January 1999 and December 2003 198 patients with SAH were admitted within three days after symptoms onset into the Department of Neurosurgery, University Hospital Zurich and were treated with aneurysm clipping. In 1999 a standardized protocol for detection and treatment of CVS was established. Patients data, imaging studies and characteristics of treatment were prospectively analyzed. Neurological outcome was assessed after 3 and 12 months in the outpatient clinic by an independent neurologist using the Glasgow Outcome Scale (GOS) [24]. Those patients who did not show up at control were contacted and asked about their functional status.

Structured treatment

Aneurysm clipping was performed with the standard microsurgical technique described by Yasargil [64]. Only patients having undergone aneurysm clipping within three days after SAH were included. All patients were treated with nimodipine for 21 days. Patients were kept flat in bed as long as cerebral autoregulation, examined with transcranial Doppler (TCD), was defect. Before the patients developed signs of CVS daily fluid balance was aimed to be positive, adjusting fluid intake by intravenous infusion of crystalloids and hydroxylethyl-starch solution (HES) 1000 ml per day. No prophylactic triple h (hypertensive hypervolemic hemodilution) therapy was initiated. Dexamethasone was given perioperative. Prophylactic antiepileptic treatment with phenytoine or valproate was initiated in SAH patients with Hunt and Hess grade 3 and higher. In patients with SAH Hunt and Hess grade 1 to 3, sedation was stopped immediately after surgery. In patients with severe SAH Hunt and Hess grade 4 to 5, a ventricular catheter (NMT Neuroscience, Frankfurt, Germany or Raumedic, Rehau, Germany) was inserted to provide continuous intracranial pressure (ICP) monitoring and drainage of cerebrospinal fluid (CSF) if necessary. If a ventricular catheter could not be placed within the ventricular system because of massive brain edema, a subdural (NMT Neuroscience, Frankfurt, Germany) or an intraparenchymatous (Raumedic, Rehau, Germany) ICP probe was inserted. With elevated ICP (>15 mmHg) treatment with intermittent CSF drainage, osmotherapy (Mannitol 20% and hypertonic NaCl-hydroxyethyl-starch solution), mild hyperventilation (target $PaCO_2$ values adapted to jugular bulb oximetry) and tris-hydroxy-methyl-aminomethane (THAM) buffer was initiated. Patients with persistant ICP-values > 15 mmHg were eligible for treatment with barbiturate coma combined with mild hypothermia. Medical therapy, barbiturate coma and hypothermia treatment were performed according to a standardized algorithm for treatment of elevated ICP [31].

Detection of cerebral vasospasm

TCD blood flow measurements were performed daily. "Symptomatic CVS" was defined in the absence of sedation and poor neurological grade by the occurrence of DIND (decrease in consciousness, new focal neurological deficits). Before "symptomatic CVS" was suspected, hypoxia, electrolyte imbalance and hydrocephalus were excluded by a further CT scan. CVS in all patients were confirmed by digital subtraction angiography. If the neurological state could not be properly assessed (e.g. sedation or poor neurological grade), patients were additionally monitored with jugular bulb oxymetry, lactate measurements from the jugular bulb [20], daily cerebral blood flow (CBF) measurements [33] and/or perfusion CT examinations. If jugular bulb O_2-desaturation occurred, arteriovenous differences of lactate (avDL) were – 0.2 umol/dl or less, CBF-values decreased by more than 20% and/or differences in territorial or hemispheric transit times occurred in perfusion CT, "symptomatic CVS" was suspected and digital subtraction angiography was performed. All patients with new ischemic infarctions – in comparison with the postoperative CT examination – were classified likewise to have "symptomatic CVS".

Treatment of cerebral vasospasm

If signs of CVS occurred, patients were treated according to a multimodal structured treatment protocol (Table 1).

Hypertensive hypervolemic hemodilution (triple h) therapy was induced if TCD mean blood flow velocities increased (mean middle cerebral artery (MCA) blood flow velocities > 140 cm/sec or increase up to >50 cm/sec within 24 hours) and/or the patient developed symptomatic CVS. Contraindications to initiate triple h therapy were heart failure, valvular heart disease, symptomatic coronary heart disease, cardiac arrhythmias and aortic aneurysms. Triple h therapy was guided with a new system to monitor systemic hemodynamics [36]. A 13 cm long 4-F arterial thermistor catheter (PV-2015L13, Pulsion Medical Systems, Munich) was inserted into the femoral artery and connected to the pulse contour analysis computer (PICCO Pulsion Medical Systems, Munich). Thermodilution measurements with calibration of cardiac index (CI) and determination of global enddiastolic volume index (GEDVI), intrathoracic blood volume index (ITBVI) and extravascular lung water index (EVLWI) were performed every six hours. In addition to the conventional parameters (mean arterial pressure (MAP) > 105 mmHg, central venous pressure (CVP) 8–12 mmHg and hematocrit 28–32%) triple h therapy was adapted to the following target values: CI > 4l/min/m², ITBVI 900–1000 ml/m² and EVLWI < 10 ml/kg. Triple h therapy was induced by administration of crystalloid and colloid infusions. Dobutamine and norepinephrine were adjusted to maximize cardiac function. Excessive natriuresis and diuresis (osmolarity in urine > osmolarity in serum, sodium in serum < 140 mmol/l) was inhibited with fludrocortisone 0.2 mg/day, excessive water diuresis (osmolarity in urine < osmolarity in serum, sodium in serum > 140 mmol/l) with desmopressine 1–4 × 2 ug i.v. per day.

Endovascular treatment: If patients with DIND did not improve or worsened despite triple h therapy digital subtraction angiography and endovascular treatment with percutaneous balloon angioplasty and/or superselective papaverine infusion (totale dose of 300 mg) into the vasospastic vessels were performed [17, 25]. Contraindications for endovascular treatment were the presence of incompletely clipped aneurysms, ischemic infarctions or space-occupying brain edema in CT.

Barbiturate coma, hypothermia: Symptomatic CVS, resistant to the above treatment or reoccurring after two to three spasmolysis sessions were treated with barbiturate coma and/or hypothermia, if ever possible, as a combined treatment. Barbiturate coma with thiopental (loading dose of 10 mg/kgBW, followed by continuous infusion) was induced at the same time as induction of hypothermia and was adapted to a burst suppression pattern in continuous EEG-monitoring. Cooling of the patients (target brain temperature 33 °C) was accomplished by using cooling blankets (Bair Hugger, Augustine Medical, Saint Prarie; MN, USA and Blanketrol, CSZ, Cincinnatti; OH, USA) or endovascular cooling catheters (Cool Line Catheter and Coolgard System; Alsius Corporation, Irvine, CA, USA) [31]. Patients were excluded if they initially suffered from congestive heart failure, neurogenic pulmonary edema, severe aspiration pneumonia, other infections or Raynaud's phenomenon. Hypothermia only was performed if specific contraindications for thiopental were present such as liver failure, hyperkaliemia or hypernatriemia. Barbiturate coma and hypothermia were continued until signs of CVS decreased. Barbiturate coma and hypothermia were terminated earlier if signs of severe infection, cardiovascular instability, liver failure (barbiturate coma), severe electrolyte disturbances (barbiturate coma) or coagulation disorders (hypothermia) were observed.

Outcome measurements

Neurological outcome was assessed after three and 12 months in the outpatient clinic by a neurologist using the Glasgow Outcome Score (GOS) [24], GOS 1 denominating death, GOS 2 vegetative state (unable to interact with the environment), GOS 3 severe disability (unable to live independently but able to follow commands), GOS 4 moderate disability (capable of living independently but unable to return to work or school) and GOS 5 mild or no disability (able to return to work or school). Those patients who did not show up at control were contacted and asked about their functional status.

Results

From 198 patients treated with aneurysm clipping within three days after SAH, TCD mean blood flow velocities increased in 105 patients (52.5%). 79 patients developed symptomatic CVS (39.9%). Characteristics of patients with symptomatic CVS are given in Table 2. The majority of patients with symptomatic CVS suffered from severe SAH. 50 patients (63.3%) had Hunt and Hess grades 3 to 5 and 69 patients (87.4%) belonged to the Fisher grades 3 and 4. Treatment characteristics are given in Table 3. 78 patients (98.7%) were treated with triple h therapy. In one patient with symptomatic CVS triple h therapy was not initiated because of heart failure. In 45 (57.7%) of the 78 patients triple h therapy had a sustained positive effect and symptoms of CVS decreased, making further therapy steps such as spasmolysis, barbiturate coma and hypothermia unnecessary. 33 patients (41.8%), despite of therapeutic triple h therapy, did not improve or worsened. These patients were subjected to digital subtraction angiography and percutaneous angioplasty and/or superselective papaverine infusion. Due to reoccurrence of CVS five patients were treated twice and two patients three times with spasmolysis. 13

Table 1. *Structured treatment protocol Department of Neurosurgery, University Hospital Zurich*

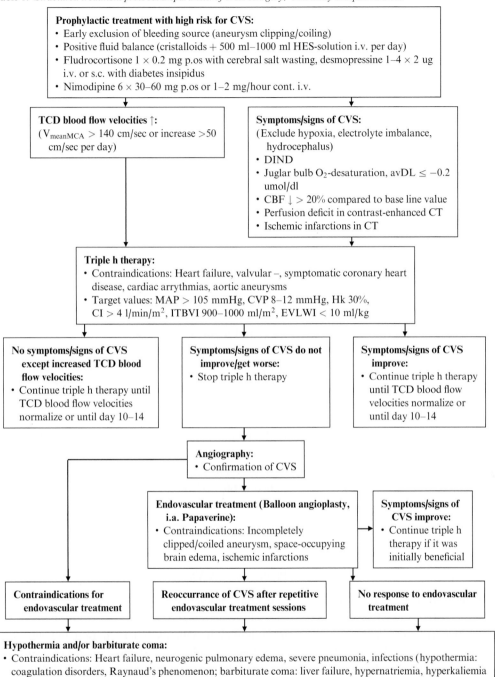

Prophylactic treatment with high risk for CVS:
- Early exclusion of bleeding source (aneurysm clipping/coiling)
- Positive fluid balance (cristalloids + 500 ml–1000 ml HES-solution i.v. per day)
- Fludrocortisone 1×0.2 mg p.os with cerebral salt wasting, desmopressine $1–4 \times 2$ ug i.v. or s.c. with diabetes insipidus
- Nimodipine $6 \times 30–60$ mg p.os or $1–2$ mg/hour cont. i.v.

TCD blood flow velocities ↑:
($V_{meanMCA} > 140$ cm/sec or increase >50 cm/sec per day)

Symptoms/signs of CVS:
(Exclude hypoxia, electrolyte imbalance, hydrocephalus)
- DIND
- Juglar bulb O_2-desaturation, avDL ≤ -0.2 umol/dl
- CBF ↓ $> 20\%$ compared to base line value
- Perfusion deficit in contrast-enhanced CT
- Ischemic infarctions in CT

Triple h therapy:
- Contraindications: Heart failure, valvular –, symptomatic coronary heart disease, cardiac arrythmias, aortic aneurysms
- Target values: MAP > 105 mmHg, CVP $8–12$ mmHg, Hk 30%, CI > 4 l/min/m², ITBVI $900–1000$ ml/m², EVLWI < 10 ml/kg

No symptoms/signs of CVS except increased TCD blood flow velocities:
- Continue triple h therapy until TCD blood flow velocities normalize or until day 10–14

Symptoms/signs of CVS do not improve/get worse:
- Stop triple h therapy

Symptoms/signs of CVS improve:
- Continue triple h therapy until TCD blood flow velocities normalize or until day 10–14

Angiography:
- Confirmation of CVS

Endovascular treatment (Balloon angioplasty, i.a. Papaverine):
- Contraindications: Incompletely clipped/coiled aneurysm, space-occupying brain edema, ischemic infarctions

Symptoms/signs of CVS improve:
- Continue triple h therapy if it was initially beneficial

Contraindications for endovascular treatment

Reoccurrance of CVS after repetitive endovascular treatment sessions

No response to endovascular treatment

Hypothermia and/or barbiturate coma:
- Contraindications: Heart failure, neurogenic pulmonary edema, severe pneumonia, infections (hypothermia: coagulation disorders, Raynaud's phenomenon; barbiturate coma: liver failure, hypernatriemia, hyperkaliemia
- Duration: Until signs of CVS improve or early discontinuation in case of severe side effects

CVS Cerebral vasospasm; *TCD* transcranial Doppler; $V_{meanMCA}$ mean blood flow velocity in the middle cerebral artery; *AvDL* arteriovenous difference of lactate; *DIND* delayed ischemic neurologic deficit; *CBF* cerebral blood flow; *MAP* mean arterial pressure; *CVP* central venous pressure; *Hk* hematocrit; *CI* cardiac index; *ITBVI* intrathoracic blood volume index; *EVLWI* extravascular lung water index.

patients had contraindications for endovascular treatment (eight patients with space-occupying brain edema and five with ischemic infarctions in CT scans) and 13 patients suffered from resistant or reoccurring CVS to repetitive spasmolysis. These patients were treated with barbiturate coma and/or hypothermia, 23 with combined treatment and three patients with hypothermia only. From these patients with refractory

Table 2. *Patient characteristics*

	Number of patients with symptomatic CVS (n = 79; 100%)
Age; mean (SD)	50.9 (11.9)
Gender	
– Male	17 (21.5%)
– Female	62 (78.5%)
GCS before surgery; mean (SD)	10.0 (4.6)
Grading	
– H & H grade 5	10 (12.7%)
– H & H grade 4	25 (31.6%)
– H & H grade 3	15 (19.0%)
– H & H grade 2	27 (34.2%)
– H & H grade 1	2 (2.5%)
– Fisher grade 4	42 (53.2%)
– Fisher grade 3	27 (34.2%)
– Fisher grade 2	8 (10.1%)
– Fisher grade 1	2 (2.5%)

n Number; *GCS* Glasgow Coma Scale; *H & H* Hunt and Hess grade.

Table 3. *Treatment characteristics*

	Number of patients with symptomatic CVS (n = 79; 100%)
Triple h therapy	78 (98.7%)
Spasmolysis	33 (41.8%)
– Once	26 (32.9%)
– Twice	5 (6.3%)
– Three times	2 (2.6%)
Hypothermia combined with barbiturate coma	23 (29.1%)
Hypothermia only	3 (3.8%)

n Number; *Triple h* hypertensive hypervolemic hemodilution.

CVS 13 patients (50%) survived with good functional outcome (GOS 4 and 5), 6 patients (23.1%) survived severely disabled and 7 patients (26.9%) died.

Of the total of 198 patients having suffered from aneurysmal SAH, six patients (3%) died from CVS and 16 patients (8.1%) suffered from permanent additional deficits from CVS (Table 4). 13 patients survived severely disabled or in a vegetative state (GOS 3 and 2 in 6.5%). In patients with symptomatic CVS good functional outcome (GOS 4 and 5) could be achieved in 52 of 79 patients (65.8%). 13 of the patients (16.5%) survived severely disabled and 14 (17.7%) died, six due to multiple infarctions, due to rebleeding and seven due to severe infections with acute respiratory distress syndrome or sepsis.

Table 4. *Patient outcome*

	Number of patients with symptomatic CVS (n = 79; 100%)
Died of CVS	6 (7.6%)
Permanent additional deficits because of CVS	16 (20.3%)
GOS	
– 5	36 (45.6%)
– 4	16 (20.2%)
– 3	13 (16.5%)
– 2	0 (0%)
– 1	14 (17.7%)

n Number; *cvs* cerebral vasospasm; *GOS* Glasgow Outcome Scale.

Discussion

In the cooperative aneurysm study 7.2% of the patients died from CVS and 6.3% survived with severe disability from CVS [30]. It is difficult to compare reports of management results because of different patient populations regarding the prognostic factors for poor outcome, in addition to variations in timing and methods for quantification of outcome. In our series, applying a step by step multimodal treatment protocol in 198 patients with aneurysmal SAH, 3% died from CVS and 6.5% survived severely disabled or in a vegetative state from CVS. From 79 patients with symptomatic CVS, good functional outcome could be obtained in 66% of the cases.

Recommendations for a structured treatment protocol

Prediction of CVS

In clinical practice not only treatment, but the accuracy of prediction and detection of symptomatic CVS, most difficult in patients under sedation and with poor neurological grade, is a very most important aspect influencing the outcome of patients after SAH. Recently, Claassen *et al.* revised the Fisher scale according to the risk to develop CVS [12]. The highest risk of developing DIND occurs in patients with thick basal cistern blood and the presence of blood in the lateral ventricles. After SAH, the complex changes of cerebral hemodynamics and oxygenation pattern with the development of DIND are underestimated if TCD-monitoring and angiography are considered singularly [1]. The role of TCD in predicting symptomatic CVS is limited to the cases where very high mean blood flow velocities are detected [61]. Moreover, to control the treatment of CVS, TCD values are influenced by triple h therapy [40]. Discrepancies between radiographic findings and DIND may depend on the relationship between local cerebral oxygen-requirement and -delivery, which only can be determined if CBF and cerebral oxygen extraction can be estimated. Jugular bulb oximetry reflects the balance between CBF and the cerebral metabolic rate of oxygen ($CMRO_2$). It represents, nevertheless, only global cerebral perfusion. The sensitivity of $SjvO_2$ to detect smaller ischemic areas secondary to CVS of single vessels is limited [33]. In cases of distal arterial narrowing, new techniques applying near infrared spectroscopy (NIRS) with a indocyanine green (ICG) dye dilution mode measuring regional values of local cortical perfusion may be more sensitive, especially in detecting microvascular or "distal" vasospasm [32, 35]. Daily TCD blood flow velocities-checks during the highest vasospasm risk period (between 4 and 10 days postbleed), however, may warn of spasm development [1, 38] and allow more aggressive prophylactic treatment of threatening CVS with triple h therapy. Cerebral angiography with direct visualization of proximal CVS and prolonged transit time of the contrast flow remains the golden standard procedure to diagnose CVS. Angiography should be routinely performed after aneurysm clipping within 14 days after ictus and in case of occurrence of symptomatic CVS at an earlier date. Shortcomings of angiography include the lack in detecting micovascular vasospasm and the risks of the procedure including catheter-induced vasospasm or vessel dissection. Advantages lie in the potential for endovascular intervention.

Pharmacologic approaches

Nimodipine, a specific blocker of the L-type voltage-gated calcium channels, has been tested in several controlled trials [2, 46]. But not the originally anticipated direct effects on vascular smooth muscle cells, but the neuroprotective effects may be of some clinical benefit in patients who never experience vasospasm, macroscopically visible in angiography [42]. Barker and Ogilvie showed in a later metanalysis improvements in good and fair outcomes, as well as reductions of death rate and CT detected infarcts with nimodipine [6]. The modified steroid free radical scavenger tirilazad mesylate, inhibiting iron-dependendent lipid perxidation and scavering free radicals, has been investigated in four large controlled trials [28]. After first promising results later metanalysis showed only post hoc positive effects in patients with poor grades [15]. Many other medical treatment options are under investigation and can not be discussed in detail within this limited context. First pilot studies with high dose magnesium sulphate, with its vascular protection properties, showed promising results [10, 60]. After randomization of 60 patients in a controlled clinical study our own results showed that with magnesium sulfate infusion (dosage of 16 mmol in 15 mins. i.v., thereafter 64 mmol/24 h continuously i.v., adapted to a target magnesium level in serum of $2\times$ baseline value for 14 days) had to be interrupted because of severe hypotension in 40% of the patients (unpublished data). The complex regulatory mechanisms of vascular smooth vessel tone after SAH are under extensive research and may lead to further promising treatment options like nitric oxide donors or selective endothelin-1 antagonists [14, 49, 65].

Triple h therapy

Benefits of triple h therapy have never been unequivocally demonstrated by randomized controlled trials [52]. In early studies patients with volume expansion showed less DIND and better outcome compared to control patients who were kept dehydrated [51], whereas in more recent studies no effect of hypervolemia on either CBF or DIND was found if control patients already receiving over 3000 ml fluids per day [37]. Dorsch therefore concludes that adequate fluid loading might be the most important aspect of early treatment and CVS prophylaxis and that it is reasonable to reserve the more vigorous loading and induced hypertension for when DIND occurs [14]. Therefore, as a prophylactic treatment in patients with high risk for CVS, fluid balance has to be carefully observed and kept positive within 1000–1500 ml per day and hematocrit is aimed to be 30%, providing the optimal level of reduced blood viscosity and improving CBF while still maintaining adequate serum oxygen carrying capacity [23]. The usefulness of triple h therapy, however, reversing secondary neurological deficits in 59% of our patients, is obvious in our daily clinical practice. Therefore, according to our treatment protocol, if TCD blood flow velocities increase and/or the patients develop symptoms of CVS triple h therapy is aggressively initiated. If triple h therapy fails to improve DIND or if the patients worsen during triple h therapy, other treatment options have to be applied and, avoiding harmful side effects, triple h therapy can be reset. In order to guide triple h therapy and achieve as high efficiency as possible and to avoid volume overload with consecutive pulmonary edema as the most severe complication [5, 29, 57] extended monitoring of systemic hemodynamics is needed. Target values have to be defined, aimed at consequently and documented for quality control. Monitoring of mean arterial pressure (MAP), central venous pressure (CVP) and pulmonary artery occlusive wedge pressure (PAOP) are conventionally used to control triple h therapy [29], although their limitations to estimate intravascular volume state are well recognized [50]. Moreover, pulmonary artery catheterization as an invasive method is controversially discussed in the literature [13]. Recently an alternative method based on transpulmonary double-indicator dilution for assessment of intravascular volume has been established [22]. Global enddiastolic volume (GEDV) and intrathoracic blood volume (ITBV) have been reported to reflect the intravascular volume status more adequately than CVP or PAOP. Further, extravascular lung water (EVLW) is a reliable predictor for early pulmonary edema [22]. Own experiences showed that the new monitoring system might be the optimal instrument to guide triple h therapy [36]. Excessive natriuresis and diueresis may occur in the context of "cerebral salt wasting" most often in patients with ruptured aneurysms of the anterior communicating artery [63] and may be aggravated by fluid and volume load with triple h therapy. Polyuria may anticipate effective intravascular volume expansion. Mori et al. showed that the inhibition of natriuresis with fludrocortisone reduces the sodium and water intake required for hypervolemia and prevents hyponatriemia. Therefore, with a high osmolarity in urine and a normal to low sodium in serum, fludrocortisone 0.2 mg/day may be supplemented with triple h therapy. In our institution, on the other hand, excessive water diuresis (low osmolarity in urine, high sodium in serum), similar to a constellation of diabetes insipidus, is treated with desmopressine $1-4 \times 2$ ug i.v. per day to avoid hypernatriemia [43].

Endovascular treatment

Indications, technology and side effects of endovascular treatment are described in detail in the subsequent article. For the neurointensivist the following aspects are to be emphasized. Balloon angioplasty and papaverine spasmolysis are performed in general anaesthesia. Symptomatic CVS leads to reduced O_2 delivery in the affected vascular territories with acute ischemia. General anaesthesia, reducing metabolic requirements of the brain, may counteract this O_2 imbalance until blood flow in vasospastic vessels is restored by a successful endovascular intervention. Respiratory arrest with vertebral artery injections and seizures are described during spasmolysis. Furthermore, in a patient with CVS, most often being confused and agitated, anaesthesia ensures that the patient does not move during the intervention. As a side effect of papaverine, with its vasodilatatory capacity, systemic hypotension may occur, which has to be treated aggressively with volume expansion, dobutamine and norepinephrine. According to our experience, maintenance of induced hypertension, high cardiac output and hypervolemia during and after the procedure are most important issues, in order to increase the efficiency of the endovascular intervention and to reduce the reoccurrence rate of CVS. Development of elevated ICP is described after papaverine instillation in patients with bilateral diffuse vasospasm [3]. Therefore brain edema and elevated ICP are considered as contraindications for papaverine treatment and ICP monitoring is recommended in patients at risk.

Other vasodilators for intra-arterial and systemic treatment are under examination. Arakawa et al. published a small case series treated with the cardiac inotrope milrinone, a phosphodiesterase inhibitor like papaverine [4]. Its use is limited by the side effect of severe systemic hypotension. In our clinical practice, we apply low dosages of milrinone through continuous intravenous infusion to augment hyperdynamic therapy by enhancing cardiac performance if cardiac output is diminished because of high systemic vascular arterial resistance in combination with catecholamines. Fasudil hydrochloride, a enzyme protein kinase C inhibitor, intraarterialy infused, has been shown to reduce symptomatic CVS [55]. Its use, at present, is limited to Japan.

Barbiturate coma, hypothermia

Animal and clinical studies have shown that hypothermia has the potential to limit the extent of secondary brain damage [7, 11, 39, 47]. Several positive effects relevant in SAH have been demonstrated, e.g. temperature dependent reduction of cerebral oxygen metabolism [20, 34], stabilization of the blood-brain barrier

[56], decreased release of neurotransmitters [26], attenuation of free radical production, and decreased postischemic edema formation [47].

Numerous neuroprotective mechanisms, partly similar to hypothermia, could be shown for barbiturates [9, 62]. The application of thiopental boli with temporary clipping is wide spread in neuroanesthesia [53]. In 1980 Kassell applied barbiturate coma in 12 patients with refractory CVS [27]. With limited resources in intensive care the results were disappointing. 11 patients died from uncontrollable intracranial hypertension, cardiac arrythmias or infections. In three patients, treated with combined barbiturate coma and hypothermia severe acid base and electrolyte disturbances occurred. With improved supportive intensive care, Finfer *et al.* in 1999 published the results of 11 patients with angioplasty resistant CVS treated with barbiturate coma, 10 of them surviving with good functional outcome [18]. Hypothermia has been applied with temporary clipping during aneurysm surgery [21] and in patients after severe SAH, brain edema and elevated ICP [19, 44]. Only a small case series treated with hypothermia (32 °C–34 °C) because of refractory CVS is described by Nagao [45]. Among eight patients five survived with good functional outcome and two patients survived moderately disabled.

In the present series 26 patients were treated with barbiturate coma and/or hypothermia. 13 patients had contraindications for endovascular treatment (space-occupying brain edema or ischemic infarctions) and 13 patients suffered from resistant or reoccurring CVS after repetitive spasmolysis. From these 23 patients, with most resistant CVS, 50% survived with a good functional outcome.

However, one has to be aware of the potentially hazardous side effects of hypothermia and barbiturate coma. From 21 patients with high grade SAH and refractory intracranial hypertension, treated with long term hypothermia/barbiturate coma up to 16 days, all patients developed severe infections [19]. It is known from animal and clinical studies, that hypothermia, as well as barbiturates, predispose to bacterial infections [8, 58]. Biggar *et al.* showed in pigs, that hypothermia impairs neutrophil circulation and their release from the bone marrow. Hypothermia may also cause bone marrow suppression and platelet sequestration in the spleen [41, 48, 54]. In addition, it has been shown in trauma patients, that leukocytes and neutrophils are reversibly and significantly decreased in thiopental coma [8]. Furthermore, patients treated with long

term hypothermia develop thrombocytopenia, defects in the platelet's ability to produce thromboxane B2 with possible bleeding complications [59]. Platelets have to transfused early and amply. Because of acid base and electrolyte disturbances (hypernatriemia and hyperkaliemia) as well as negative cardiac inotropic effects barbiturate coma have to be discontinued often. In fact, without hypothermia/barbiturate coma patients with refractory CVS might exhibit poor outcome and death. In this context, the application of aggressive treatment regimen with severe side effects and elaborate intensive care treatment are justifiable.

Conclusions

With a structured step by step treatment protocol for symptomatic CVS good functional outcome can be reached in 66% of the patients. Dorsch in a recent review concluded that with CVS as a multifactorial problem, it is likely that detection, prevention and treatment will continue to require application along several different lines [14]. In spite of the lack of definite evidence of large clinical trials, the devastating outcome of natural history of symptomatic CVS demands an aggressive CVS treatment in a structured, practically oriented multimodal treatment protocol. This policy requires close and fast multidisciplinary collaboration between neurosurgeons, neuroradiologists, competent in endovascular interventions, and specialists for neurointensive care.

References

1. Aaslid R, Huber P, Nornes H (1984) Evaluation of cerebrovascular spasm with transcranial Doppler ultrasound. J Neurosurg 60: 37–41
2. Allen GS, Ahn HS, Preziosi TJ, Battye R, Boone SC, Chou SN, Kelly DL, Weir BK, Crabbe RA, Lavik PJ, Rosenbloom SB, Dorsey FC, Ingram CR, Mellits DE, Bertsch LA, Boisvert DP, Hundley MB, Johnson RK, Strom JA, Transou CR (1983) Cerebral arterial spasm – a controlled trial of nimodipine in patients with subarachnoid hemorrhage. N Engl J Med 308: 619–624
3. Andaluz N, Tomsick TA, Tew JM Jr, van Loveren HR, Yeh HS, Zuccarello M (2002) Indications for endovascular treatment therapy for refractory vasospasm after aneurysmal subarachnoid hemorrhage. Experience at the University of Cincinnati. Surg Neurol 58: 131–138
4. Arakawa Y, Kikuta K, Hojo M, Goto Y, Ishii A, Yamagata S (2001) Milrinone for the treatment of cerebral vasospasm after subarachnoid hemorrhage: report of seven cases. Neurosurgery 48: 723–730
5. Awad IA, Carter LP, Spetzler RF, Medina M, Williams FC Jr (1987) Clinical vasospasm after subarachnoid hemorrhage:

response to hypervolemic hemodilution and arterial hypertension. Stroke 18: 365–372

6. Barker FG, Ogilvie CS (1996) Efficacy of prophylactic nimodipine for delayed ischemic deficit after subarachnoid hemorrhage: a metaanalysis. J Neurosurg 84: 405–414

7. Bernard SA, Gray TW, Buist MD, Jones BM, Silvester W, Gutteridge G, Smith K (2002) Treatment of comatose survivors of out-of-hospital cardiac arrest with induced hypothermia. N Engl J Med 346: 557–563

8. Biggar WD, Bohn D, Kent G (1983) Neutrophil circulation and release from bone marrow during hypothermia. Infect Immun 40: 708–712

9. Blaustein MP, Ector AC (1975) Barbiturate inhibition of calcium uptake by depolarized nerve terminals in vitro. Mol Pharmacol 11: 369–378

10. Boet R, Mee E (2000) Magnesium sulfate in the management of patients with Fisher Grade 3 subarachnoid hemorrhage: a pilot study. Neurosurgery 47: 602–607

11. Busto R, Dietrich WD, Globus MY, Ginsberg MD (1989) Postischemic moderate hypothermia inhibits CA1 hippocampal ischemic neuronal injury. Neurosci Lett 101: 299–304

12. Claassen J, Bernardini GL, Kreiter K, Bates J, Du YE, Copeland D, Connolly ES, Mayer SA (2001) Effect of cisternal and ventricular blood on risk of delayed cerebral ischemia after subarachnoid hemorrhage. The Fisher scale revisted. Stroke 32: 2012–2020

13. Dalen JE, Bone RC (1996) Is it time to pull the pulmonary artery catheter? JAMA 276: 916–918

14. Dorsch NW (2002) Therapeutic approaches to vasospasm in subarachnoid hemorrhage. Review. Curr Opin Crit Care 8: 128–133

15. Dorsch NW, Kassell NF, Sinkula MS (2001) Metaanalysis of trials of tirilazad mesylate in aneurysmal SAH. Acta Neurochir (Wien) [Suppl] 77: 233–235

16. Dorsch NW (1994) A review of cerebral vasospasm in aneurysmal subarachnoid haemorrhage. Part II: management. J Clin Neurosci 1: 78–92

17. Fandino J, Kaku Y, Schuknecht B, Valavanis A, Yonekawa Y (1998) Improvement of cerebral oxygenation patterns and metabolic validation of superselective intraarterial infusion of papaverine for the treatment of cerebral vasospasm. J Neurosurg 89: 93–100

18. Finfer SR, Ferch R, Morgan MK (1999) Barbiturate coma for severe, refractory vasospasm following subarachnoid haemorrhage. Intensive Care Med 25: 406–409

19. Gasser S, Khan N, Yonekawa Y, Imhof HG, Keller E (2003) Long-term hypothermia in patients with severe brain edema after poor-grade subarachnoid hemorrhage: feasibility and intensive care complications. J Neurosurg Anesthesiol 15: 240–248

20. Hegner T, Krayenbuhl N, Hefti M, Yonekawa Y, Keller E (2001) Bedside monitoring of cerebral blood flow in patients with subarachnoid hemorrhage. Acta Neurochir (Wien) [Suppl] 77: 131–134

21. Hindman BJ, Todd MM, Gelb AW, Loftus CM, Craen RA, Schubert A, Mahla ME, Torner JC (1999) Mild hypothermia as a protective therapy during intracranial aneurysm surgery: a randomized prospective pilot trial. Neurosurgery 44: 23–33

22. Hoeft A, Schorn B, Weyland A, Scholz M, Buhre W, Stepanek E, Allen SJ, Sonntag H (1994) Bedside assessment of intravascular volume status in patients undergoing coronary bypass surgery. Anesthesiology 81: 76–86

23. Janjua N, Mayer SA (2003) Cerebral vasospasm after subarachnoid hemorrhage. Review. Curr Opin in Crit Care 9: 113–119

24. Jennett B, Snoek J, Bond MR, Brooks N (1981) Disability after severe head injury: observations on the use of the Glasgow Outcome Scale. J Neurol Neurosurg Psychiatry 44: 285–293

25. Kaku Y, Yonekawa Y, Tsukahara T, Kazekawa K (1992) Superselective intra-arterial infusion of papaverine for the treatment of cerebral vasospasm after subarachnoid hemorrhage. J Neurosurg 77: 842–848

26. Karibe H, Sato K, Shimizu H, Tominaga T, Koshu K, Yoshimoto T (2000) Intraoperative mild hypothermia ameliorates postoperative cerebral blood flow impairment in patients with aneurysmal subarachnoid hemorrhage. Neurosurgery 47: 594–601

27. Kassell NF, Peerless SJ, Drake CG, Boarini DJ, Adams HP (1980) Treatment of ischemic deficits from cerebral vasospasm with high dose barbiturate therapy. Neurosurgery 7: 593–597

28. Kassell NF, Haley EC Jr, Apperson-Hansen C, Alves WM (1996) Randomized, double-blind, vehicle-controlled trial of tirilazad mesylate in patients with aneurysmal subarachnoid hemorrhage: a cooperative study in Europe, Australia, and New Zealand. J Neurosurg 84: 221–228

29. Kassell NF, Peerless SJ, Durward QJ, Beck Dw, Drake CG, Adams HP (1982) Treatment of ischemic deficits from vasospasm with intravascular volume expansion and induced arterial hypertension. Neurosurgery 11: 337–343

30. Kassell NF, Torner JC, Haley EC Jr, Jane JA, Adams Hp, Kongable GL (1990) The international cooperative study on timing of aneursym surgery. Part 1: overall management results. J Neurosurg 73: 18–36

31. Keller E, Imhof HG, Gasser S, Terzic A, Yonekawa Y (2003) Endovascular cooling with heat exchange catetheters: A new method to induce and maintain hypothermia. Intensive Care Med 29: 939–943

32. Keller E, Nadler A, Alkhadi H, Kollias SS, Yonekawa Y, Niederer P (2003) Non invasive measurement of regional cerebral blood flow and regional cerebral blood volume by near infrared spectroscopy and indocyanaine green dye dilution. Neuroimage 20: 828–839

33. Keller E, Steiner T, Fandino J, Schwab S, Hacke W (2002) Jugular venous oxygen saturation thresholds in trauma patients may not extrapolate to ischemic stroke patients: lessons from a preliminary study. J Neurosurg Anesthesiol 14: 130–136

34. Keller E, Wietasch G, Ringleb P, Scholz M, Schwarz S, Stingele R, Schwab S, Hanley D, Hacke W (2000) Bedside monitoring of cerebral blood flow in patients with acute hemispheric stroke. Crit Care Med 28: 511–516

35. Keller E, Wolf M, Martin M, Yonekawa Y (2001) Estimation of cerebral oxygenation and hemodynamics in cerebral vasospasm using indocyaningreen dye dilution and near infrared spectroscopy: a case report. J Neurosurg Anesthesiol 13: 43–48

36. Krayenbühl NT, Hegner T, Yonekawa Y, Keller E (2000) Cerebral vasospasm after subarachnoid hemorrhage: hypertensive hypervolemic hemodilution (triple-H) therapy according to new of systemic hemodynamics parameters. Acta Neurochir (Wien) [Suppl] 77: 247–250

37. Lennihan L, Mayer S, Fink ME, Beckford A, Paik MC, Zhang H, Wu YC, Klebanoff LM, Raps EC, Solomon RA (2000) Effect of hypervolemic therapy on cerebral blood flow after subarachnoid hemorrhage: a randomized controlled trial. Stroke 31: 383–391

38. Lindegaard KF (1999) The role of transcranial Doppler in the management of patients with subarachnoid hemorrhage: a review. Acta Neurochir (Wien) [Suppl] 72: 59–71

39. Maher J, Hachinski V (1993) Hypothermia as a potential treatment for cerebral ischemia. Review. Cerebrovasc Brain Metab Rev 5: 277–300

40. Manno EM, Gress DR, Schwamm LH, Diringer MN, Ogilvy CS (1998) Effects of induced hypertension on transcranial Doppler ultrasound velocities in patients after subarachnoid hemorrhage. Stroke 29: 422–428

41. McFadden JP (1988) Hypothermia-induced thrombocytopenia. J R Soc Med 81: 677

42. Meyer FB (1990) Calcium antagonists and vasospasm. Review. Neurosurg Clin N Am 1: 367–376

43. Mori T, Katayama Y, Kawamata T, Hirayama T (1999) Improved efficiency of hypervolemic therapy with inhibition of natruiresis by fludrocortisone in patients with aneurysmal subarachnoid hemorrhage. J Neurosurg 91: 947–952

44. Nagao S, Irie K, Kawai N, Kunishio K, Ogawa T, Nakamura T, Okauchi M (2000) Protective effect of mild hypothermia on symptomatic vasospasm: a preliminary report. Acta Neurochir (Wien) [Suppl] 76: 547–550

45. Nagao S, Irie K, Kawai N, Nakamura T, Kunishiro K, Matsumoto Y (2003) The use of mild hypothermia for patients with severe vasospasm: a preliminary report. J Clin Neurosci 10: 208–212

46. Pickard JD, Murray GD, Illingworth R, Shaw MD, Teasdale GM, Foy PM, Humphrey PR, Lang DA, Nelson R, Richards P (1989) Effect of oral nimodipine on cerebral infarction and outcome after subarachnoid haemorrhage: British aneurysm nimodipine trial. BMJ 298: 36–42

47. Piepgras A, Elste V, Frietsch T, Schmiedek P, Reith W, Schilling L (2001) Effect of moderate hypothermia on experimental severe subarachnoid hemorrhage, as evaluated by apparent diffusion coefficient changes. Neurosurgery 48: 1128–1135

48. Pina-Cabral JM, Ribeiro-da-Silva A, Almeida-Dias A (1985) Platelet sequestration during hypothermia in dogs treated with sulphinpyrazone and ticlopidine – reversibility accelereated after intra-abdominal rewarming. Thromb Haemost 54: 838–841

49. Pluta RM, Thompson BG, Afshar JK, Boock RJ, Juliano B, Oldfield EH (2001) Nitric oxide and vasospasm. Acta Neurochir (Wien) [Suppl] 77: 67–72

50. Raper R, Sibbald WJ (1986) Misled by the wedge? The Swan-Ganz catheter and left ventricular preload. Chest 89: 427–434

51. Rosenwasser RH, Delgado TE, Buchheit WA, Freed MH (1983) Control of hypertension and prophylaxis against vasospasm in cases of subarachnoid hemorrhage: a preliminary report. Neurosurgery 12: 658–661

52. Sen J, Belli A, Albon H, Morgan L, Petzold A, Kitchen N (2003) Triple-H therapy in the management of aneurysmal subarachnoid haemorrhage. Review. Lancet Neurol 2: 614–621

53. Shapiro HM, Galindo A, Wyte SR, Harris AB (1973) Rapid intraoperative reduction of intracranial pressure with thiopentone. Br J Anaesth 45: 1057–1062

54. Shenaq SA, Yawn DH, Saleem A, Joswiak R, Crawford ES (1986) Effect of profound hypothermia on leukocytes and platelets. Ann Clin Lab Sci 16: 130–133

55. Shibuya M, Asano T, Sasaki Y (2001) Effect of Fasudil HCl, a protein kinase inhibitor, on cerebral vasospasm. Acta Neurochir (Wien) [Suppl] 77: 201–204

56. Smith SL, Hall ED (1996) Mild pre- and posttraumatic hypothermia attenuates blood-brain barrier damage following controlled cortical impact injury in the rat. J Neurotrauma 13: 1–9

57. Solenski NJ, Haley EC JR, Kassell NF, Kongable G, Germanson T, Truskowski L, Torner JC (1995) Medical complications of aneurysmal subarachnoid hemorrhage: a report of the multicenter study, Participants of the multicenter cooperative aneurysm study. Crit Care Med 23: 1007–1017

58. Stover JF, Stocker R (1998) Barbiturate coma may promote reversible bone marrow suppression in patients iwth severe isolated traumatic brain injury. Eur J Clin Pharmacol 54: 529–534

59. Valeri CR, Feingold H, Cassidy G, Ragno G, Khuri S, Altschule MD (1986) Hypothermia-induced reversible platelet dysfunction. Ann Surg 205: 175–181

60. Veyna RS, Seyfried D, Burke DG, Zimmerman C, Mlynarek M, Nichols V, Marrocco A, Thomas AJ, Mitsias PD, Malik GM (2002) Magnesium sulfate therapy after aneurysmal subarachnoid hemorrhage. J Neurosurg 96: 510–514

61. Vora YY, Suarez-Almazor M, Steinke DE, Martin ML, Findlay JM (1999) Role of transcranial Doppler monitoring in the diagnosis of cerebral vasospasm after subarachnoid hemorrhage. Neurosurgery 44: 1237–1248

62. Waller MB, Richter JA (1980) Effects of pentobarbital and Ca2+ on the resting and K+-stimulated release of several endogenous neurotransmitters from rat midbrain slices. Biochem Pharmacol 29: 2189–2198

63. Wijdicks EF, Ropper AH, Hunnicutt EJ, Richardson GS, Nathanson JA (1991) Atrial natriuretic factor and salt wasting after aneurysmal subarachnoid hemorrhage. Stroke 22: 1519–1524

64. Yasargil MG (1984) Clinical Considerations. Surgery of the intracranial aneurysms and results, vol II. Thieme, New York Stuttgart, pp 1–32

65. Zuccarello M (2001) Endothelin: the "prime suspect" in cerebral vasospasm. Review. Acta Neurochir (Wien) [Suppl] 77: 61–65

Correspondence: Emanuela Keller, Department of Neurosurgery, University Hospital, Frauenklinikstrasse 10, 8091 Zurich, Switzerland. e-mail: emanuela.keller@usz.ch

Management of unruptured intracranial aneurysms

Acta Neurochir (2005) [Suppl] 94: 77–85
© Springer-Verlag 2005
Printed in Austria

Treatment of unruptured cerebral aneurysms; a multi-center study at Japanese national hospitals

T. Tsukahara[1]**, N. Murakami**[1]**, Y. Sakurai**[2]**, M. Yonekura**[3]**, T. Takahashi**[4]**, T. Inoue**[5]**, and Y. Yonekawa**[6]

[1] Department of Neurological Surgery and Clinical Research Center, National Hospital Organization, Kyoto Medical Center, Kyoto, Japan
[2] Department of Neurological Surgery, National Hospital Organization, Sendai Medical Center, Sendai, Japan
[3] Department of Neurological Surgery, National Hospital Organization, Nagasaki Medical Center, Nagasaki, Japan
[4] Department of Neurological Surgery, National Hospital Organization, Nagoya Medical Center, Nagoya, Japan
[5] Department of Neurological Surgery and Clinical Research Institute, National Hospital Organization, Kyusyu Medical Center, Kyusyu Medical Center, Fukuoka, Japan
[6] Department of Neurosurgery, University Hospital Zurich, Zurich, Switzerland

Summary

The treatment and natural course of unruptured cerebral aneurysms were analyzed in 615 patients with 712 unruptured cerebral aneurysms registered from seven Japanese national hospitals and Zurich University hospital. For 209 aneurysms in 181 cases, the natural course of the aneurysms was observed without surgical treatment. During the follow-up period of 3,862 months (321.8 years), 11 of these aneurysms ruptured giving a rupture rate of 3.42%/year. Five of these 11 aneurysms were less than 10 mm in diameter. Seventeen aneurysms of these 209 untreated aneurysms had blebs. Seven of these 17 aneurysms ruptured yielding the high rupture rate of 28.3%/year. The likelihood of unruptured cerebral aneurysms to rupture was not exceedingly low even when the aneurysms were smaller than 10 mm. Since the risk of rupture and morbidity in relation to surgical treatment cannot be predicted by size alone, the morphology, especially the presence of blebs, should be considered when treating unruptured cerebral aneurysms. In 434 patients, 503 cerebral aneurysms were treated surgically either by craniotomy in 472 aneurysms or endovascular coil embolization in 31 aneurysms. Surgical outcome was influenced by the presence of concurrent diseases, patient age, size and location of the aneurysms. Complications after surgical treatment of 128 incidentally found aneurysms were reported in four cases; three cases of hemiparesis and one case showing disturbance of higher brain function, with a morbidity rate of 3.1%. These results suggest that surgical treatment may be acceptable in cases of incidentally found cerebral aneurysms, especially when blebs are present.

Keywords: Unruptured cerebral aneurysm; multi-center study.

Introduction

Recently, we have more frequently encountered patients with asymptomatic unruptured cerebral aneurysms. Since subarachnoid hemorrhage (SAH) due to rupture of cerebral aneurysms is a serious disorder with high mortality and morbidity despite recent progress in SAH management, it may be reasonable to prevent potentially disastrous SAH by treating cerebral aneurysms before they rupture. A general consensus for the management of unruptured aneurysms, however, has not yet been established, since there are no prospective randomized trials of interventional treatment versus conservative management. Regarding the natural course of unruptured cerebral aneurysms Juvela *et al.* [3] reported that rupture rate was 10% within 10 years after diagnosis, 26% after 20 years and 32% after 30 years. Yasui *et al.* reported that the overall rupture rate was 2.3%/year and that the size of these aneurysms was less than 9 mm in 11 of 22 cases developing SAH. In five cases, aneurysms were smaller than 5 mm [5, 6]. In 1998, the International Study of Unruptured Intracranial Aneurysms (ISUIA) reported that the rupture rate of cerebral aneurysms smaller than 10 mm was unexpectedly low at 0.05%/year [2]. Although there were criticisms that a rather large number of patients with unruptured aneurysms were excluded from the study after surgeons indicated a high likelihood of rupture, and only the remaining patients were followed to analyze the natural history [1], this report had a rather large impact on the general public. Treatment indications for unruptured cerebral aneurysms have been markedly influenced by the report. In 1999, a multi-center study for the treatment of unruptured cerebral aneurysms was organized to re-evaluate treatment by accumulating basic data on the natural

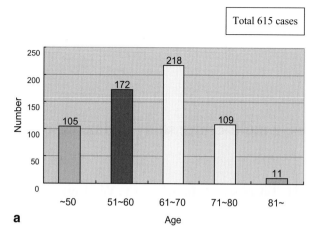

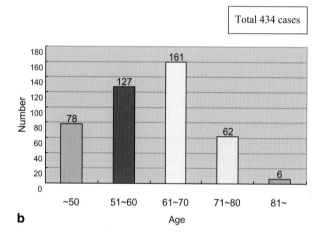

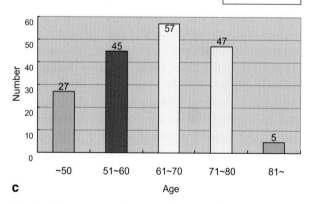

Fig. 1. (a) Ages of all patients with aneurysms. (b) Ages of patients with treated aneurysms. (c) Ages of patients with untreated aneurysms

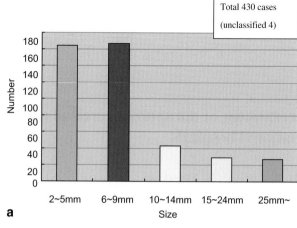

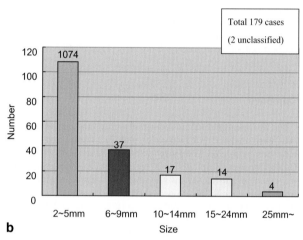

Fig. 2. (a) Sizes of treated aneurysms. (b) Sizes of untreated aneurysms

course of unruptured cerebral aneurysms and the surgical outcome after treatment. This multi-center study was supported by a Health Science Research Grant from the Japanese Ministry of Health, Labor and Welfare. This paper reports the results of the study.

Materials and methods

Between 1999 and 2001, a total of 615 patients with 712 unruptured cerebral aneurysms were registered in seven Japanese national hospitals and Zurich University hospital in Switzerland. For 209 aneurysms in 181 cases, the natural course of the aneurysms was observed without surgical treatment. Other cerebral aneurysms were treated surgically either by craniotomy in 472 cases or by endovascular coil embolization in 31 cases. Age distribution of all registered patients, surgically treated and untreated patients are shown in Fig. 1a–c, respectively. Patients aged 60–69 years comprised the peak in each group, although younger patients tended to receive surgical treatment while the older group remained untreated. Size of the cerebral aneurysms is shown in Fig. 2a (surgically treated group) and 2b (untreated group). Aneurysms were larger in treated patients.

The locations of cerebral aneurysms are shown in Fig. 3a (surgically treated group) and 3b (untreated group); Patients with unrup-

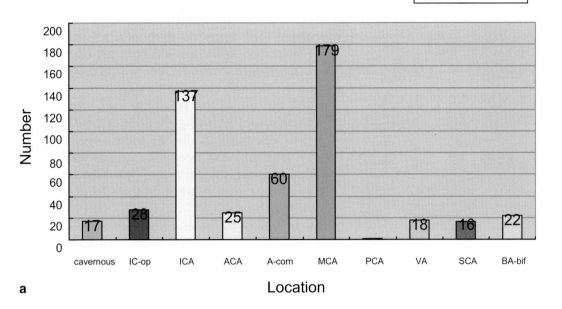

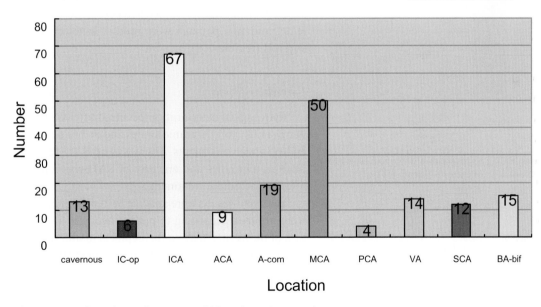

Fig. 3. (a) Locations of treated aneurysms. (b) Locations of untreated aneurysms

tured cerebral aneurysms were also categorized into four groups by clinical manifestations (Fig. 4a and b): group I; unruptured cerebral aneurysms accompanied by ruptured aneurysm (38 untreated and 93 treated cases), group II; unruptured cerebral aneurysms with other intracranial lesions (50 untreated and 115 treated cases), group III; symptomatic unruptured cerebral aneurysms (19 untreated and 98 treated cases), group IV; incidentally found unruptured cerebral aneurysms (74 untreated and 128 treated cases). In our study, a total of 202 patients were registered as incidental aneurysms in group IV. Aneurysmal size was as follows: 2 to 5 mm in 72 cases, 6 to 9 mm in 74 cases, 10 to 14 mm in 32 cases, 15 to 24 mm in 16 cases, larger than 25 mm in six cases and unknown in 2 cases. The percentage of incidentally detected aneurysms measuring less than 10 mm was 72.3% (146 cases). In one of 202 cases, aneurysmal size increased

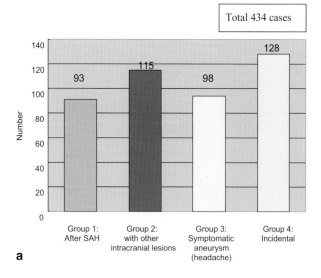

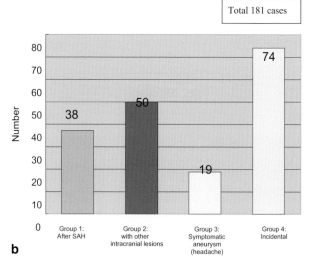

Fig. 4. (a) Conditions leading to diagnosis of the aneurysms. (b) Conditions leading to diagnosis of untreated aneurysms

over 48 months and clipping of the aneurysm was performed. Of 202 incidental cases, 128 cases were treated surgically and 74 cases were not treated.

Results

Natural course

For 209 aneurysms in 181 cases, the natural course of aneurysms was observed without treatment. During an overall follow-up period totaling 3,862 months (321.8 years), 11 of these aneurysms ruptured, giving a rupture rate of 3.42%/year. Although larger aneur-

ysms tend to show a higher rupture rate with subsequent SAH, five of these 11 aneurysms were smaller than 10 mm and two were even smaller than 5 mm (Fig. 5). Risk of rupture was not determined by size alone. Their shape had much more influence on the rupture rate. Aneurysms with blebs caused SAH with a much higher rupture rate. The rupture rate of aneurysms with blebs smaller than 10 mm was 39%, and two aneurysms with blebs even smaller than 5 mm caused SAH (Fig. 6). Eight of these 11 aneurysms were found incidentally and classified in group IV. The remaining three cases were as follows: two were symptomatic aneurysms (headache and visual disturbance) and one was accompanied by cerebral ischemic disease.

In eight of the 74 untreated cases of group IV, the aneurysms ruptured. In four cases, the size of aneurysms was larger than 10 mm, and in four cases the size was less than 10 mm. In two patients with multiple aneurysms measuring less than 5 mm each and with blebs, anterior communicating aneurysms (Acom) and IC-PC aneurysms, which were the smallest of multiple aneurysms, caused SAH. The outcome after rupture was poor. Three patients died immediately after rupture, one patient remained in a persistent vegetative state, and two patients were mildly disabled despite surgical treatment.

Surgical outcome

Neurological deterioration occurred after treatment in 52 (11.0%) of 472 craniotomies and in 3 (9.6%) of 31 endovascular treatments. There was no SAH reported after craniotomies and one case of SAH was reported after endovascular treatment.

Treatment results were analyzed after the aneurysms were grouped according to patient age, size and location of the aneurysms and their clinical manifestations.

Age (Fig. 7a); Outcome of patients aged 80 or more was worse, although the number of surgically treated patients in that age group was small.

Size (Fig. 7b); A higher number of patients with neurological deterioration was reported among patients with an aneurysm larger than 15 mm, although a higher number of neurological improvements was also observed among patients with larger aneurysm.

Location (Fig. 7c); A higher number of patients with neurological deterioration was reported among patients with aneurysms involving the basilar bifurcation compared to those with aneurysms at other sites.

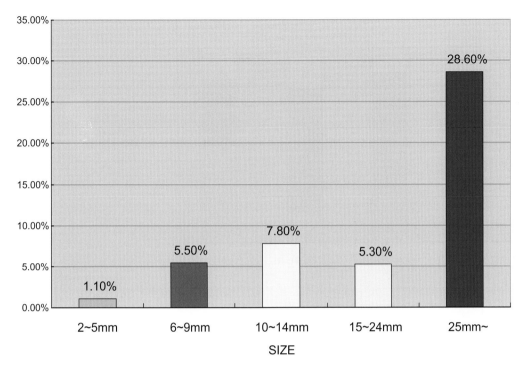

Fig. 5. Rupture rate per year

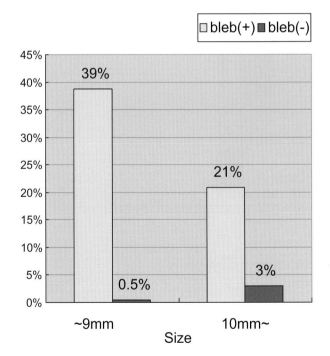

Fig. 6. Rupture rate per year with respect to the form of aneurysms

Clinical manifestation (Fig. 7d); In groups I and II, the preoperative medical condition of patients and accompanying diseases significantly influenced patient outcome. In group III, cranial nerve palsies caused by aneurysms smaller than 10 mm were improved postoperatively in nine cases. However, neurological deficits caused by aneurysms larger than 25 mm more frequently worsened after surgery.

Outcome after surgery in group IV is shown in figure 6. The outcome was evaluated by Glasgow outcome scale (GOS) 124 of 128 patients showed good recovery with a mortality of 0% and morbidity of 3.1% (Fig. 8). Two patients were severely disabled by cerebral infarction after surgery on a 2–5 mm MCA aneurysm and 15–24 mm ICA aneurysm, respectively, two patients were also mildly disabled by cerebral infarction after surgery on 10–14 mm and 15–24 mm ICA aneurysms, respectively. The other 11 patients, although they are estimated to have good recovery by GOS, subjectively experienced neurological worsening. Five patients had visual field defect after surgery for IC-ophthalmic aneurysms. Two patients had oculomotor nerve palsy after surgery on IC-PC aneurysms. Two patients with intracerebral hemorrhage of the frontal base, and one with chronic subdural hematoma, experienced impairment of higher brain function after surgery on Acom aneurysms. One patient also showed impairment of higher brain function after surgery on MCA aneurysm.

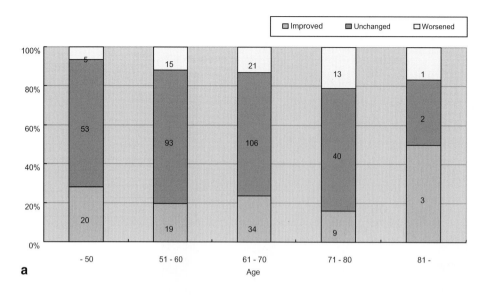

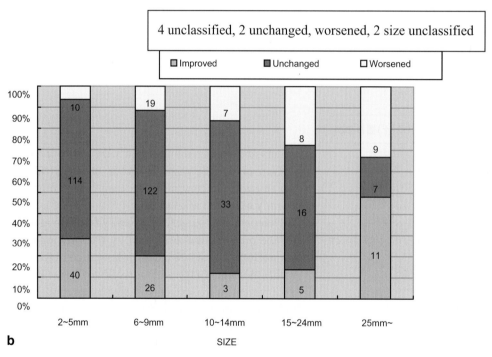

Fig. 7. (a) Surgical outcome with respect to patient age. (b) Surgical outcome with respect to aneurysm size.

Discussion

Decision-making regarding the treatment of unruptured cerebral aneurysms should be based on the natural history and risk of treatment options. At present, however, both the natural course of unruptured cerebral aneurysm and outcome after treatment have not always been clear. Cranial examination using MRI or MR angiography has found asymptomatic cerebral aneurysms in over 2% of total examinees [4]. These incidental cerebral aneurysms, which were classified as group IV in our study, detected on cranial imaging differed in nature from symptomatic aneurysms or asymptomatic unruptured aneurysms accompanied by other cerebral lesions. Therefore, management of these aneurysms should be considered separately. In our study, for 209 aneurysms in 181 cases, the natural course of the aneurysms was observed without surgical

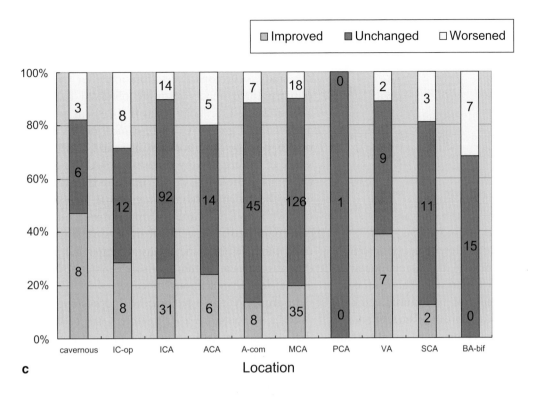

c

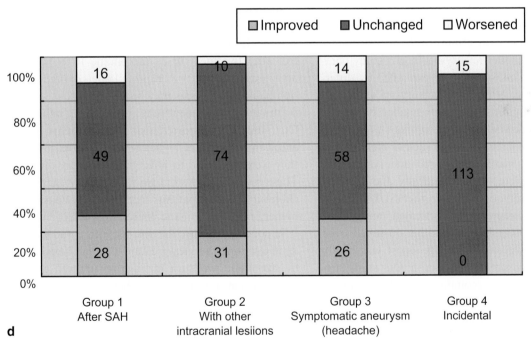

d

Fig. 7. (c) Surgical outcome with respect to aneurysm location. (d) Surgical outcome with respect to diagnostic conditions

treatment. During the total follow-up period of 3,862 months (321.8 years), 11 of these aneurysms ruptured giving a rupture rate of 3.42%/year. This rupture rate is comparable to that in previous studies. Six of these 11 aneurysms were larger than 10 mm and two were

fusiform aneurysms of vertebro-basilar arteries. The remaining two were giant aneurysms of the IC-ophthalmic and basilar tip. These aneurysms were observed via the natural course without treatment because of the high risk of surgical treatment. Prognosis

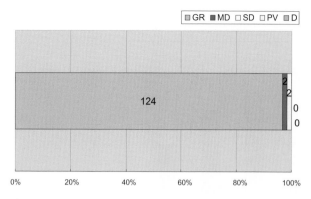

Fig. 8. Surgical outcome of aneurysms discovered incidentally

of these aneurysms is unfortunately rather poor so that we cannot discuss their management simultaneously with that of other smaller aneurysms. The main controversy in the management of unruptured cerebral aneurysms involves the management of smaller aneurysms. In our study, five of 144 aneurysms smaller than 10 mm ruptured and two ruptured aneurysms with blebs were less than 5 mm. These follow-up results suggested that the rupture rate of smaller aneurysms is not extremely low and aneurysms with an irregular shape such as a bleb have a considerably higher rupture rate than those with a uniform shape. The higher rupture rate of smaller aneurysms in our study compared to that in ISUIA, may be explained by differences in the nature of untreated aneurysms and surgical indications. In our study, many smaller aneurysms tended to be followed without treatment even if the aneurysm had an irregular shape such as blebs. However, in ISUIA, many unruptured aneurysms with irregular shape were treated surgically and thus excluded from observation. Before the ISUIA report, many Japanese neurosurgeons treated unruptured aneurysms with irregular shape rather positively even when small. However, the ISUIA report was highly influential on such surgical indication. Our study suggested that we need to recommend surgical treatment for small unruptured aneurysms with irregular shape if the surgical risk is considered low.

Conclusions

When we estimate the outcome after surgical treatment of unruptured cerebral aneurysm, we must evaluate not only the mortality or morbidity rate but also the quality of life for the patient, including issues related to higher brain function such as cognitive impairment, for example. Since the outcome after treatment varied with the state of the patient before treatment, the results of treatment should be analyzed considering the preoperative neurological status of the patient. In our study, neurological deterioration after treatment of unruptured aneurysms were observed in 10.9%; 17% in group I, 8.7% in group II, 14.3% in group III and 11.7% in group IV. These clinical results depend on preoperative conditions. So in group I or III, the severity of the accompanying diseases, SAH in group I and other neurological disease in group II or III, influenced the patient outcome. In group II, two patients died within one year after treatment due to other diseases unrelated to the cerebral aneurysms. Apparently unruptured cerebral aneurysms accompanied by conditions such as brain tumor or severe systemic diseases are outside the indications for surgery.

In group IV, since patients had no accompanying diseases, the outcome after treatment was better than that of other patient groups. In this group, 124 of 128 patients (96.9%) showed good recovery, while two cases were mildly disabled and two cases were severely disabled when postoperative quality of life was evaluated by the Glasgow outcome scale. However, 11.7% of patients had some neurological disorder after surgery. In our study, five patients had visual field defect after treatment of asymptomatic IC-ophthalmic aneurysms. Since the rupture rate of these IC-ophthalmic aneurysms may be relatively low, surgical treatment of these aneurysms are outside of indication. Our study also reported that some patients experienced impairment of higher brain function, although they were estimated to have good recovery on GOS. These results suggest that we must evaluate the surgical results of these patients more precisely considering higher brain function and neuropsychological aspects.

In conclusion, since the risk of rupture and morbidity in relation to surgical treatment cannot be predicted by size alone, we must manage unruptured cerebral aneurysms in consideration of their morphology, location and condition of the patient.

Acknowledgment

Treatment and natural course were observed in unruptured cerebral aneurysms registered from Departments of Neurosurgery of seven Japanese national hospitals; Kyoto National Hospital, Sendai National Hospital, National Nagasaki Medical Center, Nagoya National Hospital, National Kyusyu Medical Center, Osaka National Hospital and Minami Wakayama National Hospital and the Department of Neurological Surgery, Zurich University, Switzerland.

This study was supported by Health Sciences Research Grants from Japanese Ministry of Health, Labor, and Welfare.

References

1. Ausman JI (1999) The New England Journal of medicine report on unruptured intracranial aneurysms: a critique. Surg Neurol 51: 227–229
2. ISUIA Investigators (1998) Unruptured intracranial aneurysms: risks of rupture and risks of surgical intervention. N Engl J Med 339: 1725–1733
3. Juvela S, Porras M, Heiskanen O (1993) Natural history of unruptured intracranial aneurysms: a long-term follow-up study. J Neurosurg 79: 174–182
4. Nakagawa T, Hashi K (1994) The incidence and treatment of asymptomatic, unruptured cerebral aneurysms. J Neurosurg 80: 217–223
5. Yasui N, Magarisawa S, Suzuki A *et al* (1996) Subarachnoid hemorrhage caused by previously diagnosed, previously unruptured intracranial aneurysms: a retrospective analysis of 25 cases. Neurosurgery 39: 1096–1100
6. Yasui N, Suzuki A, Nishimura H *et al* (1997) Long-term follow-up study of unruptured intracranial aneurysms. Neurosurgery 40: 1155–1159

Correspondence: Tetsuya Tsukahara, Department of Neurosurgery, National Hospital Organization, Kyoto Medical Center, 1-1 Mukaihata-cho, Fukakusa, Fushimi-ku, Kyoto, 612-8555 Japan. e-mail: ttsukaha@kyotolan.hosp.go.jp

Acta Neurochir (2005) [Suppl] 94: 87–91
© Springer-Verlag 2005
Printed in Austria

Endovascular treatment of unruptured cerebral aneurysms

T. Terada, M. Tsuura, H. Matsumoto, O. Masuo, T. Tsumoto, H. Yamaga, and **T. Itakura**

Department of Neurological Surgery, Wakayama Medical University, Wakayama, Japan

Summary

76 consecutive patients with 78 unruptured cerebral aneurysms underwent endovascular therapy from July 1999 to May 2004 in our institute. For the wide-necked aneurysms, the remodeling technique, double microcatheter technique, or stent-assisted coil embolization was used, while a parent artery occlusion or covered stent was applied for the giant or fusiform aneurysms. Immediate angiographical results demonstrated 33 complete occlusions, 26 neck remnants, and 14 dome fillings. Four cases were treated with parent occlusion or stenting only, and one case was not treated with embolization but with clipping due to the rupture of the aneurysm during coil embolization. Immediate angiographic findings demonstrated that in aneurysms between 5 to 10 mm, the rate of complete occlusion was 48%, that of neck remnants 33%, and that of dome fillings 27%. In aneurysms between 11 to 25 mm, the rate of complete occlusion was 14%, that of neck remnants 28%, and that of dome fillings was 58%. In the angiographic follow-up results, all aneurysms smaller than 5 mm showed complete occlusion. In aneurysms between 5 to 10 mm, 74% of the aneurysms showed complete occlusion, and 21% showed neck remnants, and 5% showed dome filling. In aneurysms between 10 to 24 mm, 25% showed complete occlusion, while 75% showed dome filling. The overall mortality rate was 0% and the morbidity rate was 3.7% (2 major strokes, 1 minor stroke) at 30-days after embolization. In the clinical follow-up study, one case of a large basilar tip aneurysm caused a fatal rupture 28 months after the initial embolization. Endovascular therapy was performed on the unruptured aneurysms and was found to be an acceptable treatment, except for durability in cases of large aneurysms.

Keywords: Embolization; detachable coil; unruptured aneurysm; remodeling technique; stent.

Introduction

The efficacy of coil embolization for ruptured cerebral aneurysms has been proven by a randomized controlled trial [6]. However, the efficacy of endovascular therapy for unruptured cerebral aneurysms is still unknown [1], although several papers reported the superiority of embolization over direct surgery in a short-term follow-up period [2, 5, 6]. Coil embolization has shown a short-term clinical and angiographical efficacy as a therapeutic alternative to the surgical treatment of intracranial aneurysms [2, 5, 6]. However, the long-term effect of coil embolization to prevent growth or rupture of unruptured aneurysms has not been proven. We report the results of coil embolization in 76 patients with 78 aneurysms, including clinical outcome, morbidity-mortality rate, and long-term follow-up data.

Materials and methods

76 patients with 78 unruptured cerebral aneurysms underwent coil embolization at Wakayama Medical University and its branch hospitals from July 1999 to May 2004. The male/female ratio was 24/52 and mean patient's age was 59.4 years with a range of 24–79 years.

Patients were classified into three groups: 55 patients had unruptured aneurysms discovered incidentally during angiography or magnetic resonance angiography (MRA). 15 patients had unruptured aneurysms associated with a ruptured one. Eight patients had unruptured aneurysms with a mass effect, such as cranial nerve palsy etc.

Location of the aneurysms is shown in Table 1. There were 41 aneurysms located in the anterior circulation and 37 in the posterior circulation. The most common location of the aneurysms in our series was basilar tip (n = 22).

The aneurysms were classified into five groups by size, as follows: less than 5 mm, 5–10 mm, 11–24 mm, >25 mm, and the fusiform

Table 1. *Location of aneurysms*

Anterior circulation		Posterior circulation	
– Paraclinoid	18	– BA tip	22
– ICPC	5	– BA trunk	7
– MCA	4	– VA	8
– Acom	8	Total	37
– Cav-pet	2		
– IC top	2		
– IC-Ach	1		
– IC trunk	1		
Total	41		

type. There were 14 aneurysms less than 5 mm, 50 that were 5–10 mm, 7 that were 11–24 mm, 4 that were >25 m, and 3 fusiform aneurysms.

Coil embolization was performed based on the following criteria.

$$Age <= 70 \text{ years}$$

$$Aneurysm >= 5 \text{ mm}$$

Coil embolization was chosen for basilar tip, basilar trunk, and paraclinoid aneurysms.

For aneurysms in other location, coil embolization was chosen if the shape of the aneurysm was suitable for coil embolization using a single microcatheter and usual coils only (simple technique).

Method of embolization

The procedure was performed under general anesthesia and systemic heparinization. A microcatheter was navigated into the aneurysm under the road mapping mode and a detachable coil (mainly a GDC) was delivered sequentially and deployed into the aneurysm until tight packing was achieved. For wide-necked aneurysms, a remodeling technique [9] using compliant balloons such as the Commodore (J&J) or Hyperform (MTI), double microcatheter technique or stent-assisted coil embolization was used. 62 aneurysms were embolized using these simple techniques. 13 cases were treated using the remodeling technique, two with the stent-assisted technique, and two with the double microcatheter technique. For aneurysms with mass effect, parent occlusion using coils or balloons or a covered stent was deployed across the neck of the aneurysm.

Clinical and angiographic follow-up was performed as follows. Angiographical follow-up was performed every 6 months until 24 months after embolization, and an MRA was performed every year from 2 years after embolization. The angiographical data was classified into the following three categories: complete occlusion, neck remnant, and dome filling.

Results

Immediate angiographic results demonstrated 33 complete occlusions, 26 neck remnants, and 14 dome fillings. Four cases were treated with parent occlusion or stenting only, and one case was not treated with embolization but with clipping.

Immediate angiographic results were analyzed according to the size of aneurysm. In aneurysms smaller than 5 mm, the rate of complete occlusion was 36%, that for the neck remnants 36%, and that for the dome filling aneurysms 28%. In aneurysms between 5 to 10 mm, the rate of complete occlusion was 48%, that for the neck remnants 33%, and that for the dome fillings 27%. In aneurysms between 11 to 25 mm, the rate of complete occlusion was 14%, that for the neck remnants 28%, and that for the dome fillings 58%.

Angiographic follow-up results demonstrated that all aneurysms smaller than 5 mm showed complete occlusion. In aneurysms between 5 to 10 mm, 74% of the aneurysms showed complete occlusion, and 21%

showed neck remnants, and 5% showed dome filling. In aneurysms between 10 to 24 mm, 25% showed complete occlusion, while 75% showed dome filling.

As for complications during the procedure, one aneurysm was perforated with the first GDC coil. An immediate angiography demonstrated extravasation of the contrast medium. Heparin was immediately reversed. Then, the coil that penetrated the aneurysmal wall was deployed in extra and intraaneurysmal space. However, the entire lumen of the aneurysm was not packed. Therefore, the patient was moved to the operation room and surgical clipping was performed for the partially embolized MCA aneurysm. The patient was discharged without any new neurological deficits after surgery. Five thrombo-embolic complications appeared in 82 aneurysms. The overall mortality rate was 0%, and the morbidity rate was 3.7% (2 major strokes, 1 minor stroke) at 30-days after embolization.

In the clinical follow-up study, one case of a large basilar tip aneurysm caused a fatal rupture 28 months after initial embolization. In this case, the patient had not visited the hospital for 28 months after embolization. He finally came to our hospital 28 months after embolization due to abdominal pain. At that time, a plain craniogram was examined, and a change in the shape of the embolized coil was found. An angiography was scheduled, but the day before admission he suffered a massive subarachnoid hemorrhage and died. The rupture rate of all aneurysms in our series was 1.3% in the follow-up period of mean 3.2 years. Therefore, the annual rupture rate in our series was 0.4%.

Representative cases

A 67-year-old male was admitted to our hospital for the treatment of unruptured basilar tip aneurysm of $10 \times 8 \times 8$ mm in size, which was found on angiography for the diagnosis of cerebral infarction (Fig. 1 a,b). Coil embolization was performed under general anesthesia. The aneurysm was wide-necked, and a remodeling technique was used for the coil embolization. A Commodore double lumen balloon catheter was introduced from the left vertebral artery and a microcatheter for coil embolization (Prowler-14) was introduced from the right vertebral artery. A GDC-18 coil (8 mm $\times$ 20 cm) was introduced into the aneurysm under dilatation of the balloon placed from the left posterior cerebral artery to the basilar artery. After deployment of the first coil to preserve the bilateral pos-

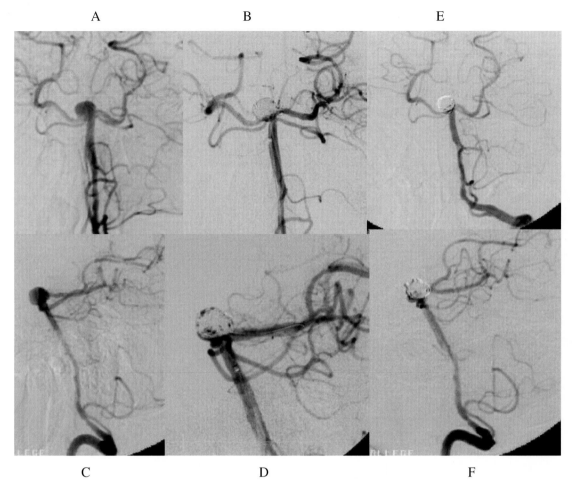

Fig. 1. Angiographic findings of case 1. (A) AP view of the vertebral angiography. A wide-necked aneurysm was demonstrated. (B) Lateral view of the vertebral angiography. (C) AP view of the vertebral angiography after coil embolization. Bilateral posterior cerebral arteries were preserved. (D) Lateral view of the vertebral angiography. (E) AP view of the vertebral angiography one year after initial embolization. Dome filling was not demonstrated. (F) Lateral view of the vertebral angiography one year after initial embolization

terior cerebral arteries, packing coils were introduced into the framing coil (Fig. 1 c,d). Embolization was completed under the condition of dome filling. On the follow-up angiogram one year after embolization, the aneurysm had been obliterated keeping the bilateral posterior cerebral arteries patent (Fig. 1 e,f).

A 50-year-old male had a small intracerebral hemorrhage. On CT, an isodensity mass was found in the interpeduncular cistern. Angiography revealed a large unruptured basilar tip aneurysm 14 × 10 × 11 mm in size (Fig. 2 a,b). The neck of the aneurysm was broad, and bilateral posterior cerebral arteries had branched from the dome of the aneurysm. The double microcatheter technique was used to embolize this aneurysm. GDC-18 coils 12 mm × 30 cm and 10 mm × 30 cm were deployed into the aneurysm

from microcatheters introduced from the bilateral vertebral arteries. The aneurysm was embolized but the dome of the aneurysm was partially filled with contrast medium to keep the bilateral posterior cerebral arteries patent (Fig. 2 c,d). The patient had not visited our hospital until 28 months after the procedure, at which time deformity of the initially embolized coil was found (Fig. 2 e,f). The evening of the day of his visit to the hospital, a massive subarachnoid hemorrhage occurred and he died.

Discussion

Aneurysmal SAH has a 30-day mortality rate of 45% and an approximately 50% rate of disabilities among survivors. The prevention of SAH has been

A   B   E

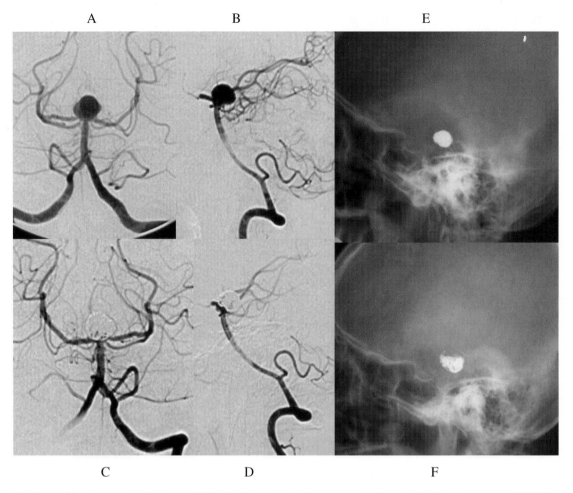

C   D   F

Fig. 2. Radiological findings of case 2. (A,B) Vertebral angiography demonstrated wide-necked basilar tip aneurysm. (C,D) The aneurysm was embolized and left the bilateral posterior cerebral arteries patent. (E) Plain craniogram after initial coil embolization. (F) Plain craniogram 28 months after initial embolization

promoted as the most effective strategy for reducing the morbidity and mortality rate. Recently, the largest study of unruptured cerebral aneurysms, the International Study of Unruptured Intracranial Aneurysms, reported a rupture rate of 0.05% for unruptured aneurysms < 10 mm in diameter and no history of SAH, and 0.5% for those with previous SAH. In aneurysms > 10 mm, the rupture rate was approximately 1% [3]. More recently, the ISUIA published a slightly higher rate of rupture of unruptured cerebral aneurysms after detailed evaluation of aneurysma location [3].

For treating unruptured cerebral aneurysms, coil embolization has proven to be effective in early and clinical evaluations. Johnston *et al.* [4] reported the results of surgical clipping and coil embolization of unruptured cerebral aneurysms. A morbidity rate of

18.5% was found in the surgical group and 10.6% in the endovascular group, and the mortality rate was 2.3% and 0.4%, respectively. We treated 78 unruptured cerebral aneurysms, on which direct surgery was difficult to perform. Therefore, many aneurysms in the posterior circulation and paraclinoid area were included in our series. Morbidity and mortality rates at 30-days were 3.7% and 0%, respectively. These results are acceptable for the treatment of unruptured cerebral aneurysms. However, the biggest problem with coil embolization is recanalization after embolization. In smaller aneurysms of <10 mm, the recanalization rate was lower than 25%, while in large aneurysms of >=11 mm, the recanalization rate was 75%. Of the large aneurysms, one aneurysm caused a fatal subarachnoid hemorrhage 28 months after embolization.

Various types of new coils have been developed to

solve this problem, such as the Matrix coil [9], hydro-coil, or bFGF core coils [5], which are supposed to induce fibrosis inside the aneurysm to prevent recanalization.

References

1. Bederson JB, Awad IA, Wiebers DO, Piepgras D, Haley EC Jr, Brott T, Hademenos G, Chyatte D, Rosenwasser R, Caroselli C (2000) Recommendations for the management of patients with unruptured intracranial aneurysms: a statement for healthcare professionals from the Stroke Council of the American Heart Association. Stroke 31: 2742–2750
2. Gonzalez N, Murayama Y, Nien YL, Martin N, Frazee J, Duckwiler G, Jahan R, Gobin YP, Vinuela F (2004) Treatment of unruptured aneurysms with GDCs: clinical experiences with 247 aneurysms. AJNR Am J Neuroradiol 25: 577–583
3. International Study of Unruptured Intracranial Aneurysms Investigators Unruptured intracranial aneurysms – risk of rupture and risks of surgical intervention (1998). N Engl J Med 339: 1725–1733
4. Johnston SC, Dudley RA, Gress DR, Ono L (1999) Surgical and endovascular treatment of unruptured cerebral aneurysms at university hospitals. Neurology 52: 1799–1805
5. Matsumoto H, Terada T, Tsuura M, Itakura T, Ogawa A (2003) Basic fibroblast growth factor released from a platinum coil with a polyvinyl alcohol core enhances cellular proliferation and vascular wall thickness: an in vitro and in vivo study. Neurosurgery 53: 402–408
6. Molyneux A, Kerr R, Stratton I, Sandercock P, Clarke M, Shrimpton J, Holman R, International Subarachnoid Aneurysm Trial (ISAT) Collaborative Group (2002) International subarachnoid aneurysm trial (ISAT) of neurosurgical clipping versus endovascular coiling in 2143 patients with ruptured intracranial aneurysms: a randomised trial. Lancet 26: 1267–1274
7. Moret J, Cognard C, Weill A, Castaings L, Rey A (1997) Reconstruction technique in the treatment of wide-neck intracranial aneurysms. Long-term angiographic and clinical results. A propos of 56 cases. J Neuroradiol 24: 30–44
8. Murayama Y, Vinuela F, Duckwiler GR, Gobin YP, Guglielmi G (1999) Embolization of incidental cerebral aneurysms by using the Guglielmi detachable coil system. J Neurosurg 90: 207–214
9. Murayama Y, Vinuela F, Tateshima S, Song JK, Gonzalez NR, Wallace MP (2001) Bio-absorbable polymeric material coils for embolization of intracranial aneurysms: a preliminary experimental study. J Neurosurg 94: 454–463

Correspondence: Tomoaki Terada, 811-1 Kimiidera, Wakayama City, 641-0012, Japan. e-mail: teradato@wakayama-med.ac.jp

Acta Neurochir (2005) [Suppl] 94: 93–96
© Springer-Verlag 2005
Printed in Austria

Management of ruptured aneurysms combined with coexisting aneurysms

H.-G. Imhof and **Y. Yonekawa**

Department of Neurosurgery, University Hospital Zurich, Zurich, Switzerland

Summary

In patients suffering from subarachnoid haemorrhage (SAH) and presenting with multiple intracranial aneurysms (MIA) two questions have to be decided on: 1st when is the ideal moment to eliminate the ruptured aneurysm and 2nd when to treat the coexisting aneurysms.

In our series we retrospectively analysed 124 SAH-patients presenting with a total of 323 aneurysms.

In 57 patients the ruptured aneurysm and all coexisting aneurysms were clipped during the first operation, whereas in 9 patients only some of the coexisting aneurysms (group-A; age in median 55 years) were clipped besides the ruptured one. In 55 patients (group-B; age in median 55 years) the first operation was restricted to clipping the ruptured aneurysm, dealing with the coexisting aneurysm subsequently. Immediately after admission 3 patients passed away. One of the 64 patients waiting (average 60 days, median 14 days) for the subsequent clipping of the not yet secured aneurysms suffered a SAH. Six to 12 months after the initial SAH, 78% of the cases in both groups reached a Glasgow Outcome Score of 4 or 5.

Even if in patients with coexisting unruptured intracranial aneurysms the elimination of each and every aneurysm is recommended, the advantages of an unstaged procedure versus the additional strain caused by the prolongation of the procedure, e.g. approach over the midline, 2 or more craniotomies, and the risk of additional ischemic damage to the brain, caused by increased manipulation of cerebral arteries and brain tissue, have to be carefully considered. This is of special importance in dealing with patients in higher Hunt and Hess grades.

Keywords: Aneurysm surgery; intracranial aneurysms; management outcome; multiple aneurysms; subarachnoid hemorrhage.

Introduction

Eliminating a ruptured aneurysm is a prophylactic procedure preventing rebleeding and facilitating the treatment of delayed vasospasm. Unless a space occupying haematoma or an acute hydrocephalus can be drained, the procedure does not improve the actual condition of the patient, but is apt to hurt the brain even more, as it reacts especially sensitive to additional damage.

In patients suffering from multiple intracranial aneurysms (MIA) not only the ideal moment to eliminate the ruptured aneurysm has to be decided on but also when to treat the coexisting aneurysms.

The aim of this study is a retrospective analysis of our policy dealing with MIA.

Material and method

Evaluation of the records of all the patients having been treated for ruptured intracranial aneurysms in the Neurosurgical Department of the University-Hospital Zurich between 1997 and 2003, established 124 patients presenting with subarachnoid haemorrhage (SAH) and MIA (Table 1).

At time of entering the Neurosurgical Department of the University-Hospital Zurich 60,4% of patients presented with a Glasgow Coma Score of 13–15, 26,6% with 8 points or less (Table 2). Table 3 shows the degree of haemorrhage according to the Fisher-Scale. Immediately after arriving in the Neurosurgical Department and before a treatment could start 3 patients died.

The localisation of the 124 ruptured aneurysms and the 199 coexisting aneurysms is shown in Table 4. 81 patients suffered from 2 intracranial aneurysms, 25 from 3 aneurysms and 18 patients from 4 or more intracranial aneurysms.

Table 1. *Population (n = 124)*

Age	Men	Females	Total
30–39	3	7	10
40–49	7	26	33
50–59	11	29	40
60–69	4	27	31
70–79	0	8	8
80–89	0	2	2
	25	*99*	124

Table 2. *Initial Glasgow Coma Score*

3 to 8	33	(26,6%)
9 to 11	5	(4,0%)
13 to 15	75	(60,4%)
Unknown	11	(8,8%)
	124	

Table 3. *Fisher Grading*

0	3	(2,4%)
1	10	(8,0%)
2	20	(16,1%)
3	27	(21,7%)
4	64	(51,6%)
	124	

Table 4. *Locations of the aneurysms (n = 323)*

	Ruptured (n = 124)		Non ruptured (n = 199)		Total	%
MCA	37	(29,8%)	72	(36,2%)	109	33,7%
ICA	29	(23,4%)	75	(37,7%)	104	32,2%
Acoma	34	(27,4%)	13	(6,5%)	47	14,5%
BA	7	(5,6%)	8	(4,0%)	15	4,6%
PICA	6	(4,8%)	7	(3,5%)	13	4%
dist. ACA	9	(7,3%)	14	(7,0%)	23	7,1%
PCA	2	(1,6%)	5	(2,5%)	7	2,2%
Others	0		5	(2,5%)	5	1,5%
	124		199		323	

Results

In 85 patients (69%) the ruptured aneurysm was clipped within 72 hours after the SAH, in 28 of them as an emergency to evacuate a space occupying intracerebral haematoma.

Sequence of clipping of the ruptured and the coexisting aneurysms

In 66 (55%) patients several or all the aneurysms were clipped in one session (group A), in 55 (45%) patients initially only the ruptured aneurysm was eliminated whereas the coexisting aneurysms were secured later on. Immediately after admission 3 patients passed away.

Table 5 and Table 6 show the initial ("time of entering the Neurosurgical Department") Glasgow Coma Score (GCS), respectively Fisher Grade, for patients of group A ("simultaneous") and group B ("staged").

Group A (simultaneous procedure): In 57 (this is in 47% of 124 patients) of the 66 (55%) patients not only the ruptured but all the diagnosed aneurysms were clipped within the initial session. In 50 of these 57 patients this could be achieved by performing one craniotomy only – 38 of the coexisting aneurysms were located ipsilateral to the ruptured one, in 12 patients the coexisting aneurysms could be reached by passing the midline. In 7 patients 2 craniotomies were done in the initial session (Table 7). Finally, in 9

Table 5. *Sequence of clipping/Initial Glasgow Coma Score (n = 121)*

	Group A (simultaneous)		Group B (staged)	
GCS-3–8	17	25,7%	16	29%
GCS 9–12	4	6%	4	7,3%
GCS 13–15	42	63,6%	30	54,5%
Unknown	3	4,5%	5	9%
	66		55	

Table 6. *Sequence of clipping/Fisher Grade (n = 121)*

Grading	Group A (simultaneous)		Group B (staged)	
Fisher 0	3	(4,5%)	2	(3,6%)
Fisher 1	9	(13,6%)	3	(5,4%)
Fisher 2	11	(16,6%)	6	(16,5%)
Fisher 3	15	(22,7%)	15	(27,2%)
Fisher 4	28	(42,4%)	29	(52,7%)
	66		55	

Table 7. *Locations of the aneurysms/Sequence of clipping/operative approach/ (n = 112*)*

Unrupt. Aneurysms	Group A (simultaneous)		Group B (staged)	
Ipsilateral	38	(66,7%)	14	(25,4%)
Contralateral	12	(21%)	31	(56,3%)
2 Craniotomies necessary	7	(12,3%)	10	(18,1%)
	57*		55	

* In an other 9 patients presenting with 34 Aneurysms, initially the ruptured and several (but not all) coexisting aneurysms were clipped. Only 2 of these 9 patient had the coexisting aneurysms ipsilateral to the ruptured one.

patients presenting with 34 aneurysms, the ruptured and several (but not all) coexisting aneurysms were also clipped within the initial session.

Group B (staged procedure): In 55 (45%) patients only the ruptured aneurysm was secured initially, whereas the coexisting aneurysms were secured later on. In 7 cases several aneurysms were left due to bad condition several aneurysms were left untouched in 7 of these 55 patients.

Outcome (6 to 12 months after the initial SAH): Table 8 shows the Glasgow Outcome Score (GOS) in patients undergoing 1, 2 or several sessions. About 78% of the cases of each group reached a GOS of 4 and 5 .

With an GCS of 9 or higher at time of entering the Neurosurgical Department 87% of patients reached a Glasgow Outcome Score GCS of 4 and 5.

Table 8. *Sequence of clipping/Glasgow Outcome Score (n = 121)*

GOS	Group A (simultaneous)		Group B (staged)	
1	2	(3,5%)	2	(3,6%)
2	2	(3,5%)	3	(5,4%)
3	8	(14%)	7	(12,7%)
4	22	(38,6%)	21	(38,2%)
5	23	(40,4%)	22	(40%)
	57		55	

Table 9. *Correlation initial GCS/GOS*

GCS	GOS4/5
GCS-3–8	54,5%
GCS 9–12	87,5%
GCS 13–15	86,1%
Unknown	37,5%

Discussion

To prevent rebleeding and to facilitate the treatment of possibly arising delayed vasospasm, ruptured cerebral aneurysms should be eliminated from circulation as early as possible, ideally without adding further damage to the brain [2, 3, 5, 13, 14, 27].

About one third of patients suffering from a ruptured cerebral aneurysm are found to have additional asymptomatic aneurysms [8, 12, 16, 20]. In patients with MIA the aneurysms located at the bifurcation, such as the anterior communicating artery and the middle cerebral artery, bleed easily to contrast with lateral aneurysms such as those found at the branching and bending points on the internal carotid artery [23].

Coexisting aneurysms of all sizes in patients with SAH due to another treated aneurysm carry a higher risk for future haemorrhage than similar sized aneurysms without a SAH history and have to be considered for treatment [1].

Actually, in treating ruptured aneurysms, early operation (day 0–3) is generally accepted, at least in patients in good condition [17, 21]. Even if there is no clear evidence advocating early or late surgical treatment after aneurysmal rupture [3], ultra early surgery and a nonselective policy need not necessarily generate a large number of dependent survivors, even among elderly poor-grade patients [4, 14].

In patients with coexisting unruptured intracranial aneurysms the elimination of all the aneurysms is recommended [5, 7, 29], at best within one session [18, 24, 26] and within one week from onset [15]. An unstaged procedure has several advantages over a staged one:

- In case of difficulties in identifying the ruptured aneurysm clipping all the coexisting aneurysms prevents further bleedings [9].
- It allows an aggressive treatment of delayed cerebral ischemia without risking the rupture of unsecured coexisting aneurysms.

- The patient need not be confronted with the possibilities of suffering further bleedings or subsequent procedures.

These advantages have to be balanced against the additional strain caused by the prolongation of the procedure, e.g. approach over the midline, 2 or more craniotomies, and the risk of additional ischemic damage to the brain, caused by increased manipulation of cerebral arteries and brain tissue. This is of special importance in dealing with patients in higher HH-grades.

Our retrospective analysis includes 124 patients (80% women) suffering from subarachnoid haemorrhage, presenting a total of 323 aneurysms. Women seem to present a higher percentage of MIA than men [10, 12, 16]. The highest rate of rupture was found in aneurysms located at the Acom (72%), followed by aneurysms of the BA (46%) and finally of the ICA.

In 57 patients all the coexisting aneurysms were clipped within the same session as the ruptured one, whereas in 9 patients only some of the coexisting aneurysms (group-A; age in median 55 years) were clipped at the same time. In 55 patients (group-B; age in median 55 years) the first operation saw only the clipping of the ruptured aneurysm, the coexisting aneurysms being treated subsequently.

1 of the 64 patients waiting (average 60 days, median 14 days) for the subsequent clipping of the not yet secured aneurysms suffered a SAH.

In spite of the differences of the stress caused by the one-step procedure in comparison with a staged procedure – 20% of patients in group A needed an approach over the midline to the contralateral side, in an other 14% 2 craniotomies had to be done – about 78% of the cases in both groups reached a GOS of 4 or 5, 6 to 12 months after the initial SAH . There is no striking difference in age between group A and group B (53,5 years and 56 years respectively). Concerning GCS at time of entering the Neurosurgical Department and Fisher-Grade, there are more patients with a high GCS and a low Fisher-Grade in group A (Table 5 and 6).

One of the reasons for reaching a GOS of 4 or 5 in about 78% of our population might be the fact, that in patients with low GCS and high Fisher Grading we are given to proceed stepwise in securing the aneurysms. Another one might be our attitude to decide during surgery about how to handle the coexisting aneurysms. In patients presenting a tight, swollen brain, it is wise not to persist in a one-step procedure, the same is true when clipping of the ruptured aneurysm turns out to be unexpectedly difficult [6, 8, 18, 19].

Nevertheless, deciding on a staged procedure, demands careful inspection of the aneurysms as to eliminate the appearance of a recent ruptured aneurysm and the risk of subsequent bleedings from untreated aneurysms has to be realised [22, 26, 28].

References

1. Bederson JB, Awad IA, Wiebers DO, Piepgras D, Haley EC Jr, Brott T, Hademenos G, Chyatte D, Rosenwasser R, Caroselli C (2000) Recommendations for the management of patients with unruptured intracranial aneurysms: a statement for healthcare professionals from the Stroke Council of the American Heart Association. Stroke 31: 2742–2750
2. Chyatte D, Fode NC, Sundt TM Jr (1988) Early versus late intracranial aneurysm surgery in subarachnoid hemorrhage. J Neurosurg 69: 326–331
3. de Gans K, Nieuwkamp DJ, Rinkel GJ, Algra A (2002) Timing of aneurysm surgery in subarachnoid hemorrhage: a systematic review of the literature. Neurosurgery 50: 336–342
4. Elliott JP, Le Roux PD (1998) Subarachnoid hemorrhage and cerebral aneurysms in the elderly. Review. Neurosurg Clin N Am 9: 587–594
5. Findlay JM (1997) Current management of aneurysmal subarachnoid hemorrhage guidelines from the Canadian Neurosurgical Society. Can J Neurol Sci 24: 161–170
6. Grigorian AA, Marcovici A, Flamm ES (2003) Intraoperative factors associated with surgical outcome in patients with unruptured cerebral aneurysms: the experience of a single surgeon. J Neurosurg 99: 452–457
7. Heiskanen O (1981) Risk of bleeding from unruptured aneurysm in cases with multiple intracranial aneurysms. J Neurosurg 55: 524–526
8. Hernesniemi J, Rinne J (2003) Multiple aneurysms. Surg Neurol 60: 136–137
9. Hino A, Fujimoto M, Iwamoto Y, Yamaki T, Katsumori T (2000) False localization of rupture site in patients with multiple cerebral aneurysms and subarachnoid hemorrhage. Neurosurgery 46: 825–830
10. Inagawa T (1991) Surgical treatment of multiple intracranial aneurysms. Acta Neurochir (Wien) 108: 22–29
11. International Study of Unruptured Intracranial Aneurysms Investigators (1998) Unruptured intracranial aneurysms – risk of rupture and risks of surgical intervention. N Engl J Med 339: 1725–1733
12. Kaminogo M, Yonekura M, Shibata S (2003) Incidence and outcome of multiple intracranial aneurysms in a defined population. Stroke 34: 16–21
13. Kassell NF, Torner JC, Jane JA, Haley EC Jr, Adams HP (1990) The international cooperative study on the timing of aneurysm surgery. Part 2: surgical results. J Neurosurg 73: 37–47
14. Laidlaw JD, Siu KH (2002) Ultra-early surgery for aneurysmal subarachnoid hemorrhage: outcomes for a consecutive series of 391 patients not selected by grade or age. J Neurosurg 97: 250–259
15. Mizoi K, Suzuki J, Yoshimoto T (1989) Surgical treatment of multiple aneurysms: Review of experience with 372 cases. Acta Neurochir (Wien) 96: 8–14
16. Nehls DG, Flom RA, Carter LP, Spetzler RF (1985) Multiple intracranial aneurysms: determining the site of rupture. J Neurosurg 63: 342–348
17. Ohman J, Heiskanen O (1989) Timing of operation for ruptured supratentorial aneurysms: a prospective randomized study. J Neurosurg 70: 55–60
18. Orz Y, Osawa M, Tanaka Y, Kyoshima K, Kobayashi S (1996) Surgical outcome for multiple intracranial aneurysms. Acta Neurochir (Wien) 138: 411–417
19. Rinne J, Hernesniemi J, Niskanen M (1995) Management outcome for multiple intracranial aneurysms. Neurosurgery 36: 31–38
20. Rinne J, Hernesniemi J, Puranen M, Saari T (1994) Multiple intracranial aneurysms in a defined population: prospective angiographic and clinical study. Neurosurgery 35: 803–808
21. Solomon RA, Onesti ST, Klebanoff L (1991) Relationship between the timing of aneurysm surgery and the development of delayed cerebral ischemia. J Neurosurg 75: 56–61
22. Swift DM, Solomon RA (1992) Unruptured aneurysms and postoperative volume expansion. J Neurosurg 77: 908–910
23. Ujiie H, Sato K, Onda H, Oikawa A, Kagawa M, Takakura K, Kobayashi N (1993) Clinical analysis of incidentally discovered unruptured aneurysms. Stroke 24: 1850–1856
24. Ulrich P, Perneczky A, Muacevic A (1997) Surgical strategy in cases of multiple aneurysms. Zentralbl Neurochir 58: 163–170
25. Vajda J, Juhasz J, Pasztor E, Nyary I (1988) Contralateral approach to bilateral and ophthalmic aneurysms. Neurosurgery 22: 662–668
26. Vajda J (1992) Multiple intracranial aneurysms: a high risk condition. Acta Neurochir (Wien) 118: 59–75
27. Whitfield PC, Kirkpatrick PJ (2001) Timing of surgery for aneurysmal subarachnoid haemorrhage. (Review). Cochrane Database Syst Rev: CD001697
28. Wiebers DO, Whisnant JP, Hoston J, Meissner I, Brown RD Jr, Piepgras DG, Forbes GS, Thielen K, Nichols D, O'Fallon WM, Peacock J, Jaeger L, Kassell NF, Kongable-Beckman Gl, Torner JC, International Study of Unruptured Intracranial Aneurysms Investigators (2003) Unruptured intracranial aneurysms: natural history, clinical outcome, and risks of surgical and endovascular treatment. Lancet 362: 103–110
29. Winn HR, Almaani WS, Berga SL, Jane JA, Richardson AE (1983) The long-term outcome in patients with multiple aneurysms. Incidence of late hemorrhage and implications for treatment of incidental aneurysms. J Neurosurg 59: 642–651

Correspondence: Hans-Georg Imhof, Department of Neurosurgery, Neurochirurgische Universitätsklinik Zurich, Frauenklinikstrasse 10, 8091 Zurich, Switzerland. e-mail: hgimhof@nch.unizh.ch

Acta Neurochir (2005) [Suppl] 94: 97–101
© Springer-Verlag 2005
Printed in Austria

Surgical treatment of unruptured cerebral aneurysms in the elderly

K. Suyama[1], **M. Kaminogo**[2], **M. Yonekura**[1], **H. Baba**[1], and **I. Nagata**[2]

[1] Department of Neurosurgery, National Hospital Organization, Nagasaki Medical Center, Nagasaki, Japan
[2] Department of Neurosurgery, Nagasaki University School of Medicine, Nagasaki, Japan

Summary

We retrospectively analyzed the prevalence and surgical outcomes of unruptured cerebral aneurysms in the elderly for the past five years. Between 1998 and 2002, we collected data from 575 subjects with unruptured aneurysms who had no history of subarachnoid hemorrhage (SAH). One hundred and eighty-two of these patients (31.7%) were aged ≥70 years and they had 233 aneurysms. The proportion of older patients among all subjects increased significantly from 21.4% in 1998 to 40.3% in 2002.

Unruptured aneurysms found in the elderly had a predominance of female, higher frequency of multiple aneurysms, and lower frequency of anterior communicating artery aneurysms when compared with those in the younger patients. The majority of intradural aneurysms detected in the elderly were less than 10 mm in diameter (84.8%). One hundred and eleven out of 224 intradural aneurysms in the elderly were treated (49.6%); most aneurysms were directly clipped, while only 13 aneurysms including six basilar artery aneurysms were coiled endovascularly. Among the 83 elderly subjects who underwent direct surgery, perioperative complication appeared in seven subjects (morbidity 8.4%, mortality 1.2%). No SAH occurred postoperatively and conservatively during 1–5 years of follow-up.

Since the rupture rate of small unruptured aneurysms without SAH history is reported to be low, surgical indication should be considered with care particularly in the elderly.

Keywords: Unruptured cerebral aneurysms; elderly patients; outcome; subarachnoid hemorrhage.

Introduction

Recent epidemiological studies have revealed that the incidence of subarachnoid hemorrhage (SAH) in the elderly has been increasing, and that overall outcome of SAH is poor [16, 17, 23, 32]. Whether the incidence of SAH is parallel to the prevalence of unruptured cerebral aneurysms and whether incidentally detected aneurysms result in fatal rupture remains uncertain. We have to face the fact that an increasing number of unruptured aneurysms even in the elderly are discovered owing to advancements in non-invasive neuroimaging techniques such as magnetic resonance angiography (MRA) and computed tomography angiography (CTA) [32].

Indications for surgical treatment of unruptured aneurysms are generally thought to depend on age, physical and neurological status, patient psychological factors, and location, size, and shape of aneurysms [21, 26, 30, 31, 36]. Increased surgical risks and reduced life expectancy among the elderly would decrease the surgical benefits, and even minor perioperative complications may cause serious problems [3, 5, 21]. Therefore, justification for surgery of unruptured aneurysm in the elderly has not yet been established.

Beginning in January 1998, we collected records in our database for consecutive patients with unruptured cerebral aneurysms diagnosed at our university hospital or affiliated hospitals. In the present study, we retrospectively collected data for the past five years on subjects with newly diagnosed unruptured aneurysms that were not associated with SAH, to clarify trends in the prevalence and management of unruptured aneurysms in the elderly.

Materials and methods

Between January 1998 and December 2002, 575 subjects with unruptured intracranial aneurysms newly diagnosed by MRA and/or CTA were enrolled in this study. When needed, catheter angiography was performed for confirmation of the MRA or CTA findings and for planning the optimal treatment, i.e. neck clipping or endovascular coiling. Subjects were classified into two age groups, ≥70 years old and <70 years old, according to the criteria of the Japan Geriatric Neurosurgery Society. No patient with a history of SAH was included in the study. Trends for the prevalence and management of unruptured aneurysms among the elderly were analyzed and compared with those in the younger subjects.

Aneurysms detected were classified as small (<5 mm), medium (5–9 mm), large (10–24 mm) or giant (≥25 mm) on the basis of the maximal diameter. Surgical outcome was assessed according to the

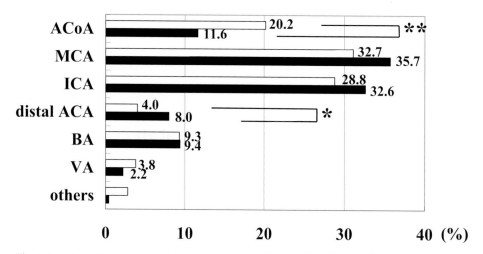

Fig. 1. Location of the unruptured intradural aneurysms. Horizontal bar indicates frequency of aneurysms detected. White column and black column indicate subjects aged <70 years and those aged ≥70 years, respectively. *P < 0.05, **P < 0.01. *ACoA* Anterior communicating artery; *MCA* middle cerebral artery; *ICA* internal carotid artery; *distal ACA* distal anterior cerebral artery; *BA* basilar artery; *VA* vertebral artery

Glasgow Outcome Scale [14] three months after surgery. Any neurological deficit occurring within 30 days of surgery was considered a surgical complication.

The proportion of elderly among all subjects with unruptured aneurysms in each year from 1998 to 2002, and differences in frequencies between the groups were compared with chi-square test. A value of P < 0.05 was considered significant.

Results

Of 575 subjects with unruptured intracranial aneurysms, 182 (31.7%) were aged ≥70 years and had 233 aneurysms (198 in the anterior circulation; 26 in the posterior circulation; 9 in the cavernous portion of the internal carotid artery). The frequency of female increased progressively with age, comprising 73.1% of the elderly subjects. The proportion of elderly patients increased yearly from 21.4% in 1998, reaching 40.3% in 2002 (P < 0.01).

In subjects aged <70 years, the most frequent reason for the diagnosis of unruptured aneurysm was non-specific symptoms such as chronic headache, dizziness and vertigo. Incidental detection at the brain check-up [24] was the second most frequent reason and frequency was significantly higher than that in the elderly (31.8% vs. 17.0%, P < 0.01). On the other hand, unruptured aneurysms in the elderly were mostly diagnosed during routine imaging for other cerebrovascular diseases including symptomatic cerebral infarction, and frequency was much higher than that in the younger subjects (35.2% vs. 17.5%, P < 0.01).

A total of 620 intradural aneurysms were detected in this study, of which 12.6% were located in the posterior circulation. The most frequently found location was the middle cerebral artery (32.7%), followed by the internal carotid artery (30.2%). The anterior communicating artery was only 17.1%. As shown in Fig. 1, the frequency of the anterior communicating artery aneurysm was much lower in the elderly (11.6% vs. 20.2%, P < 0.01) while that of the distal anterior cerebral artery aneurysm was slightly but significantly higher in the elderly (8.0% vs. 4.0%, P < 0.05).

In the elderly subjects as well as the younger patients intradural aneurysms with size 5–9 mm in diameter were most frequently found. Frequencies of aneurysms < 5 mm and aneurysms < 10 mm in the elderly were not significantly different from those found in the younger subjects (42.4% vs. 36.9%, 84.8% vs. 83.4%, respectively).

The frequency of female subjects and of multiple aneurysms were significantly higher in the elderly (Table 1). Family history of either SAH or unruptured cerebral aneurysm within the second-degree relatives was not significantly different between the two groups. In the elderly, the frequency of the treatment for intradural aneurysms was 52.0% in the anterior circulation, and 30.8% in the posterior circulation. Thirty-one of 95 (32.6%) small aneurysms, 60 of 95 (63.2%) medium aneurysms, 19 of 31 (61.3%) large aneurysms, and 1 of 3 (33.3%) giant aneurysms were surgically treated. Small aneurysms less than 5 mm in diameter were less frequently treated in the elderly than the younger subjects (32.6% vs. 47.3%, P < 0.05); however, aneurysms ≥ 5 mm in diameter were similarly treated between the two groups.

Table 1. *Comparison of frequencies in subjects with unruptured aneurysms between <70 years and ≥70 years of age*

	Total (%)	<70 y.o. (%)	≥70 y.o. (%)	p value
Number of subjects	575	393	182	
Female subjects	363 (63.1)	230 (58.5)	133 (73.1)	0.0008
Multiple aneurysms	93 (16.2)	52 (13.2)	41 (22.5)	0.0049
Family history	38 (6.6)	26 (6.6)	12 (6.6)	0.9920
Intradural aneurysms	620 (100)	396 (100)	224 (100)	
Treated aneurysms	352 (56.8)	241 (60.9)	111 (49.6)	0.0063
Craniotomy	307 (49.5)	209 (52.8)	98 (43.8)	0.0308
Endovascular	45 (7.3)	32 (8.1)	13 (5.8)	0.2938

Family history, family history of either SAH or unruptured cerebral aneurysm within second-degree relatives; craniotomy, direct clipping of the aneurysm; endovascular, endovascular coiling.

Table 2. *Surgical complications after direct clipping of the unruptured aneurysm in the elderly*

Age/sex	Aneurysm location	Aneurysm size (mm)	Outcome (GOS)	Cause of poor condition
74 F	PCoA	10–24	MD	postoperative ICA stenosis
73 M	MCA	<5	MD	perforator injury (hemiparesis)
72 F	PCoA	5–9	D	poor general condition
77 M	MCA	<5	MD	chronic subdural hematoma
77 M	MCA	5–9	SD	perforator injury (hemiparesis)
77 F	ACoA	5–9	MD	perforator injury (mild dementia)
72 F	PCoA	<5	MD	oculomotor palsy

M Male; *F* female; *PCoA* posterior communicating artery; *MCA* middle cerebral artery; *ACoA* anterior communicating artery; *ICA* internal carotid artery; *GOS* Glasgow Outcome Scale; *MD* moderate disability; *SD* severe disability; *D* death.

Of 224 intradural aneurysms detected in the elderly, more than half were conservatively followed up, 43.8% were treated by craniotomy, while 5.8% or only 13 aneurysms including six basilar artery aneurysms were treated endovascularly (Table 1). Treatment (clipping or endovascular coiling) for intradural aneurysms was less frequently performed in 111 of 224 in the elderly (49.6%), compared with 241 of 396 in the younger subjects (60.9%). The frequency of craniotomy was slightly lower in the elderly, while that of endovascular treatment was not significantly different. Among 83 elderly subjects who underwent direct clipping, perioperative complication appeared in seven subjects (morbidity 8.4% at three months after surgery, mortality 1.2%, Table 2). Most complications were due to perforator injury during surgery, although those were not specifically apparent in the elderly. There was no SAH reported postoperatively and conservatively during 1–5 years of follow-up. The morbidity rate in the elderly was slightly lower than that in the younger subjects, although this difference did not reach significance (8.4% vs. 10.8%).

Discussion

There is currently insufficient evidence to recommend a standard management for unruptured cerebral aneurysms [2, 7, 10, 13, 20, 27, 29]; particularly only few data have been reported regarding management for those in the elderly without a history of SAH [4, 18]. Although treatment risks are commonly thought to be higher in the elderly [19, 25], several reports indicate that advancing age alone does not necessarily preclude good outcome in aneurysm surgery [9, 22]. In our study, morbidity rate in the elderly was not higher than that of the younger subjects. Since frequencies of treatment for aneurysms ≥ 5 mm in diameter were similar between the two groups, relatively low frequency of surgical complication in the elderly might be attributable to appropriate subject selection in performing surgery.

We had only one patient who exhibited permanent mental deterioration after clipping of the anterior communicating artery aneurysm, which is reported to occasionally appear in the elderly [1, 6, 8, 15]. Since we did not perform neuropsychological examinations in all subjects perioperatively, we might have underestimated the complication rate following surgery. Further evaluations including neuropsychological studies for overall outcomes in surgery for unruptured aneurysms are warranted especially in the elderly.

The present study demonstrated that discovery of unruptured aneurysms in the elderly has progressively increased. In addition, our data showed trends for unruptured aneurysms found in the elderly, with female predominance, higher frequency of multiple aneurysm, and lower frequency of anterior communicating artery aneurysm, which are thought to be among the most important factors in aneurysmal rupture [2, 17, 30]. Moreover, the majority of aneurysms detected were less than 10 mm in diameter, which were frequently treated even in the elderly. Although the annual rupture rate of unruptured cerebral aneurysms is still controversial [11, 12, 28, 33, 35], that of small aneurysms without a SAH history is generally considered low. Therefore, we should have further information about characteristics of small-unruptured aneurysms in the elderly to avoid unnecessary invasive procedures, and improve overall outcomes of surgery for unruptured aneurysms with appropriate subject selection.

With increasing proportion of people aged ≥70 years, the detection rate of unruptured cerebral aneurysms in the elderly has also been rising. Thus, management of unruptured aneurysms in elderly patients will be much more important in the coming years. Further prospective studies to accumulate data related both to the natural history of unruptured aneurysms [12, 34, 35] and to surgical outcomes are necessary to determine surgical indications for unruptured aneurysms in the elderly.

References

1. Bottger S, Prosiegel M, Steiger HJ, Yassouridis A (1998) Neurobehavioral disturbance, rehabilitation outcome and lesion site in patients after rupture and repair of anterior communicating artery aneurysm. J Neurol Neurosurg Psychiatry 65: 93–102
2. Brennan JW, Schwartz ML (2000) Unruptured intracranial aneurysms: Appraisal of the literature and suggested recommendations for surgery, using evidence-based medicine criteria. Neurosurgery 47: 1359–1372
3. Chang HS, Kirino T (1995) Quantification of operative benefit for unruptured cerebral aneurysms: A theoretical approach. J Neurosurg 83: 413–420
4. Chung RY, Carter BS, Norbash A, Budzik R, Putnam C, Ogilvy CS (2000) Management outcomes for ruptured and unruptured aneurysms in the elderly. Neurosurgery 47: 827–833
5. Deruty R, Pelissou-Guyotat I, Mottolese C, Amat D (1996) management of unruptured cerebral aneurysms. Neurol Res 18: 39–44
6. Fukunaga A, Uchida K, Hashimoto J, Kawase T (1999) Neuropsychological evaluation and cerebral blood flow study of 30 patients with unruptured cerebral aneurysms before and after surgery. Surg Neurol 51: 132–138
7. Hemplmann RG, Barth H, Buhl R, Mehdorn HM (2002) Clinical outcome after surgery of intracranial unruptured aneurysms: results of a series between 1991 and 2001. Acta Neurochir [Suppl] 82: 51–54
8. Hillis AE, Anderson N, Sampath P, Rigamonti D (2000) Cognitive impairments after surgical repair of ruptured and unruptured aneurysms. J Neurol Neurosurg Psychiatry 69: 608–615
9. Inagawa T, Yamamoto M, Kamiya K, Ogasawara H (1988) Management of elderly patients with aneurysmal subarachnoid hemorrhage. J Neurosurg 69: 332–339
10. Inoue T (2002) Treatment of incidental unruptured aneurysms. Acta Neurochir [Suppl] 82: 11–15
11. International Study of Unruptured Intracranial Aneurysms Investigators (1988) Unruptured intracranial aneurysms: risks of rupture and risks of surgical intervention. N Engl J Med 339: 1725–1733
12. International Study of Unruptured Intracranial Aneurysms Investigators (2003) Unruptured intracranial aneurysms: natural history, clinical outcome, and risks of surgical and endovascular treatment. Lancet 362: 103–110
13. Ishihara H, Yoshimura S, Konu L, Khan N, Yonekawa Y (2002) Surgical prognosis of unruptured cerebral aneurysms: Report of 40 cases in University Hospital Zurich. Acta Neurochir [Suppl] 82: 35–39
14. Jennet B, Bond M (1975) Assessment of outcome after severe brain damage: a practical scale. Lancet 1: 480–484
15. Jimbo H, Hanakawa K, Ozawa H, Dohi K, Sawabe Y, Matsumoto K, Nagata K (2000) Neuropsychological changes after surgery for anterior communicating artery aneurysm. Neurol Med Chir (Tokyo) 40: 83–87
16. Kaminogo M, Yonekura M (2002) Trends in subarachnoid hemorrhage in elderly persons from Nagasaki, Japan: Analysis of the Nagasaki SAH data bank for cerebral aneurysm, 1989–1998. Acta Neurochir 144: 1133–1139
17. Kaminogo M, Yonekura M, Shibata S (2003) Incidence and outcome of multiple intracranial aneurysms in a defined population. Stroke 34: 16–21
18. Kashiwagi S, Yamashita K, Kato S, Takasago T, Ito H (2000) Elective neck clipping for unruptured aneurysm in elderly patients. Surg Neurol 53: 14–20
19. Khanna RK, Malik GM, Qureshi N (1996) Predicting outcome following surgical treatment of unruptured intracranial aneurysms: a proposed grading system. J Neurosurg 84: 49–54
20. King JT Jr, Berlin JA, Flamm ES (1994) Morbidity and mortality from elective surgery for asymptomatic, unruptured, intracranial aneurysms: A meta-analysis. J Neurosurg 81: 842–937
21. King JT Jr, Glick HA, Mason TJ, Flamm ES (1995) Elective surgery for asymptomatic, unruptured, intracranial aneurysms: a cost-effectiveness analysis. J Neurosurg 83: 403–412
22. Lan Q, Ikeda H, Jimbo H, Izumiyama H, Matsumoto K (2000) Considerations on surgical treatment for elderly patients with intracranial aneurysms. Surg Neurol 53: 231–238
23. Menghini VV, Brown RD Jr, Sicks JD, O'Fallon WM, Wiebers DO (1998) Incidence and prevalence of intracranial aneurysms and hemorrhage in Olmsted County, Minnesota, 1965 to 1995. Neurology 51: 405–411
24. Nakagawa T, Hashi K (1994) The incidence and treatment of

asymptomatic, unruptured cerebral aneurysms. J Neurosurg 80: 217–223

25. Ogilvy CS, Carter BS (2003) Stratification of outcome for surgically treated unruptured intracranial aneurysms. Neurosurgery 52: 82–87

26. Orz YI, Hongo K, Tanaka Y, Nagashima H, Osawa M, Kyoshima K, Kobayashi S (2000) Risks of surgery for patients with unruptured intracranial aneurysms. Surg Neurol 53: 21–27

27. Raaymakers TW, Rinkel GJ, Limburg M, Algra A (1998) Mortality and morbidity of surgery for unruptured intracranial aneurysms: A meta-analysis. Stroke 29: 1531–1538

28. Tsutsumi K, Ueki K, Morita A, Kirino T (2000) Risk of rupture from incidental cerebral aneurysms. J Neurosurg 93: 550–553

29. Tukahara T, Murakami N, Sakurai Y, Yonekura M, Takahashi T, Inoue T (2002) Treatment of unruptured cerebral aneurysms – a multi-center study of Japanese national hospitals. Acta Neurochir [Suppl] 82: 3–10

30. Weir B, Disney L, Karrison T (2002) Size of ruptured and unruptured aneurysms in relation to their sites and the ages of patients. J Neurosurg 96: 64–70

31. Weir B, Amidei C, Kongable G, Findlay JM, Kassell NF, Kelly J, Dai L, Karrison T (2003) The aspect ratio (dome/neck) of ruptured and unruptured aneurysms. J Neurosurg 99: 447–451

32. Yamashita K, Kashiwagi S, Kato S, Takasago T, Ito H (1997) Cerebral aneurysms in the elderly in Yamaguchi, Japan. Analysis of the Yamaguchi Data Bank of cerebral aneurysm from 1985 to 1995. Stroke 28: 1926–1931

33. Yasui N, Suzuki A, Nishimura H, Suzuki K, Abe T (1997) Long-term follow-up study of unruptured intracranial aneurysms. Neurosurgery 40: 1150–1160

34. Yonekura M (2002) Importance of prospective studies for deciding on a therapeutic guideline for unruptured cerebral aneurysm. Acta Neurochir [Suppl] 82: 21–25

35. Yonekura M (2004) Small unruptured aneurysm verification (SUAVe study, Japan) – interim report. Neurol Med Chir (Tokyo) 44: 213–214

36. Yoshimoto T, Mizoi K (1997) Importance of management of unruptured cerebral aneurysms. Surg Neurol 47: 522–526

Correspondence: Kazuhiko Suyama, Department of Neurosurgery, National Hospital Organization, Nagasaki Medical Center, 2-1001-1 Kubara, Omura 856-8562, Japan. e-mail: ksuyama@nmc.hosp.go.jp

Intracranial arteriovenous malformations and Dural AVM, AVF

Acta Neurochir (2005) [Suppl] 94: 105–110
© Springer-Verlag 2005
Printed in Austria

Three cases of AVM at eloquent areas finally treated with conventional microsurgical method

Y. Yonekawa[1], **H.-G. Imhof**[1], **M. Bjeljac**[1], **M. Curcic**[2], and **N. Khan**[1]

[1] Department of Neurosurgery, University Hospital Zurich, Zurich, Switzerland
[2] Department of Anesthesiology, University Hospital Zurich, Zurich, Switzerland

Summary

Three special cases of AVM finally treated with conventional microsurgical method are presented. Two cases of medium sized AVMs were located at the central region, one of them was primarily treated with Gamma-knife followed by endovascular embolization having been complicated with growing cyst formation followed ultimately by microsurgical removal. The AVM of another case was embolized three times, followed by removal of the residual nidus under awake surgery. The third AVM located at the hypothalamus in the vicinity of the optic nerve was considered unsuitable for embolization and Gamma-knife therapy, and therefore removed by microsurgery using special approaches after a trial of embolization.

In terms of microsurgical removal, preoperative embolization, embolization material, awake surgery and selection of special approaches are discussed.

Keywords: Arteriovenous malformation; gamma-knife; cyst formation; eloquent area; embolization; awake surgery; approach.

Introduction

The introduction and use of additional modalities other than the classical microsurgical removal in the treatment of arterio-venous malformations AVMs such as embolization and stereotactic radiosurgery have changed the overall management of AVMs especially in terms of the currently practised indications, timing and combination treatment of these malformations. Three cases of AVMs located at eloquent areas and/or at functionally important structures finally treated with microsurgical removal are presented with special discussion on cyst formation after Gamma-knife therapy and several technical points inherent to surgical removal of AVMs. The significance of presurgical embolization, awake surgery and selection of special surgical approach is emphasized.

Case reports

Case 1 RT (Fig. 1). This 28 years old male had an intracerebral hematoma at the age of four in 1984 due to an AVM and underwent surgical evacuation of the hematoma. The medium size (6 cm) AVM was mainly located at the postcentral gyrus with a main feeder of the Rolandic artery and with drainers of the vein of Rolando and the vein of Labbé. He was primarily treated with Gamma-knife twice in 1987 and 1990 resulting in partial occlusion. The AVM presented with partial and generalized epileptic seizures which had recently become resistant to medication. Follow-up MRI in 2001 displayed increase in the size of AVM surrounded by two cysts. A cyst formation was noticed anterior to the nidus already at the time of check-up a year earlier. Another cyst of 3 cm in size was newly detected postero-supero-medial to the nidus without any neurological deterioration. The patient was hospitalized in 2002 due to neurological deterioration with increased spastic hemiparesis on the left side along with some sensory disturbance as a consequence of growth of the cyst with space occupying effect. The AVM was partially embolized followed by microsurgical removal of the AVM along with extirpation of both cysts in March 2003. Postoperative course was uneventful. Pathology of the cyst revealed to be gliosis containing a lot of calcification and some hyalinization. At the time of postoperative following up on 16. April 2004, the patient was doing well with slight hemiparesis but without any focal epileptic seizure under antiepileptic medication. Neuroimagings of MRI and MRA displayed complete removal of AVM nidus and cysts without any midline shifts.

Case 2 MC (Fig. 2). This 35 year old female suffered from slight weakness of the right extremity associated with dizziness, tinnitus and right sided ptosis three years ago (1999). AVM of 3 × 4 cm was found located at the postcentral gyrus and the inferior parietal lobule with main feeder of the Rolandic artery and with drainers of veins of Rolando. The first embolization procedure in 1999 at another institution resulted in partial embolization and was complicated with a right sided hemiparesis, which recovered almost completely within three months. The patient decided to have the AVM removed surgically due to the constant psychological stress. After an additional two staged embolization in our institution resulting in 80–90% occlusion of the nidus in 2003, microsurgical removal of the residual nidus was performed under awake surgery on 17. July 2003. The surgery was complicated with hemiparesis on the right side appearing 48 hours after surgery. Follow-up CT scan showed a small intracerebral hemorrhage probably of congested venous origin, which was not

Case RT 1980 M

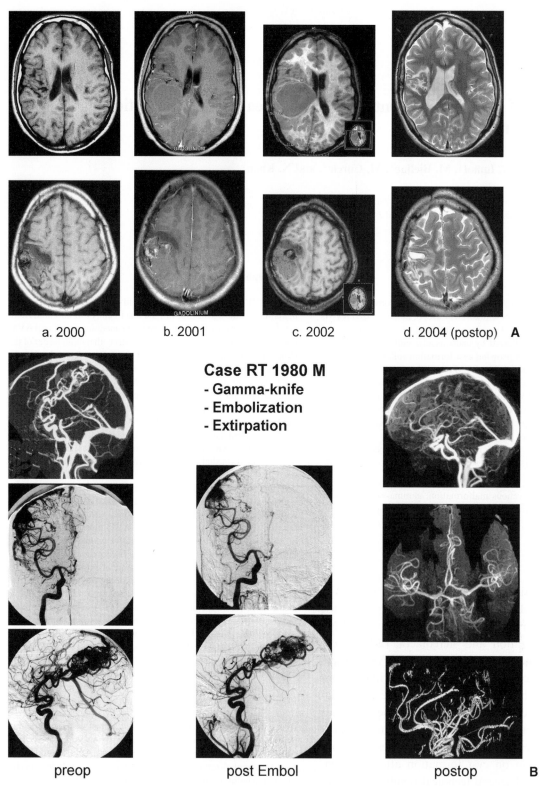

a. 2000   b. 2001   c. 2002   d. 2004 (postop) **A**

Case RT 1980 M
- Gamma-knife
- Embolization
- Extirpation

preop   post Embol   postop   **B**

Fig. 1. (A) (a) 2000: 13 years after the first Gamma-knife therapy and 10 years after the second Gamma-knife therapy. Cyst formation at the post central gyrus and presumably beginning of another cyst fromation at the inferior parietal lobule at the very vicinity of the residual AVM nidus. (b) 2001: enlargement of the nidus and the cyst. (c) 2002: remarkable growth of the cyst with space occupying effect. (d) 2004: status after the removal of the cyst and the residual AVM. (B) Left column: MR angiogram and the conventional digital angiogram DSA displays the residual AVM after twice a Gamma-knife therapy. Middle column: DSA shows preoperative embolization of ca. 50% of the nidus. Right column: Postoperative follow-up MRA displays complete resection of the AVM corresponding with MRI picture of d.2004

Case MC 1960 F

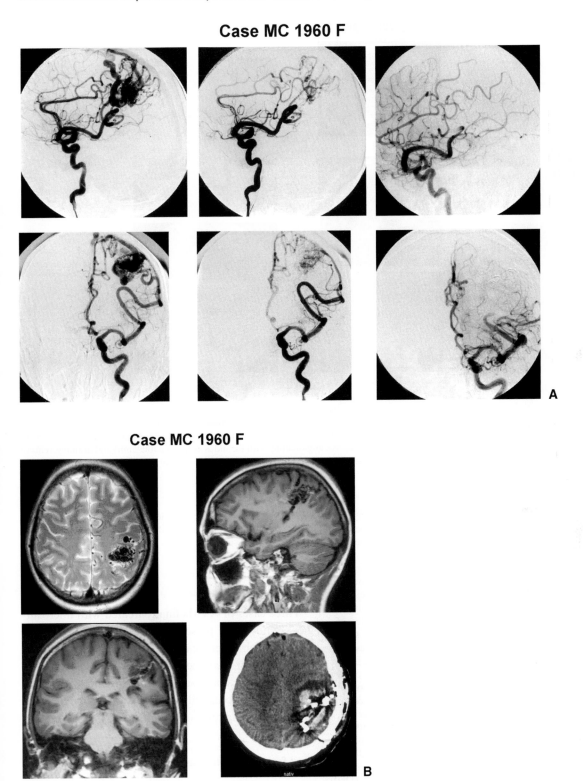

Case MC 1960 F

Fig. 2. (A) Left column: DSA 3 years after a partial embolization of the AVM. Middle column: after 3rd embolization resulted in ca. 80–90% occlusion of the AVM. Right column: State of complete removal of the nidus after awake surgery. (B) MRI before surgical removal of the partially embolized AVM. CT scan shows venous hemorrahge occurring 2 days after surgery

Case WP 1963 M

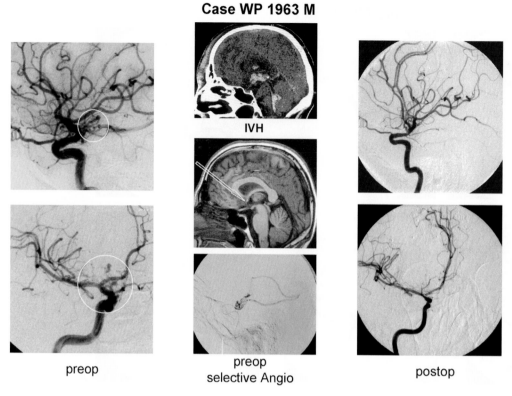

IVH

preop

preop
selective Angio

postop

Fig. 3. Left column: Circles indicate the AVM nidus containing aneurysmatic components. Middle column: the sagittal CT view shows hematocephalus in which the third ventricle and the fourth ventricle are full of hematoma due to rupture of the AVM. Arrow indicates the access to the nidus via the RCCLTA. Bottom images indicates a super-selective angiography with the nidus at the hypothalamus and draining veins of the internal cerebral vein and the vein of Rosenthal. Right column: Follow-up DSA shows complete removal of the AVM

seen on CT scan taken the next day after surgery. Follow-up angiography displayed complete removal of the AVM. The hemiparesis subsided almost completely at the time of follow-up three months later and the patient returned to previous work.

Case WP (Fig. 3). 37 year old male suffered from SAH for the first time in 2001. The patient underwent partial embolization for the small AVM detected in the right hypothalamus at that time. The AVM bled again in April 2004 into the third and the fourth ventricle. The patient presented with generalized seizure associated with loss of consciousness. On angiography a small nidus of 1 cm with some aneurysmatic components was found in the right hypothalamus and in the very vicinity of the right optic nerve and the chiasm. The nidus was fed by direct branches of the right internal carotid artery and drained into the vein of Rosenthal and into the internal cerebral vein. After another trial of embolization, which was abandoned for fear of the risk of visual disturbances and hypothalamic dysfunction, direct microsurgical removal was performed in April 2004 with the right pterional approach plus selective extradural anterior clinoidectomy SEAC in combination with a transrostrum corporis callosi–lamina terminalis approach TRCLTA. Part of the nidus located at the lateral eminence under the right optic tract could be removed by the former approach and the remaining nidus with extension into the right hypothalamus with aneurysmatic component was removed by the latter TRCLTA after an additional right sided frontal craniotomy. Careful treatment in the intensive care unit was necessary for a couple of weeks: long lasting disturbance in consciousness, diabetes insipidus associated with electrolyte disturbances due to hematocephalus and hypothalamic syndrome. It took several months for the

patient to recover (outcome of moderate disability) with some recent memory disturbances but with neither visual disturbance nor hemiparesis.

Discussion

Three cases of AVMs finally treated with microsurgical removal are presented. These are specific examples in which other treatment modalities were primarily applied for years because of the AVM location in eloquent cortical and subcortical sites and of their difficult surgical accessibility. Discussion will be focussed on the following topics.

Cyst formation after Gamma-knife therapy of AVMs

Among complications of Gamma-knife therapy, cyst formation due to gliosis and spongy degeneration of the brain tissue has been reported to be rather infrequent and to be benign, so that need of surgical treatment seems to be exceptional [4, 6–8, 10]. Our case with medium sized AVM submitted to Gamma-knife therapy twice resulted in partial obliteration of the nidus and in cyst formation after 10 years showing that a careful follow-up is mandatory and for a long time duration. Once this complication is found out especially in the presence of residual nidus, opimal timing of removal of the residual AVM and the cyst should not be overlooked.

Preoperative embolization and embolization material

It is now evident that endovascular embolization alone itself can complete AVM treatment in considerable cases [10]. On the other hand, there is so far to date no publication known to prove systematically the benefit of presurgical partial embolization in a large series of AVM patients. We support, however, the view that preoperative embolization makes microsurgical removal easier: less intraoperative bleeding due to partial embolization, decreased numbers of feeding arteries from the depth. For this purpose, merits of embolization with liquid material such as EVAL was reported [4], but embolization with bucrylate turned out to have several advantages, although a rigid or solid mass of embolized AVM interferes in its preparation in the depth. Piece by piece removal of embolized AVM is possible and some demarcation layer between partially embolized AVMs and their surrounding tissue due to ischemia and/or heating effect at the time of polymerization makes nidus preparation easier [2].

Awake surgery

Awake surgery is common for the microsurgical removal of gliomas in eloquent areas, this has been developed especially for epilepsy surgery [3, 6]. Awake surgery for the AVM of our case 2 revealed to be effective, although the case was complicated with small bleeding. This may be due to venous congestion [1]. One could check motor and sensory functions at the time of temporary occlusion of some perinidal feeding branches of the Rolandic artery and at the time of stimulation of the cortex around the AVM nidus. Case No 1 would have been treated with success with the same method namely preoperative embolization and awake surgery without any use of Gamma-knife therapy. Awake surgery for small and medium sized AVMs in an eloquent area should be seriously taken into consideration as treatment option with or without presurgical embolization.

Selection of approaches

The case No 3 of rather small hypothalamic AVM with repeated intraventricular bleeding is considered to be inappropriate for endovascular embolization or Gamma-knife therapy because the feeding arteries also supply important structures and also the close proximity of the optic nerve to the hypothalamus. For the safe surgical removal some special approaches were necessary. Use of the additional SEAC procedure [11] to the pterional approach enabled to have access to the nidus of AVM at the eminentia lateralis by increased mobilization of the optic nerve and of the internal carotid artery (hence enlarging the opticocarotid triangle) determining feeding arteries and non feeding arteries originating directly from the ICA. Transrostrum corporis callosi–lamina terminalis approach TRCLA [9] enabled us to have access to the nidus with aneurysmatic component in the right hypothalamus. This is a specific case example in which selection of the appropriate surgical approach for safe removal of an AVM was crucial.

Conclusion

Three cases of microsurgical removal of AVMs at eloquent areas and/or functionally important structures are presented. Strategical consideration on the use of preoperative embolization, awake surgery and selection of approaches are discussed along with special mention of cyst formation as a complication of Gamma-knife therapy which required surgical removal.

References

1. Al-Rodhan NR, Sundt TM Jr, Piepgras DG, Nichols DA, Rufenacht D, Stevens LN (1993) Occlusive hyperemia: a theory for the hemodynamic complications following resection of intracerebral arteriovenous malformations. J Neurosurg 78: 167–175
2. Iwama T, Yoshimura K, Keller E, Imhof HG, Khan N, Leblebicioglu-Könü D, Tanaka M, Valavanis A, Yonekawa Y (2003) Emergency craniotomy for intraparenchymal massive hematoma after embolization of supratentorial arteriovenous malformations. Neurosurgery 53: 1251–1260
3. Ojemann G, Ojemann J, Lettich E, Berger M (1989) Corical language localization in left, dominant hemisephere. An electrical stimulation mapping investigation in 117 patients. J Neurosurg 71: 316–326
4. Taki W, Yonekawa Y, Iwata H, Uno A, Yamashita K, Amemiya H (1990) A new liquid material for embolization of arteriovenous malformations. AJNR 11: 163–168

5. Tanaka T, Kobayashi T, Kida Y (1998) Two cases of cyst formation after Gamma-knife surgery for AVM. Surg Cereb Stroke (Jpn) 26: 15–19
6. Taylor MD, Bernstein M (1999) Awake craniotomy with brain mapping as the routine surgical approach to treating patients with supratentorial intraaxial tumors: a prospective trial of 200 cases. J Neurosurg 90: 35–41
7. Yamamoto M, Ide M, Jimbo M, Takakura K, Hirai T, Lindquist C, Karlsson B (1996) Gamma knife radiosurgery in medium-sized arteriovenous malformations. Surg Cereb Stroke (Jpn) 24: 465–473
8. Yamamoto M, Jimbo M, Hara M, Saito I, Mori K (1996) Gamma-knife radiosurgery for arteriovenous malformations: long-term follow-up results focusing on complications occurring more than 5 years after irradiation. Neurosrugery 38: 906–914
9. Yonekawa Y (2003) Radical removal of craniopharygiomas – Consideration on approaches and their consequences. 13th meeting of Japan society for hypothalamic and pituitary tumors. Matsue, Japan February 5. 2002
10. Yonekawa Y, Fandino J, Taub E (2001) Surgical therapy. In: Fisher M, Bogousslavsky J (eds) Current review of cerebrovascular disease. Current Medicine, Philadelphia, pp 219–232
11. Yonekawa Y, Ogata N, Imhof HG, Olivecrona M, Strommer K, Kwak TE, Roth P, Groscurth P (1997) Selective extradural anterior clinoidectomy for supra- and parasellar processes. Technical note. J Neurosurg 87: 636–642

Correspondence: Yasuhiro Yonekawa, Neurochirurgische Universitätsklinik Zurich, Frauenklinikstresse 10, 8091 Zurich, Switzerland. e-mail: yasuhiro.yonekawa@usz.ch

Acta Neurochir (2005) [Suppl] 94: 111–114
© Springer-Verlag 2005
Printed in Austria

Early surgery for ruptured cerebral arteriovenous malformations

J. Kuhmonen[1]**, A. Piippo**[1]**, K. Väärt**[1]**, A. Karatas**[1]**, K. Ishii**[1]**, P. Winkler**[2]**, M. Niemelä**[1]**, M. Porras**[3]**, and J. Hernesniemi**[1]

[1] Department of Neurosurgery, Helsinki University Central Hospital, Helsinki, Finland
[2] Department of Neurosurgery, Ludwig-Maximilians-University of Munich, Munich, Germany
[3] Department of Radiology, Helsinki University Central Hospital, Helsinki, Finland

Summary

Acute surgery on cerebral arteriovenous malformations (AVMs) has seldom been reported or used. We reviewed 49 patients of ages 2 months to 78 years (mean 32.8 years), 32 male (65%) and 17 female (35%), treated acutely (within 4 days of bleed) in Helsinki Neurosurgery during 1997–2002. The following variables were assessed in regards to the outcome (Glasgow outcome score; GOS; 2–3 months after bleed): age, sex, Hunt and Hess Grade (HH), Spetzler-Martin Grade (SMG), location of AVM, size of intraparenchymal haematoma (ICH), and presence of intraventricular haemorrhage (IVH).

Most of the patients were in a poor clinical condition on admission (two thirds were HH 4–5). 45 (92%) patients underwent extirpation of AVM and evacuation of ICH, within 4 days after bleed. Over 55% had good functional outcome. GOS correlated significantly with HH (p = 0.001), age (p = 0.006), and IVH (p = 0.049). On the other hand, SMG, location of AVM, and size of haematoma did not significantly predict the outcome. Microneurosurgery with preoperative embolization has made possible the excision of 90% of AVMs. It is our experience that it can be done acute and early, and it saves lives as compared to natural history of cerebral AVMs or late surgery, and accelerates rehabilitation of the patients.

Keywords: Arteriovenous malformation; vascular malformation; subarachnoid haemorrhage; intracerebral haematoma, acute surgery.

Introduction

Arteriovenous malformations (AVMs) are relatively rare but, nevertheless, a major cause of haemorrhagic stroke in the young population. It has been suggested that 45–70% of the adult AVM patients present with an acute intracranial haemorrhage [1, 3, 10, 12]. Several previous studies of the natural history of AVMs have estimated that there is a 2 to 4% annual risk of haemorrhage from an AVM [1, 3, 8, 12], and a risk of recurrent haemorrhage of 7 to 14% per year initially, declining to a prehaemorrhage level after 5 years [3, 8].

While most ruptured cerebral aneurysms are operated on acutely since more than 25 years, acute surgery on cerebral AVMs has seldom been reported or used. It has been claimed to be contraindicated and dangerous leading to persistent deficits [11, 14]. On the other hand, surgery has the clear advantage of enabling a complete removal of an AVM in one session, and thus, abolishing the risk of the most dreaded event, recurrent haemorrhage. The aim of this review of acutely operated patients with ruptured cerebral AVM was to find predicting factors for the outcome.

Materials and methods

Out of more than 1000 cerebral AVMs treated during years 1932–2004 in Helsinki and Kuopio, we reviewed all patients with ruptured cerebral AVM that were operated within 4 days after haemorrhage between 1997 and 2002 in the Department of Neurosurgery, Helsinki University Central Hospital. During this time period, altogether 179 cerebral AVMs were operated on, 100 of them unruptured. The 49 patients scrutinised – being close to one sixth of more than 300 cerebral AVMs operated on by the senior author (JH) [5] – 32 male (65%) and 17 female (35%), had a mean age of 32.8 years (range 0.2–78 years). Data were obtained from medical records and radiographic studies including demographics, Hunt and Hess Grade (HH) [7] at admission, Glasgow outcome score (GOS; GR = good recovery; MD = moderate disability; SD = severe disability; V = vegetative; D = dead) [9] 2–3 months after haemorrhage, size of intraparenchymal haematoma (ICH), presence of intraventicular haemorrhage (IVH), location of AVM, Spetzler-Martin Grade (SMG) [15], and operative treatment.

45 (92%) patients underwent craniotomy and extirpation of AVM, and evacuation of ICH, if necessary. Of the remaining four patients (8%), three were acutely treated with ventricular drainage (one pa-

tient primarily in Thailand) and one patient had trephination and evacuation of ICH primarily in Estonia. All patients had preoperatively head CT, DSA and/or CTA, and most patients also a MRI. Embolization was used if feasible in association to DSA. A postoperative angiography was always performed and repeated, if necessary.

Data were analyzed with the SPSS for Windows (release 9.0.1.1999, SPSS Inc.). Univariate association of continuous variables was tested by Spearman rank (r_s) correlation coefficients. Analysis of factors that may contribute to the outcome was undertaken by unconditional logistic regression. Maximum-likelihood stepwise forward elimination procedures were used, with selection of variables based on the magnitude of their probability values (<0.05). A two-tailed p-value < 0.05 was considered significant.

Results

Most of the patients were HH 4 and 5 at admission: 13 (27%) and 19 (39%), respectively. Size of ICH was smaller than 2.5 cm in 10 patients (20%), 2.5–5 cm in 27 patients (55%), and more than 5 cm in 12 patients (25%). Twenty-one patients (43%) had a complicating IVH. Twenty-one (43%) of the AVMs were SMG 2, almost 60% of the AVMs were grades 1 and 2. More than half of the patients had good functional outcome (GOS GR or MD) 2–3 months after bleed. The outcome correlated significantly with HH (p = 0.001), age (p = 0.006), and IVH (p = 0.049). The correlations of GOS with HH, SMG, size of ICH, and IVH are shown in Table 1. Figure 1 demonstrates radiological findings of two patients. Only one postoperative angiography showed a small residual AVM, this was not re-treated during the follow up time.

Discussion

These data of 49 patients with ruptured AVM, operated acutely after haemorrhage show that most of the patients were in a poor clinical condition on arrival (two thirds were HH 4–5). Almost 80% of the patients had a significant ICH, and more than 40% also a complicating IVH. In 92% of the patients AVM was acutely extirpated. Over 55% of the patients had good functional outcome 2–3 months after bleed. Factors that clearly predicted the outcome were HH and age. Also, presence of IVH correlated with GOS.

We evaluated the outcome 2–3 months after bleed. A longer recovery period is required to detect more final outcome. The follow up of the patients will be extended up to one year in our next studies.

Earlier studies have considered variables such as SMG (AVM size, location in the eloquent areas, and

Table 1. *The Glasgow outcome score (GOS)*

GOS						
HH	*GR*	*MD*	*SD*	*V*	*D*	*Total*
1	3	0	0	0	0	3
2	4	3	2	0	0	9
3	3	0	2	0	0	5
4	4	3	5	0	1	13
5	5	2	4	3	5	19
Total	19	8	13	3	6	49
SMG						
1	6	0	1	1	0	8
2	9	1	9	0	2	21
3	1	6	3	1	2	13
4	2	1	0	1	2	6
5	1	0	0	0	0	1
Total	19	8	13	3	6	49
ICH Ø						
<2.5 cm	4	3	1	0	2	10
2.5–5 cm	12	3	8	0	4	27
>5 cm	3	2	4	3	0	12
Total	19	8	13	3	6	49
IVH	5	4	6	2	4	21

GR Good recovery; *MD* moderate disability; *SD* severe disability; *V* vegetative; *D* dead: 2–3 months after haemorrhage in correlation with Hunt and Hess *(HH)* and Spetzler-Martin Grades *(SMG)*, size (Ø) of intraparenchymal haematoma *(ICH)*, and presence of intraventricular haematoma *(IVH)*.

deep venous drainage) [6, 11, 15] and patient's clinical condition at the time of surgery [4, 6, 13, 16] to influence the management outcome. However, morbidity and mortality rates have varied in some previous studies because of patient selection (exclusion of patients in primarily poor condition [2]). We included all admitted patients consecutively in our series. One recent study has suggested an independent effect of age on the risk of AVM surgery [4]. Our data shows age to have significant influence on the outcome. It is the primary severity of the bleed, not SMG, location of AVM, and size of ICH, that significantly influences the outcome. This might be due to our aggressive and acute treatment, i.e., within 4 days of bleed, careful evacuation of ICH, when needed, and 98% success in excising AVM totally in the same session.

Microneurosurgery with preoperative embolization has made possible the excision of 90% of arteriovenous malformations; and it is our experience that it can be done early to save lives and to accelerate rehabilitation of the patients. A few surgeons specialising in the surgery of AVMs and aneurysms should be available in every country.

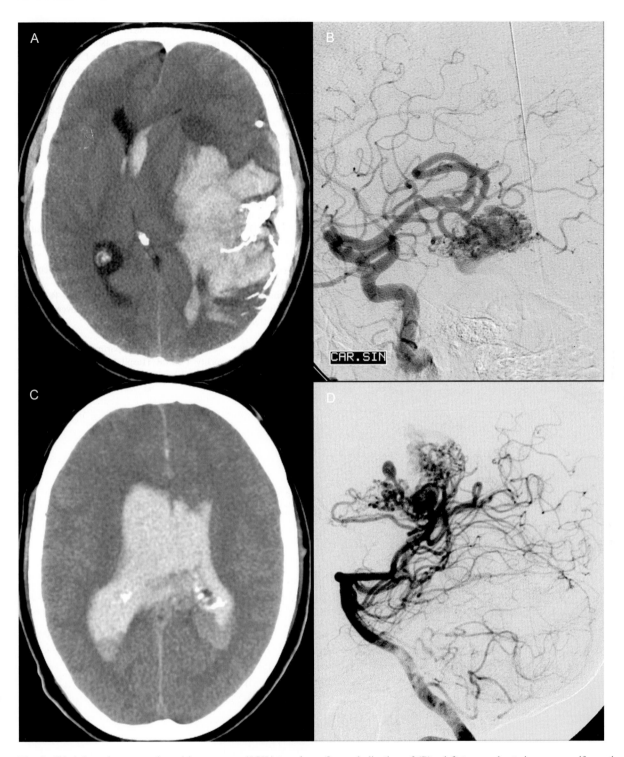

Fig. 1. (A) A huge intraparenchymal haematoma *(ICH)* two days after embolization of (B) a left temporal arteriovenous malformation *(AVM)* in 39-year-old male. Preoperatively Hunt and Hess Grade *(HH)* was 5. ICH was evacuated and AVM extirpated, resulting in vegetative state at 3 months after bleed, and finally severe disability. (C–D) 38-year-old male admitted deeply unconscious *(HH 5)* to hospital. (C) CT scan showing massive intraventricular haematoma. (D) Vertebral angiography revealed a trigonal AVM, which was extirpated. Unfortunately the patient did not survive

References

1. Crawford PM, West CR, Chadwick DW, Shaw MD (1986) Arteriovenous malformations of the brain: natural history in unoperated patients. J Neurol Neurosurg Psychiatry 49: 1–10
2. Davis C, Symon L (1985) The management of cerebral arteriovenous malformations. Acta Neurochir (Wien) 74: 4–11
3. Graf CJ, Perret GE, Torner JC (1983) Bleeding from cerebral arteriovenous malformations as a part of their natural history. J Neurosurg 58: 331–337
4. Hartmann A, Pile-Spellman J, Stapf C, Sciacca RR, Faulstich A, Mohr JP, Schumacher HC, Mast H (2002) Risk of endovascular treatment of brain arteriovenous malformations. Stroke 33: 1816–1820
5. Hernesniemi J, Keränen T (1990) Microsurgical treatment of arteriovenous malformations of the brain in a defined population. Surg Neurol 33: 384–390
6. Heros RC, Korosue K, Diebold PM (1990) Surgical excision of cerebral arteriovenous malformations: late results. Neurosurgery 26: 570–578
7. Hunt WE, Hess RM (1968) Surgical risk as related to time of intervention in the repair of intracranial aneurysms. J Neurosurg 28: 14–20
8. Itoyama Y, Uemura S, Ushio Y, Kuratsu J, Nonaka N, Wada H, Sano Y, Fukumura A, Yoshida K, Yano T (1989) Natural course of unoperated intracranial arteriovenous malformations: study of 50 cases. J Neurosurg 71: 805–809
9. Jennett B, Bond M (1975) Assessment of outcome after severe brain damage: a practical scale. Lancet 1: 480–484
10. Karlsson B, Lindquist C, Johansson A, Steiner L (1997) Annual risk for the first hemorrhage from untreated cerebral arteriovenous malformations. Minim Invasive Neurosurg 40: 40–46
11. Luessenhop A, Rosa L (1984) Cerebral arteriovenous malformations. Indications for and results of surgery, and the role of intravascular techniques. J Neurosurg 60: 14–22
12. Ondra SL, Troupp H, George ED, Schwab K (1990) The natural history of symptomatic arteriovenous malformations of the brain: a 24-year follow up assessment. J Neurosurg 73: 387–391
13. Pelletieri L (1979) Surgical versus conservative treatment of intracranial arteriovenous malformations. A study in surgical decision-making. Acta Neurochir [Suppl] 29: 1–86
14. Troupp H, Marttila I, Halonen V (1970) Arteriovenous malformations of the brain. Prognosis without operation. Acta Neurochir (Wien) 22: 125–128
15. Spetzler R, Martin N (1986) A proposed grading system for arteriovenous malformations. J Neurosurg 65: 476–483
16. Steinmeier R, Schramm J, Müller HG, Fahlbusch R (1989) Evaluation of prognostic factors in cerebral arteriovenous malformations. Neurosurgery 24: 193–200

Correspondence: Juha Hernesniemi, Department of Neurosurgery, Helsinki University Central Hospital, Topeliuksenkatu 5, 00260 Helsinki, Finland. e-mail: juha.hernesniemi@hus.fi

Acta Neurochir (2005) [Suppl] 94: 115–122
© Springer-Verlag 2005
Printed in Austria

Cranial and spinal dural arteriovenous malformations and fistulas: an update

H.-J. Steiger[1], **D. Hänggi**[1], and **R. Schmid-Elsaesser**[2]

[1] Department of Neurosurgery, Heinrich-Heine-University, Düsseldorf, Germany
[2] Department of Neurosurgery, Ludwig-Maximilians-University Munich, Munich, Germany

Summary

Awareness of a potential arteriovenous fistula is critical for diagnosis of cranial as well as spinal fistulas. The natural history of cranial and spinal dural arteriovenous fistulas has been clarified during the last decade and interdisciplinary therapies have experienced a substantial development recently. The classification of Cognard & Merland is now the most widely accepted one for cranial dural AVF. It is based on the degree of flow reversal in the sinuses and cortical veins and reflects well the natural history of the different lesions and serves as basis for therapeutic indications. Several studies have defined the annual bleeding risk of cranial dural fistulas between 1.8 and 15%, depending on the pattern of venous drainage and initial symptomatology. Surgical, endovascular and radiosurgical methods must be selectively chosen for the treatment. The risk associated with surgical or endovascular treatment of benign fistulas is higher than the risk of eliminating fistulas that have already led to cortical venous reflux. Transvenous endovascular occlusion or surgical disconnection of draining veins is the treatment of first choice for cranial and spinal dAVF with venous flow reversal. Benign cranial dural arteriovenous fistulas are a developing indication for radiosurgery.

Keywords: Dural arteriovenous fistula; classification; microsurgery; embolisation; radiosurgery.

Cranial arteriovenous fistulas

Cranial and spinal arteriovenous shunts correspond to two types of lesions: (1) Direct fistulas (carotid-cavernous, carotid-jugular, vertebro-vertebral) and (2) indirect or dural arteriovenous fistulas (dAVF). Direct arteriovenous fistulas most commonly affect the cavernous sinus. According to the angiographic classification of Barrow *et al.* these direct internal carotid artery-cavernous sinus fistulas (CCF) are classified as a CCF Type A [2]. These direct fistulas are usually the result of a head trauma, with or without clinically evident basilar skull fracture, or penetrating injuries. Rupture of an intracavernous ICA aneurysm can also produce a direct Type A fistula. The other

types of CCF are indirect truly dural arteriovenous fistulas in the dura around the cavernous sinus. Barrow *et al.* described three types of indirect fistulas depending on the dural vascular supply from the ICA and ECA respectively (Types B, C, D).

More generally, intracranial dAVFs represent arteriovenous shunts from a dural arterial supply to a dural venous drainage channel (see Fig. 1). The nidus of arteriovenous shunting is contained within the leaflets of the dura mater, the wall of a dural sinus, the falx, or the tentorium [1]. Unlike pial arteriovenous malformations, dAVFs seldom have a discrete nidus. Instead, they are composed of numerous arteriovenous

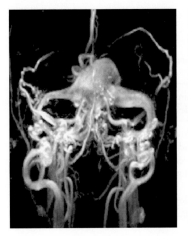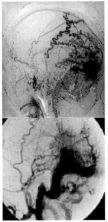

Fig 1. (left) MRA of a dural arteriovenous fistula of the confluens sinuum, showing varicose dilatation of the confluens, venous drainage mainly via the transverse sinuses and arterial supply by both carotid systems and the vertebral arteries; (right) arterial and venous phase of external carotid angiography showing multiple dilated scalp arteries, retrograde leptomeningeal venous flow and flow reversal and thrombosis in the superior sagittal sinus. This 18-year-old man presented with intracranial hypertension. He was cured by multiple endovascular and surgical interventions resulting in complete resection of the confluens

microfistulas with thickened dural arteries and dilated draining channels. The feeding arteries are dural arteries and therefore mainly branches of the external carotids system. Most frequent feeders are the occipital, tentorial, and middle meningeal arteries. Dural AVFs occasionally obtain blood also from the internal carotid or vertebral system.

Epidemiology and clinical characteristics

Most frequently the transverse or sigmoid sinus (60%) is affected. The next common sites are the cavernous sinus (15%), the tentorial incisura (10%), and the superior sagittal sinus and dural convexity (10%), followed by fistulas in the anterior and middle cranial fossa (10%).

The natural history of dAVFs is highly variable [16, 17]. Fistulas can be asymptomatic or present with benign or aggressive symptoms. Cognard *et al.* reviewed the symptoms and progression of dAVFs, and correlated the findings with various angiographic patterns [4]. They found that lesions that drain into a sinus with antegrade flow rarely cause aggressive symptoms, such as intracranial hypertension, epilepsy or neurological deficits (see Table 1). They observed an increasing percentage of aggressive symptoms with retrograde flow in the sinus and/or cortical veins, and that the risk of haemorrhage was associated with cortical venous

drainage. Particularly dAVFs with direct cortical venous drainage and venous ectasia were likely to present with aggressive symptoms (97%) and haemorrhage (66%). The bleeding rate of dAVFs was clarified by analysis of major case series only recently. Brown and collaborators defined in 1994 by a prospective non-selected follow-up study the average bleeding risk as 1.8%/year [3]. Satomi and coworkers from Toronto confirmed in 2002 that benign cranial dural arteriovenous fistulas have indeed a good outcome under conservative management with only 2% conversion to cortical drainage during follow-up [23]. Van Dijk and coworkers showed in 2002 that the clinical course of cranial dural arteriovenous fistulas with long-term persistent cortical venous reflux is unfavourable with a 10%/year mortality and a total of 15% annual events [31]. Duffau *et al.* described in 1999 a subgroup of intracranial dural arteriovenous fistulas which is prone to early re-bleeding [7].

Treatment options

When patients present with minor complaints of noise in the head or headaches, often no treatment needs to be offered. However, pulsatile tinnitus, headache or mastoid pain can be so severe that they limit quality of life. In these cases the potential risk and benefit of treatment has to be considered carefully. In patients with progressive disabling symptoms and in those who are at increased risk for haemorrhage according to the angiographic pattern of the dAVF, definite treatment is warranted.

Many treatment strategies for dAVFs have been described in the literature. Accepted treatment options include microsurgery, embolisation and radiosurgery or combinations of these methods [24, 25].

Table 1. *Cognard & Merland classification of cranial dural arteriovenous fistulas [4, 6]*

	Haemodynamic characteristics	Risk of aggressive symptoms	Risk of haemorrhage
Type I	antegrade flow in sinuses and bridging veins	1%	0%
Type II a	retrograde flow in sinus	37%	0%
Type II b	retrograde flow in bridging veins	30%	20%
Type II a+b	retrograde flow in sinus and bridging veins	67%	6%
Type III	direct fistula in bridging vein	76%	40%
Type IV	direct fistula in varicose bridging vein	97%	66%
Type V	spinal venous drainage	100%	46%

Microneurosurgery

Sundt and Piepgras published the first systematic series regarding surgical treatment of arteriovenous malformations of the lateral and sigmoid dural sinuses [27]. The preferred surgical treatment was complete excision coupled with packing of the sigmoid sinus. The operative approach was illustrated and discussed in detail. Results and complications were reviewed in 27 patients whose symptomatology had progressed under conservative management; 22 of these cases harboured primary lesions and five had recurrences. There were 22 excellent, one good, and two poor results (both of the latter from blindness that preceded surgery). There were two deaths, both in patients previously operated on with incomplete removal or obliteration of the dAVF by attempted embolisation.

Surgical excision, with or without prior embolisation, remains the most versatile and effective therapeutic option for complete elimination of dAVFs. Simple ligature of feeding vessels produced success rates of only 0 to 8% and can no longer be recommended [15]. It is agreed that curative treatment of dAVFs generally involves excision of the diseased venous segment. However, surgical excision of dAVFs is associated with notable mortality and morbidity, especially when the transverse-sigmoid sinus or the tentorium are involved. Surgical resection of these dAVFs carries the risk of aggravating the underlying venous hypertension. Elimination of the arterial supply has been advocated if the sinus continues to provide a major route of venous drainage. However, arterial occlusion alone usually leads to recurrence. En bloc resection of the diseased sinus along with the nidus can be performed when the sinus is thrombosed or there is prominent collateral venous drainage. Arterialized red draining veins can be taken with impunity, but radical resection may be limited when disease involves major dural sinuses or bridging veins, especially when these venous channels are still patent with antegrade drainage [24].

Apart from formal resection permanent clinical and angiographic cure can be expected by complete obliteration of the venous outflow. Thompson and co-workers as well as Collice et al. described interruption of leptomeningeal drainage for cranial dural AV fistulas with pure leptomeningeal drainage [5, 12, 30]. For fistulas with a pure leptomeningeal drainage this mode of therapy has become the method of choice (see Figs. 2 and 3). If only the retrograde leptomeningeal outflow is obliterated in sinus fistulas with secondary cortical reflux (Cognard Type 2 b and 2 a+b) conversion of an aggressive fistula into a benign one can be expected from obliteration of the leptomeningeal drainage [32].

In our opinion, surgery is indicated when embolisation is impossible or results in subtotal occlusion and when life-threatening or debilitating symptoms such as haemorrhage, retrograde venous drainage, intracranial hypertension, focal deficit, or epilepsy are present. Pulsatile tinnitus, headache, and mastoid pain may also indicate the need for therapy. Subtotal occlusion of a fistula by surgery or embolisation alone is not protective against further complications, especially haemorrhage. The goal of treatment is to achieve a rapid and complete anatomical cure.

Endovascular treatment

Successful endovascular transarterial occlusion of dAVFs has been reported. However, long-term follow-up review of patients often was lacking. If followed long enough, embolised dAVFs have been shown to recanalise [24, 25, 33]. Only for lesions of the cavernous sinus, embolisation was already prior to the advent of transvenous techniques recommended as the primary treatment by almost all authors. The reported success rates are some 60% for transarterial approaches. For lesions in other locations, it is now quite clear that transarterial embolisation may significantly decrease flow through a dAVF, but arterial embolisation is unlikely to result in complete and permanent obliteration of the fistula. Transvenous or combined transvenous-arterial approaches seem to be more efficacious for dAVFs that remain patent after transarterial therapy or that cannot be reached arterially. Halbach and co-workers pioneered transvenous embolisation of dural fistulas involving the transverse and sigmoid sinuses [11]. Today the higher efficacy of transvenous embolisation compared to transarterial embolisation is generally accepted. However, the risks and long-term results of transvenous obliteration are still unknown. Roy and Raymond emphasized that the occlusion must be precise [22]. An erroneous occlusion could reroute the fistulous output and overload an intracerebral vein. Cavernous dural fistulas with a venous access route can be treated by this technique without significant risk of harm. However, dAVFs in other locations must be carefully evaluated to ensure that the embolisation does not interfere with normal venous drainage of the adjacent brain. This is particularly true for low-risk fistulas, in which the brain still uses the involved sinus for venous drainage.

Radiosurgery

Lewis et al. reported on nine patients with tentorial dAVFs treated with transarterial embolisation combined with stereotactic radiosurgery. Five of the seven patients who underwent radiosurgery had a residual dAVF after a mean follow-up period of 24 months and one patient suffered transient radiation injury to the brain stem [13]. Link et al. developed a treatment strategy that includes radiosurgery followed by partic-

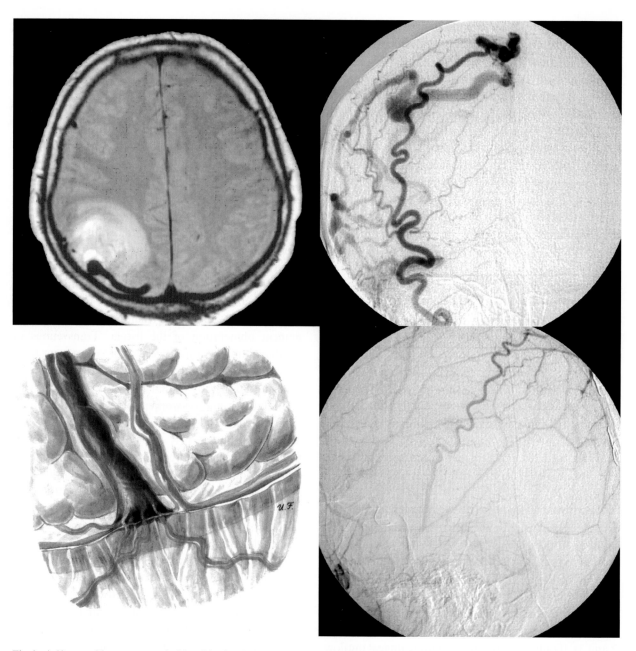

Fig. 2. A 59-year-old man presented with sudden headache and hemianopia. MRI showed a right parietal haemorrhage and a dilated bridging vein. Right external carotid angiography showing direct fistula into a varicose leptomeningeal vein and cortical reflux. Outflow of the leptomeningeal vein into the superior sagittal sinus is thrombosed. Intraoperative view after right parietal craniotomy showing multiple dural arteries entering the leptomeningeal vein. Curative therapy consisted of coagulation and division of this vein. Postoperative right external carotid angiography showing elimination of the fistula

ulate embolisation for selected patients with symptomatic dAVFs who are not good surgical candidates [14]. They treated 29 patients with dAVFs using a Leksell Gamma-Knife unit. Within 2 days after radiosurgery, 17 patients with AVFs that exhibited retrograde venous drainage (12 patients) and/or produced intractable bruit (eight patients) underwent particulate embolisation of external carotid feeding vessels. Angiography 1 to 3 years posttreatment in 18 patients showed total obliteration of 13 fistulas (72%) and partial obliteration of five (28%). No lesion had bled after treatment. Since these pioneering reports other series have confirmed the high efficacy and the low risk of radiosurgery for dural arteriovenous fistulas [8–10,

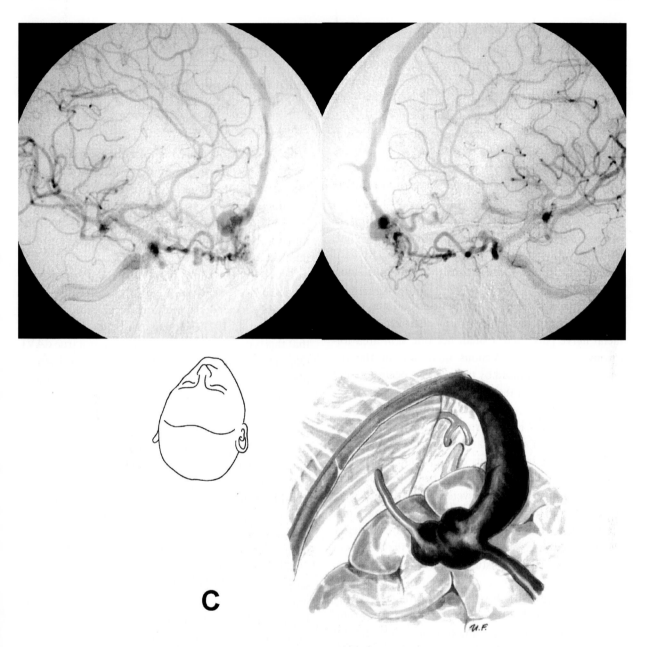

Fig. 3. A 53-year-old man presented with progressive headache. Right and left internal carotid arteriography showed fistula supplied by both anterior ethmoidal arteries and draining into a right frontopolar bridging vein. (C) After right frontal interhemispheric exposure the arterialized retrograde leptomeningeal artery was identified. Disconnection of this vein led to angiographic and clinical cure

20, 21]. The reported cure rates range between 80 and 90%.

Multidisciplinary treatment

The treatment of complex intracranial dAVFs often remains problematic. Combination of all primary treatment modalities must be used with the aim 1) to eliminate venous reflux and 2) to obliterate the fistula completely to prevent recurrence.

Personal experience (Munich/Düsseldorf, 1994–2003)

Our initial experience with treatment of 30 cranial dural fistulas including the transverse and sigmoid sinuses was summarized in 1997 by Olteanu-Nerbe *et al.* [19]. Depending on the venous drainage the fistulas were classified following Cognard's description with 18 patients Type I (main sinus with antegrade flow), 5 Type II a (main sinus with reflux into the contralateral sinus), 5 Type II b (reflux into cortical veins),

1 Type II a+b (both) and 1 of Type III (direct cortical drainage). Bruit, pulsatile tinnitus and headaches were the most common symptoms. 6 patients presented with intracranial haemorrhage, 4 with progressive neurological deficit or seizures and 3 with dementia. Arterial embolisation was performed in all cases except one, where a transvenous approach for balloon occlusion of the transverse sinus was performed. 21 patients were treated by single or repeated embolisation alone. Only in 9/21 cases did arterial embolisation result in complete occlusion of the fistula. In 12/21 patients incomplete occlusion was achieved. Following embolisation 8 patients underwent additional surgery including coagulation of the feeding arteries and arterialized veins, sinus resection and reconstruction of the sinus. Overall, 18 patients were cured, 11 improved and 1 patient was unchanged. There were a total number of 5 complications including transient stroke, transient facial nerve palsy and a small necrotic skin area following embolisation. Venous infarction of the occipital lobe was induced by transvenous occlusion and surgical resection of the transverse sinus in one patient each, respectively.

Following this initial experience we modified the general policy in so far that we limited venous occlusive surgery or transvenous embolisation to patients with venous reflux. Patients with benign fistulas and orthograde flow in the transverse/sigmoid sinus were treated by arterial embolisation and Gamma-Knife radiosurgery. This change of policy could completely eliminate major complications during in the treatment of transverse/sigmoid fistulas treated between 1997 and 2003.

Carotid-cavernous fistulas were treated during the entire period from 1994–2003 almost exclusively by endovascular embolisation. Transarterial and transvenous methods were combined. The results of the treatment of cavernous sinus fistulas were uniformly satisfactory with the only complication of transient worsening of cranial nerve deficits. Recently, we began to indicate Gamma-Knife radiosurgery for some low-flow dural fistulas of the cavernous sinus.

Direct fistulas into leptomeningeal veins (Cognard Type III–V) were almost exclusively approached surgically by interruption of the venous drainage. The more than 30 patients operated on between 1994 and 2003 were uniformly cured and only minor approach related complications had to be accepted, such as transient temporal lobe swelling after subtemporal approach or anosmia in a case of a fistula in the olfactory groove.

Spinal dural arteriovenous fistulas

Definition and aetiology

Spinal arteriovenous malformations encompass a variety of lesions with abnormal connections between the arterial and venous circulation. The normal high-resistance capillary system is missing. Spinal arteriovenous malformations have been divided by location into dural AVFs (Type I) and intradural arteriovenous malformations (AVM) (Type II–IV).

Type I (dural arteriovenous fistula) is a typical long, single-coiled vessel type of malformation that is almost invariably located on the dorsal pial surface of the spinal cord. In 1977, Kendall and Logue first reported that this type of spinal AVM was actually a true dAVF [25]. They identified AV fistulas in the dural sleeves of spinal nerve roots in nine patients who had radiographic and intraoperative findings consistent with lesions that were previously considered pial venous angiomas. Hence, these lesions were recognized as spinal dAVFs. The spinal dAVF, which is a low-flow shunt located proximally in the dural sleeve of a spinal nerve root and the adjacent spinal dura, is supplied by the dural branch of the intervertebral artery. A perimedullary vein, usually the sole venous outflow from the fistula, then carries shunted arterial blood, retrograde to the normal direction of flow, to the coronal plexus.

Spinal dAVFs can be further classified into lesions with a single arterial feeder (Type I-A) and those with multiple arterial feeders (Type I-B). The multiple feeders in Type I-B can originate from either a single or multiple levels, and they are present unilaterally or bilaterally.

Treatment

It is fortunate that the most common type of spinal AVMs is also the easiest to treat. In the past, the traditional treatment has been excision or stripping of the long, arterialized venous complex. This was a dangerous procedure because it required large exposures and carried the risk of spinal cord contusion or infarct. Furthermore, it is now recognized as unnecessary. The present surgical treatment in most cases consists of excision of the dural fistula, if this is easy to accomplish, or interruption of the arterialized veins that drain the fistula. Treatment limited to simple interruption of the vein draining the dAVF is an adequate therapy in most patients. It eliminates the underlying pathophysiology – venous hypertension – without risk to normal vessels that supply the cord, and carries a negligible risk of symptomatic recurrence. In patients with spinal dAVFs with only intrathecal perimedullary venous drainage, which includes most patients with these lesions, surgical interruption of the intradural draining vein provides lasting and curative treatment. In patients with both intra- and extradural drainage of the AVF, complete excision of the fistula or interruption of the intra- and extradural venous drainage of the fistula is indicated. In patients in whom a common vessel supplies the spinal cord and the dural AVF, simple surgical interruption of the vein draining the AVF is the treatment of choice, as it provides lasting obliteration of the fistula and it is the only treatment that does not risk arterial occlusion and cord infarction. However, it is important to realise that in Type I-B fistulas multiple arterial feeders can originate from multiple levels and also bilaterally. Since complete obliteration of the fistula is the primary goal of surgery, angiographic documentation of all feeders is critical if surgery is planned.

Several authors reported on long-term surgical results in Type I fistulas. Some 60–70% of the patients improve, 25–30% are stabilized and 5–10% appear to further deteriorate [28, 29]. After it had been recognised that excision of the dilated venous complex is not necessary, and that most patients improve after the shunt is obliterated, some authors have recommended that embolisation of the fistula should be attempted first [26]. However, failure of embolisation is not uncommon [18]. In view of these results, many authors consider surgery as the treatment of choice in spinal dAVFs, because surgery is more effective than endovascular embolisation, which should be reserved for nonsurgical candidates.

Radiosurgery is not an established method for spinal dural fistulas. In analogy with the results on cranial arteriovenous fistulas it appears likely that radiosurgery could be an effective modality. Whether introduction of this modality is useful in the light of the relative simplicity of the surgical method appears doubtful.

Personal results

Since 1994 we defended the strategy of a primary surgical therapy of cervical and thoracic dural fistulas.

These fistulas were only embolised if the patients wished a non-surgical mode of therapy and if there was no spinal cord arterial supply from the feeder artery. Lumbar and sacral fistulas were usually embolised with isobutyl-cyanoacrylate (Histarcryl ^{TM}). A total of some 40 of these patients was managed between 1994 and 2003. The overall rate of recovery corresponded to the data given in the literature. One third of the patients did not recover satisfactorily. Further deterioration was noticed in one patient. Three patients had to be operated for recanalization after embolisation and one surgical patient had to be reoperated for residual fistula after surgery.

References

1. Awad IA, Little JR, Akarawi WP, Ahl J (1990) Intracranial dural arteriovenous malformations: factors predisposing to an aggressive neurological course. J Neurosurg 72: 839–850
2. Barrow DL, Spector RH, Braun IF, Landman JA, Tindall SC, Tindall GT (1985) Classification and treatment of spontaneous carotid-cavernous sinus fistulas. J Neurosurg 62: 248–256
3. Brown RD Jr, Wiebers DO, Nichols DA (1994) Intracranial dural arteriovenous fistulae: angiographic predictors of intracranial hemorrhage and clinical outcome in nonsurgical patients. J Neurosurg 81: 531–538
4. Cognard C, Gobin YP, Pierot L, Bailly AL, Houdart E, Casasco A, Chiras J, Merland JJ (1995) Cerebral dural arteriovenous fistulas: clinical and angiographic correlation with a revised classification of venous drainage. Radiology 194: 671–680
5. Collice M, D'Aliberti G, Talamonti G, Branca V, Boccardi E, Scialfa G, Versari PP (1996) Surgical interruption of leptomeningeal drainage as treatment for intracranial dural arteriovenous fistulas without dural sinus drainage. J Neurosurg 84: 810–817
6. Davies MA, TerBrugge K, Willinsky R, Coyne T, Saleh J, Wallace MC (1996) The validity of classification for the clinical presentation of intracranial dural arteriovenous fistulas. J Neurosurg 85: 830–837
7. Duffau H, Lopes M, Janosevic V, Sichez JP, Faillot T, Capelle L, Ismail M, Bitar A, Arthuis F, Fohanno D (1999) Early rebleeding from intracranial dural arteriovenous fistulas: report of 20 cases and review of the literature. Review. J Neurosurg 90: 78–84
8. Friedman JA, Meyer FB, Nichols DA, Coffey RJ, Hopkins LN, Maher CO, Meissner ID, Pollock BE (2001) Fatal progression of posttraumatic dural arteriovenous fistulas refractory to multimodal therapy. Case report. J Neurosurg 94: 831–835
9. Friedman JA, Pollock BE, Nichols DA, Gorman DA, Foote RL, Stafford SL (2001) Results of combined stereotactic radiosurgery and transarterial embolization for dural arteriovenous fistulas of the transverse and sigmoid sinuses. J Neurosurg 94: 886–891
10. Guo WY, Pan DH, Wu HM, Chung WY, Shiau CY, Wang LW, Chiou HJ, Yen MY, Teng MM (1998) Radiosurgery as a treatment alternative for dural arteriovenous fistulas of the cavernous sinus. AJNR Am J Neuroradiol 19: 1081–1087
11. Halbach V, Higashida RT, Hieshima GB, Mehringer CM, Hardin CW (1989) Transvenous embolization of dural fistulas

involving the transverse and sigmoid sinuses. AJNR Am J Neuroradiol 10: 385–392

12. Hoh BL, Choudhri TF, Connolly ES Jr, Solomon RA (1998) Surgical management of high-grade intracranial dural arteriovenous fistulas: leptomeningeal venous disruption without nidus excision. Neurosurgery 42: 796–805

13. Lewis AI, Tomsick TA, Tew JM Jr (1994) Management of tentorial dural arteriovenous malformations: transarterial embolization combined with stereotactic radiation or surgery. J Neurosurg 81: 851–859

14. Link MJ, Coffey RJ, Nichols DA, Gorman DA (1996) The role of radiosurgery and particulate embolization in the treatment of dural arteriovenous fistulas. J Neurosurg 84: 804–809

15. Lucas CP, Zabramski JM, Spetzler RF, Jacobowitz R (1997) Treatment for intracranial dural arteriovenous malformations: a meta-analysis from the English language literature. Neurosurgery 40: 1119–1132

16. Mironov A (1994) Pathogenetical consideration of spontaneous dural arteriovenous fistulas (DAVFs). Acta Neurochir (Wien) 131: 45–58

17. Mironov A (1995) Classification of spontaneous dural arteriovenous fistulas with regard to their pathogenesis. Acta Radiol 36: 582–592

18. Morgan MK, Marsh WR (1989) Management of spinal dural arteriovenous malformations. J Neurosurg 70: 832–836

19. Olteanu-Nerbe V, Uhl E, Steiger HJ, Yousry T, Reulen HJ (1997) Dural arteriovenous fistulas including the transverse and sigmoid sinuses: results of treatment in 30 cases. Acta Neurochir (Wien) 139: 307–318

20. Pan DH, Chung WY, Guo WY, Wu HM, Liu KD, Shiau CY, Wang LW (2002) Stereotactic radiosurgery for the treatment of dural arteriovenous fistulas involving the transverse-sigmoid sinus. J Neurosurg 96: 823–829

21. Pollock BE, Nichols DA, Garrity JA, Gorman DA, Stafford SL (1999) Stereotactic radiosurgery and particulate embolization for cavernous sinus dural arteriovenous fistulae. Neurosurgery 45: 459–467

22. Roy D, Raymond J (1997) The role of transvenous embolization in the treatment of intracranial dural arteriovenous fistulas. Neurosurgery 40: 1133–1144

23. Satomi J, van Dijk JM, Terbrugge KG, Willinsky RA, Wallace MC (2002) Benign cranial dural arteriovenous fistulas: outcome of conservative management based on the natural history of the lesion. J Neurosurg 97: 767–770

24. Schmid-Elsaesser R, Steiger HJ, Yousry T, Seelos KC, Reulen HJ (1997) Radical resection of meningiomas and arteriovenous fistulas involving critical dural sinus segments: experience with intraoperative sinus pressure monitoring and elective sinus reconstruction in 10 patients. Neurosurgery 41: 1005–1018

25. Schmid-Elsaesser R (2002) General considerations and review of the literature. In: Steiger HJ, Schmid-Elsaesser R, Muacevic A, Brückmann H, Wowra B (2002) Neurosurgery of Arteriovenous Malformations and Fistulas. A Multimodal Approch. Springer, Wien New York pp 1–56

26. Song JK, Gobin YP, Duckwiler GR, Murayama Y, Frazee JG, Martin NA, Vinuela F (2001) N-butyl 2-cyanoacrylate embolization of spinal dural arteriovenous fistulae. AJNR Am J Neuroradiol 22: 40–47

27. Sundt TM Jr, Piepgras DG (1983) The surgical approach to arteriovenous malformations of the lateral and sigmoid dural sinuses. J Neurosurg 59: 32–39

28. Symon L, Kuyama H, Kendall B (1984) Dural arteriovenous malformations of the spine. Clinical features and surgical results in 55 cases. J Neurosurg 60: 238–247

29. Tacconi L, Lopez-Izquierdo BC, Symon L (1997) Outcome and prognostic factors in the surgical treatment of spinal dural arteriovenous fistulas. A long-term study. Br J Neurosurg 11: 298–305

30. Thompson BG, Doppman JL, Oldfield EH (1994) Treatment of cranial dural arteriovenous fistulae by interruption of leptomeningeal venous drainage. J Neurosurg 80: 617–623

31. van Dijk JM, TerBrugge KG, Willinsky RA, Wallace MC (2002) Clinical course of cranial dural arteriovenous fistulas with long-term persistent cortical venous reflux. Stroke 33: 1233–1236

32. van Dijk JM, TerBrugge KG, Willinsky RA, Wallace MC (2004) Selective disconnection of cortical venous reflux as treatment for cranial dural arteriovenous fistulas. J Neurosurg 101: 31–35

33. Vinuela FV, Debrun GM, Fox AJ, Kan S (1983) Detachable calibrated-leak balloon for superselective angiography and embolization of dural arteriovenous malformations. J Neurosurg 58: 817–823

Correspondence: H.-J. Steiger, Neurochirurgische Universitätsklinik, Moorenstraße 5, 40225 Düsseldorf, Germany. e-mail: steiger@uni-duesseldorf.de

Acta Neurochir (2005) [Suppl] 94: 123–126
© Springer-Verlag 2005
Printed in Austria

Hemodynamic status and treatment of aggressive dural arteriovenous fistulas

N. Kuwayama, M. Kubo, K. Tsumura, H. Yamamoto, and **S. Endo**

Department of Neurosurgery and Neuroendovascular Therapy, Toyama Medical & Pharmaceutical University, Toyama, Japan

Summary

In this study the hemodynamic status and treatment modality of aggressive dural arteriovenous fistulas (dAVFs) was evaluated.

Of 145 intracranial dAVFs treated in our clinic, there were 38 aggressive lesions presenting with hemorrhage, infarction, seizures, and symptoms of increased intracranial pressure. They included 3 (5% of all cavernous sinus lesions) cavernous sinus, 24 (44%) transverse-sigmoid and superior sagittal sinus, and 11 (46%) direct cortical types of dAVFs.

Of these 38 aggressive lesions, retrograde leptomeningeal venous drainage was disclosed in 35 lesions, and retrograde sinus drainage in 3. Eighteen cases were treated only with endovascular procedures, 7 with surgical interventions, and 13 with combined endovascular and surgical procedures. Angiographic results were complete obliteration in 66% of the cases, subtotal and partial obliteration in 34%. Clinical outcome was GR (good recovery) in 58% of cases, MD (moderate disability) in 18%, SD (severe disability) in 13%, VS (vegetative state) in 8%, and D (death) (due to acute cardiac infarction) in 3%. Symptomatic procedural complication occurred in 3 cases.

In conclusion, aggressive dural AVF resulted from retrograde leptomeningeal venous drainage. Combined surgical and endovascular treatment played the leading part in the management of this aggressive type of lesion.

Keywords: Dural arteriovenous fistula; endovascular treatment; surgical treatment.

Introduction

Dural arteriovenous fistulas (AVFs) are a rare clinical entity which accounts for 12% of intracranial arteriovenous malformations (AVMs) [14].

Unlike cerebral AVMs, dural AVFs are now considered an acquired lesion [4]. The etiology, however, still remains unknown in most cases. Clinical symptoms of the patients relate greatly to the increased venous pressure, which is considered to be the essential pathophysiology of this disease. It is well known that dural AVFs sometimes behave aggressively depending on the pattern of venous drainage [1], resulting in intracranial hemorrhage, venous infarction, increased intracranial pressure, and status epilepticus.

The purpose of this study is to evaluate the hemodynamic status and treatment modality of these aggressive dural AVFs.

Patients and method

Of 145 intracranial dAVFs which were treated in our clinic from 1990 to 2003, there were 38 aggressive lesions (26% of all cases) which presented with intracranial hemorrhage, venous infarction, convulsions, or progressive neurological deficits resulting from increased intracranial pressure.

They included 3 cavernous sinus lesions (5% of all cavernous sinus cases), 24 transverse-sigmoid and superior sagittal sinus lesions (44% of cases in these locations), and 11 direct cortical type dAVFs (46% of cases with this type) which included fistulas involving the convexity (2 cases), anterior cranial base (4 cases), craniocervical junction (4 cases), and tentorium (1 case).

Patterns of venous drainage were evaluated, focusing particularly on the retrograde leptomeningeal venous and retrograde sinus drainage (RLVD, RSD). Treatment modalities and results were also evaluated retrospectively.

Results (Table 1)

RLVD or RSD was observed in the preoperative angiogram in 60 of the 145 patients.

Among these 60 patients, 38 lesions showed the aggressive course including intracranial hemorrhage (24 cases), venous infarction (5 cases), seizures (3 cases), and symptoms of increased intracranial pressure (6 cases). Thirty-five lesions were associated with RLVD, and 3 lesions with RSD. No aggressive clinical courses were observed in the patients not associated with RLVD or RSD.

Of these 38 patients with an aggressive lesion, 18 were treated with endovascular procedures (transarterial embolization (TAE), transvenous embolization (TVE), or combination of these procedures), 7 were treated solely with surgical intervention (discontinuing the draining veins), and 13 with combined endovascu-

Table 1. *Angiographic and clinical features and results of treatment of 38 patients with aggressive dAVF*

Case	Age	Sex	Location	Presentation	Lraining pattern	Treatment	% Obliteration	Complication	GOS	Remarks
1	60	M	ACB	SDH	RLVD	operation	100		GR	
2	65	M	ACB	ICH	RLVD	operation	100		GR	
3	68	M	ACB	ICH	RLVD	operation	100		GR	
4	58	M	ACB	ICH	RLVD	operation	100		VS	poor basic condition
5	73	M	CCj	SAH	RLVD	TAE	20		VS	poor basic condition
6	52	F	CCj	SAH	RLVD	TAE	100	permanent #1	VS	retroperitoneal bleeding
7	65	M	CCj	SAH	RLVD	TAE	50	permanent #2	SD	NBCA migration
8	52	M	CCj	CI	RLVD	operation	100		SD	
9	70	M	CV	CI	RLVD	TAE	100		MD	
10	41	M	CV	ICH	RLVD	operation	100		MD	
11	60	M	Tent	SAH	RLVD	operation	100		MD	
12	48	M	CS	ICH	RLVD	surgical TVE	100		SD	
13	82	F	CS	ICH	RLVD	TVE	90		MD	
14	69	M	CS	ICH	RLVD	TAE	90		GR	
15	69	M	SSS	ICH	RLVD (bil)	surgical TVE	100		GR	
16	60	M	TS	ICH	RLVD	surgical TVE	100		GR	
17	70	M	TS	ICH	RLVD	surgical TVE	100		MD	
18	47	M	TS	ICH	RLVD	surgical TVE	100		SD	
19	63	M	TS/SSS	ICH	RLVD (bil)	surgical TVE	90		D	AMI 10 days after treatment
20	66	M	TS	ICH	RLVD	surgical TVE	100		MD	
21	56	F	TS	ICH	RLVD	TAE/operation	100		GR	
22	78	F	TS	ICH	RLVD (bil)	TVE	100		SD	poor basic condition
23	72	M	TS	ICH	RLVD	TAE	100	transient #3	GR	lower cranial nerve palsy
24	78	M	TS	ICH	RSD	TVE	100		GR	
25	61	M	TS	ICH	RLVD	TAE/operation	90		GR	
26	87	F	TS + confluence	SAH, dementia	RLVD	TAE/TVE	50		MD	poor basic condition
27	64	F	TS	CI	RLVD	surgical TVE	100		GR	
28	67	M	TS	CI	RSD	TVE	90		GR	
29	60	M	SSS	drop attack (CI)	RLVD (bil)	surgical TVE	100		GR	
30	70	M	SSS/TS	dementia	RLVD (bil)	TAE/TVE	50		GR	
31	51	M	TS (bil)	dementia	RLVD (bil)	TAE	50		GR	
32	82	F	TS (bil)	dementia	RLVD/RSD	TVE	50		GR	
33	71	F	TS	dementia	RLVD	TAE/TVE	100		GR	
34	53	M	TS	VI	RLVD	TAE	100		GR	
35	74	M	TS + confluence	VI	RSD	TAE/TVE	50		GR	
36	57	M	SSS	SE	RLVD	TAE	90		GR	
37	75	M	TS	SE	RLVD	surgical TVE	100		GR	
38	61	F	TS	SE	RLVD	surgical TVE	100		GR	

SDH Subdural hematoma, *ICH* intracerebral hematoma, *SAH* subarachnoid hemorrhage, *CI* cerebral infarction, *SE* status epilepticus, *VI* visual impairment, *RLVD* retrograde leptomeningeal drainage, *RSD* retrograde sinus drainage, *TAE* transarterial embolization, *TVE* transvenous embolization, *AMI* acute myocardial infarction, *#1* Retroperitoneal bleeding, *#2* PCA embolism due to NBCA migration, *#3* lower cranial nerve palsy.

lar and surgical procedures (11 surgical TVEs, and 2 TAEs followed by surgical intervention).

Angiographic results were complete obliteration in 25 patients (66% of aggressive lesions), subtotal oblit-

eration in 6 (16%), partial obliteration in 7 (18%). Clinical outcome was GR in 22 patients (58%), MD in 7 (18%), SD in 5 (13%), VS in 3 (8%), and D in 1 (3%, due to acute myocardial infarction). Thus, favorable angiographic results were obtained in 31 (82%), and favorable clinical outcome in 29 (76%) patients.

Symptomatic procedural complications were observed in 3 patients including one showing a transient ischemic cranial nerve symptom after glue injection, one suffering a permanent hemiparesis due to glue migration to the parent vertebral artery, and the other one with neurologic deterioration caused by a massive retroperitoneal bleeding.

Discussion

The recent development of neuroendovascular techniques enables us to treat dural arteriovenous fistulas very safely and effectively. However, we have sometimes experienced complicated lesions which were not easy to treat. These lesions sometimes behave aggressively causing intracranial hemorrhage, venous infarction, seizures, and symptoms of increased intracranial pressure. Hemodynamic features of these aggressive dAVFs are quite essential to consider the symptoms and evaluate the treatment modalities of this disease.

Aggressive clinical course

Dural AVF is a disease of which pathophysiology is thought to be based on the abnormality of the venous side [13]. Its symptoms, therefore, are also related with the abnormal venous conditions. Antegrade venous drainage usually does not behave aggressively, only sometimes causing vascular bruit (pulsatile tinnitus) which is not basically life-threatening. As clearly shown in this series, aggressive clinical courses resulted from venous hypertension caused by retrograde leptomeningeal venous or retrograde sinus drainage (RLVD, RSD).

In a review of the literature, Awad *et al.* [1] have clarified that leptomeningeal venous drainage, variceal or aneurysmal venous dilatation, and galenic drainage were significant factors as predisposition for this aggressive neurological course. Brown, *et al.* [3] reported a long-term follow-up study of 54 patients with dural AVFs and concluded that a significant predictor for intracranial hemorrhage was venous varix on a draining vein. Lesions draining into leptomeningeal veins (RLVD) also had an increased occurrence of hemorrhage. There have been several reports [2, 5, 9, 15, 16] where pure leptomeningeal drainage without involvement of dural sinus (direct cortical type in our series) was emphasized as a potential risk of bleeding. Sinus occlusion is another potential factor to modify the venous drainage. Ishii *et al.* [11] identified a subgroup of patients with a high risk of hemorrhage and dementia due to a severe venous overload through occlusive changes of transverse-sigmoid sinus. A recent report clarified the annual risk of hemorrhage (8.1%) and annual mortality rate (10.4%) in cases with long-term persistent cortical venous drainage [6]. Rebleeding risk (35% within 2 weeks) has also been emphasized in the lesions with RLVD [7].

Treatment

Transarterial embolization (TAE) with glue is effective to reduce the arterial inflow, but it is sometimes difficult to obtain complete and permanent obliteration of the shunt in this way. Transvenous embolization (TVE) [10, 17] is now recognized as one of the most effective and radical treatments of dural AVFs and may be an alternative to standard surgical treatment for many patients, particularly for the majority of the cases with cavernous sinus lesion. However, microcatheters sometimes cannot access the lesions transvenously with isolated sinus and those with pure leptomeningeal venous drainage without sinus involvement (direct cortical type). These are exactly the lesions causing the aggressive neurological course. We reported the efficacy of the direct sinus packing [8] for patients with isolated transverse-sigmoid sinus dural AVFs, and surgical transvenous embolization [12] for patients with cavernous sinus lesion draining only into the cortical veins. It is well known that transvenous catheterization is sometimes successful for lesions in which no draining access route is opacified on the angiogram. But in cases of unsuccessful percutaneous transvenous approach, the surgical TVE as reported by us is very effective to access and cure the lesion. We believe it plays the leading role in the management of aggressive dAVFs.

Conclusions

1) Of 145 cases with intracranial dural AVF, there were 38 aggressive lesions which presented with hemorrhage, infarction, seizures, and symptoms of increased intracranial pressure.

2) Retrograde leptomeningeal venous drainage was disclosed in most cases and thought to be a causative factor of the aggressive behavior.

3) Half the patients were treated solely with endo-

vascular procedure, and the remaining patients were managed surgically alone or with combined endovascular and surgical procedures.

4) Treatment results and clinical outcomes were favorable in most cases of multimodal treatment.

5) The aggressive dural AVF should be treated flexibly with endovascular, surgical, or combined procedures. The importance of teamwork between neuroradiology, neurology, neuroanesthesiology, and neurosurgery should be emphasized.

References

1. Awad IA, Little JR, Akarawi WP, Ahl J (1990) Intracranial dural arteriovenous malformations: factors predisposing to an aggressive neurological course. J Neurosurg 72: 839–850
2. Barnwell SL, Halbach VV, Dowd CF, Higashida RT, Hieshima GB, Wilson CB (1991) A variant of arteriovenous fistulas within the wall of dural sinuses. Results of combined surgical and endovascular therapy. J Neurosurg 74: 199–204
3. Brown RD Jr, Wiebers DO, Nichols DA (1994) Intracranial dural arteriovenous fistulae: angiographic predictors of intracranial hemorrhage and clinical outcome in nonsurgical patients. J Neurosurg 81: 531–538
4. Chaudhary MY, Sachdev VP, Cho SH, Weitzner I Jr, Puljic S, Huang YP (1982) Dural arteriovenous malformation of the major venous sinuses: an acquired lesion. AJNR Am J Neuroradiol 3: 13–19
5. Collice M, D'Aliberti G, Talamonti G, Branca V, Boccardi E, Scialfa G, Versari PP (1996) Surgical interruption of leptomeningeal drainage as treatment for intracranial dural arteriovenous fistulas without dural sinus drainage. J Neurosurg 84: 810–817
6. van Dijk JM, terBrugge KG, Willinsky RA, Wallace MC (2002) Clinical course of cranial dural arteriovenous fistulas with long-term persistent cortical venous reflux. Stroke 33: 1233–1236
7. Duffau H, Lopes M, Janosevic V, Sichez JP, Faillot T, Capelle L, Ismail M, Bitar A, Arthuis F, Fohanno D (1999) Early rebleeding from intracranial dural arteriovenous fistulas: report of 20 cases and review of the literature. J Neurosurg 90: 78–84
8. Endo S, Kuwayama N, Takaku A, Nishijima M (1998) Direct packing of the isolated sinus in patients with dural arteriovenous fistulas of the transverse-sigmoid sinus. J Neurosurg 88: 449–456
9. Grisoli F, Vincentelli F, Fuchs S, Baldini M, Raybaud C, Leclercq TA, Vigouroux RP (1984) Surgical treatment of tentorial arteriovenous malformations draining into the subarachnoid space. Report of four cases. J Neurosurg 60: 1059–1066
10. Halbach VV, Higashida RT, Hieshima GB, Mehringer CM, Hardin CW (1989) Transvenous embolization of dural fistulas involving the transverse and sigmoid sinuses. AJNR Am J Neuroradiol 10: 385–392
11. Ishii K, Goto K, Ihara K, Hieshima GB, Halbach VV, Bentson JR, Shirouzu T, Fukumura A (1987) High-risk dural arteriovenous fistulae of the transverse and sigmoid sinuses. AJNR Am J Neuroradiol 8: 1113–1120
12. Kuwayama N, Endo S, Kitabayashi M, Nishijima M, Takaku A (1998) Surgical transvenous embolization of a cortically draining carotid cavernous fistula via a vein of the sylvian fissure. AJNR Am J Neuroradiol 19: 1329–1332
13. Mullan S (1994) Reflections upon the nature and management of intracranial and intraspinal vascular malformations and fistulae. J Neurosurg 80: 606–616
14. Newton TH, Cronqvist S (1969) Involvement of dural arteries in intracranial arteriovenous malformations. Radiology 93: 1071–1078
15. Pierot L, Chiras J, Meder JF, Rose M, Rivierez M, Marsault C (1992) Dural arteriovenous fistulas of the posterior fossa draining into subarachnoid veins. AJNR Am J Neuroradiol 13: 315–323
16. Thompson BG, Doppman JL, Oldfield EH (1994) Treatment of cranial arteriovenous fistulae by interruption of leptomeningeal venous drainage. J Neurosurg 80: 617–623
17. Urtasun F, Biondi A, Casaco A, Houdart E, Caputo N, Aymard A, Merland JJ (1996) Cerebral dural arteriovenous fistulas: percutaneous transvenous embolization. Radiology 199: 209–217

Correspondence: Department of Neurosurgery and Neuroendovascular Therapy, Toyama Medical & Pharmaceutical University, Toyama Sugitani 2630, Toyama 930-0194, Japan. e-mail: kuwayama@ms.toyama-mpu.ac.jp

Cerebral revascularization

Acta Neurochir (2005) [Suppl] 94: 129–132
© Springer-Verlag 2005
Printed in Austria

Carotid- and vertebral-stenosis
Conventional microsurgical endarterectomy

A. Barth

Department of Neurosurgery, University Hospital of Bern, Bern, Switzerland

Summary

In the 1990's, carotid endarterectomy (CEA) has matured to a widely performed, standard intervention with well defined successive steps. The key feature of microsurgical CEA is the use of the operating microscope for magnification of the surgical field and microsuture of the arteriotomy. Further measures contributing to the success of microsurgical CEA include intraoperative monitoring of cerebral blood flow, selective shunt placement and neuroprotection during arterial cross-clamping. In experienced hands, the operation is not difficult and goes without complication in the great majority of patients. An overall complication rate of 6–8% combining mortality, major morbidity and minor morbidity is acceptable in view of the often multimorbid patients undergoing the operation. However, a rate of major morbidity/mortality not exceeding 1–2% is a realistic goal for microsurgical CEA. On the long-term, the rate of restenosis needing treatment should not exceed 1–2%. To preserve objectivity and quality control of CEA, the clinical results should be assessed independently of the surgeon by a neutral observer, ideally a neurologist.

Keywords: Carotid stenosis; carotid endarterectomy; microsurgery; operating microscope.

Introduction

Carotid endarterectomy (CEA) is a prophylactic measure destined to decrease the risk of stroke in patients with atherosclerotic disease of the internal carotid artery (ICA). The best indication for CEA is given in patients with a recently symptomatic, high-grade carotid stenosis, in whom the risk of ipsilateral stroke can reach 20–25% during the following 3 years under best medical therapy [5, 9, 12]. Other indications for CEA are asymptomatic high-grade stenoses [7, 8] and evidently symptomatic middle-grade stenoses [4]. The success of CEA depends upon the selection of patients and the rate of perioperative complications. The best candidates for surgery are those with a high risk of stroke under medical therapy and a low risk of complications after the operation [3, 13]. According to the guidelines of the American Stroke Association, the rate of perioperative complications should not exceed 6% for symptomatic stenoses and 3% for asymptomatic stenoses [6, 11]. All benefit of the operation is lost for the patient when the complication rate approaches 10%.

In this review, we present the key features of microsurgical CEA and examplify the advantages of the operation on the basis of the results obtained in the last 6 years at the Department of Neurosurgery of the University Hospital of Bern, Switzerland.

Principles of microsurgical CEA

Microsurgery of the carotid bifurcation should be performed in a quiet environment without any time stress. Three principles can be advantageously observed to create favourable conditions during the operation. The first principle consists in securing cerebral blood flow on the side of CEA during arterial clamping. Continuous transcranial ultrasonographic measurement of blood flow velocity in the ipsilateral middle cerebral artery can be used to determine the need for an intraoperative shunt. A shunt is inserted between the CCA and ICA only in case of a clear decrease of flow velocity of more than 60% after ICA clamping, indicating an insufficient collateral circulation to the ipsilateral hemisphere. The second principle consists in increasing the tolerance of the brain to ischemia. This can be achieved with a medicamentous coma monitored by intraoperative EEG (burst suppression). In the last years, intravenous propofol was prefered to the classical barbiturate thiopental because it induces less variations of blood pressure during the different steps of the operation and allows a faster recovery of anesthesia. We never observed neurotoxic

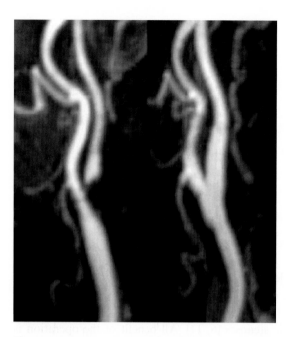

Fig. 1. MR-angiographic example of carotid bifurcation reconstruction using a primary continuous microsuture without patch. After removal of the atherosclerotic plaque, exact restoration of the anatomic contours of the bifurcation is obtained by microadaptation of the vessel wall borders

effects of propofol during such a short intraoperative administration. With the use of propofol and careful manipulation of the carotid body, the systolic blood pressure can be set at a constant value of 120–140 mm Hg independently of arterial clamping or opening. As a last measure to protect the brain against ischemia, a mild hypothermia of 33–34 °C can be induced during the time of clamping. With these different measures installed, temporary interruption of blood flow to the brain can be maintained without problem as long as deemed necessary to remove the stenosis and recanalize the carotid bifurcation. This introduces the third principle of microsurgical CEA, which consists in the use of the operating microscope with its wellknown advantages of optimal magnification and illumination of the surgical field. After removal of any residual fragments of the arteriosclerotic plaques, the microscope enables an exact anatomic reconstruction of the carotid bifurcation using a primary microsuture without patch (Fig. 1).

Steps of microsurgical CEA

Once very controversial, carotid surgery has matured to a widely performed, standard intervention with well defined successive steps. In experienced hands, the operation is not difficult and goes without complication in the great majority of patients. The different steps of microsurgical CEA have been described recently in details by J. E. Bailes [1, 2]. The first part of the operation is performed macroscopically with the help of surgical loupes. The patient is positioned supine with the neck slightly extended and the head turned to the opposite side. Potential difficulties in the exposition of the carotid arteries should be anticipated on the preoperative images by determining the exact position of the carotid bifurcation in reference to the cervical spine and by evaluating the medial or lateral projection of the initial portion of ICA. Further important preoperative information concerns the length of the stenosis and the presence of ulcerations. Preparation of the carotid vessels progresses from proximal to distal along the medial border of the sternocleidomastoid muscle with successive dissection of the CCA, superior thyroid artery, ECA, and finally ICA. The proximal limit of dissection is usually given by the omohyoid muscle and the distal limit by the digastric muscle. The nerve and vessel supply to the sternocleidomastoid muscle can be divided and the large crossing veins of the neck ligated as encountered. In contrast, the vagus and hypoglossal nerves along with the ansa cervicalis are to be preserved. Intravenous heparin (100 IE/kg) is administered at the beginning of arterial manipulation. The ICA should be dissected as high as possible in the neck, usually about 5 cm above the bifurcation, proceeding laterally to the hypoglossal nerve. The stenosed portion itself is prepared at the end, when distal control on the normal ICA is secured, in order to reduce the risk of intraoperative cerebral emboli. After induction of propofol coma, the ICA is clamped first using a large temporary aneurysm clip, followed by the CCA, ECA and superior thyroid artery. The CCA is sharply incised proximally to the bifurcation and the arteriotomy extended into the ICA a few millimeters above the upper limit of the plaque. If a shunt is necessary, 3 to 5 minutes can be invested without risk of brain ischemia to insert the distal end of the shunt well above the plaque into the normal ICA. A slow careful shunt placement diminishes the risk of arterial dissection and also cerebral emboli. The cleavage between arterial wall and atherosclerotic plaque can be identified in every case. After gross removal of the plaque, the operating microscope is used to systematically inspect the vessels of the bifurcation and to remove every residual fragment of the plaque. At the distal end of arteriotomy, the transition zone between endarterectomized and normal ICA should be as smooth as possible to avoid postoperative thrombosis. If necessary, tacking sutures can be applied on the intima. After brief opening of the clamps on ICA and CCA, the exposed arterial wall is abundantly rinced with heparinized saline. The arteriotomy is closed with a tight continuous 6-0 monofilament suture without patch beginning distally and progressing proximally. Care is taken to adapt the muscularis media at every stich to insure watertightness and to avoid postoperative rupture. Before complete closure, air is expelled out of the bifurcation and the clamps are removed in a standard fashion, beginning with the ECA, then CCA and lastly ICA. In the rule, full heparinization is not antagonized at the end of the operation as careful hemostasis and a slightly compressive dressing are sufficient to prevent postoperative wound hematoma formation.

Postoperative care

Patients are evaluated neurologically immediately after awakening and observed overnight in the recovery room for development of wound hematoma, hypertension, or new neurologic deficits. Platelet anti-aggregation is administered on a continuous basis. In patients with preoperative oral anticoagulation, increasing doses of heparin are given for 3 days before resuming oral anticoagulants when wound healing is stabilized.

Clinical results

Perioperative complications are defined as any adverse events occurring during and up to 30 days after the operation. Adverse events are usually classified as mortality, major morbidity, and minor morbidity. According to ECST [10], major neurologic morbidity is defined as a neurologic deficit persisting after 7 days. Severe postoperative heart disease such as myocard infarction also belongs to the major morbidity of CEA. In contrast, neurologic deficits lasting less than 7 days, transient heart failure, and local complications count as minor morbidity because of their transient nature. From an epidemiologic point of view, the mortality and major morbidity are the only important parameters which determine the quality and the success of the operation. To preserve objectivity and quality control of CEA, it is mandatory that the clinical results are assessed independently of the surgeon by a neutral ob-

Table 1. *Clinical results of microsurgical CEA (Department of Neurosurgery, University Hospital of Bern, Switzerland, 1998–2004)*

_	N	Percent
Operated patients	321	100%
_	_	_
Overall complications	21	6.6%
_	_	_
Major complications	3	0.9%
Mortality	1	0.3%
Neurologic deficit > 7 days	1	0.3%
Severe heart disease	1	0.3%
_	_	_
Minor complications	18	5.7%
TIA, deficit < 7 days	4	1.2%
Transient heart failure	6	1.9%
Wound abscess, hematoma	4	1.2%
Recurrent nerve paresis	3	1.1%
Epileptic seizure	1	0.3%

server, ideally a neurologist. In our hospital, a neurologic and ultrasonographic evaluation of all operated patients is performed at hospital discharge and repeated 6 weeks later. The pre-, intra-, and postoperative data are gathered prospectively and saved in a data bank according to the guidelines of the local ethic commission. During the last 6 years, 321 patients harbouring a symptomatic or asymptomatic carotid stenosis have been operated in our Department using the described microsurgical method of CEA (Table 1). The exclusion rate was 5% and concerned patients with severe preoperative neurologic deficits, dementia, unstable heart disease, or a limited life expectancy. During the first 30 days following the operation, one patient died and two patients presented severe complications, resulting in a combined major morbidity/mortality rate of 0.9%. A transient minor complication occurred in 5.7% of the patients. The overall combined morbidity/mortality rate in our series was 6.6%, which corresponds to the published standards [5, 7–9, 12]. During the observation period of 1998 to 2004, 1.5% of the patients (5/321) presented a recurrent high-grade stenosis of the operated carotid artery which needed treatment by angioplasty and stenting.

Conclusions

The indications for CEA have been well clarified in the 1990's after the publication of several large multicentric randomized trials [5, 7, 9, 12]. An overall rate of perioperative complications of 6–8% is acceptable in view of the often multimorbid patients undergoing the operation. However, most of the complications should remain of benign nature and the rate of combined major morbidity/mortality should not exceed 1–2%. The principles of microsurgery can be advantageously applied during CEA, particularly for patients at high risk of neurologic complications.

References

1. Bailes JE (2002) Carotid endarterectomy. Review. Neurosurgery 50: 1290–1295
2. Bailes JE, Spetzler RF (1996) Microsurgical carotid endarterectomy. Lippincott-Raven, Philadelphia
3. Barth A, Bassetti C (2003) Patient selection for carotid endarterectomy: how far is risk modeling applicable to the individual? Stroke 34: 524–527
4. Barnett HJ, Taylor DW, Eliasziw M, Fox AJ, Ferguson GG, Haynes RB, Rankin RN, Clagett GP, Hachinski VC, Sackett DL, Thorpe KE, Meldrum HE, Spence JD (1998) Benefit of carotid endarterectomy in patients with symptomatic moderate or severe stenosis. North American Symptomatic Carotid Endarterectomy Trial Collaborators. N Eng J Med 339: 1415–1425
5. Beneficial effect of carotid endarterectomy in symptomatic patients with high-grade carotid stenosis (1991) North American Symptomatic Carotid Endarterectomy Trialists Collaborative Group. N Engl J Med 325: 445–453
6. Biller J, Feinberg WM, Castaldo JE, Whittemore AD, Harbaugh RE, Dempsey RJ, Caplan LR, Kresowik TF, Matchar DB, Toole J, Easton JD, Adams HP Jr, Brass LM, Hobson RW 2nd, Brott TG, Sternau L (1998) Guidelines for carotid endarterectomy: a statement for healthcare professionals from a special writing group of the Stroke Council, American Heart Association. Stroke 29: 554–562
7. Endarterectomy for asymptomatic carotid artery stenosis (1995) Executive Committee for the Asymptomatic Carotid Atherosclerosis Study. JAMA 273: 1421–1428
8. Halliday A, Mansfield A, Marro J, Peto C, Peto R, Potter J, Thomas D, MCR Asymptomatic Carotid Surgery Trial (ACST) Collaborative Group (2004) Prevention of disabling and fatal strokes by successful carotid endarterectomy in patients without recent neurological symptoms: randomised controlled trial. Lancet 363: 1491–1502
9. Mayberg MR, Wilson SE, Yatsu F, Weiss DG, Messina L, Hershey LA, Colling C, Eskridge J, Deykin D, Winn HR (1991) Carotid endarterectomy and prevention of cerebral ischemia in symptomatic carotid stenosis. Veterans Affairs Cooperative Studies Program 309 Trialist Group. JAMA 266: 3289–3294
10. MCR European Carotid Surgery Trial (1991) Interim results for symptomatic patients with severe (70–99%) or with mild (0–29%) carotid stenosis. European Carotid Surgery Trialists' Collanorative Group. Lancet 337: 1235–1243
11. Moore WS, Barnett HJ, Beebe HG, Bernstein EF, Brener BJ, Brott T, Caplan LR, Day A, Goldstone J, Hobson RW (1995) Guidelines for carotid endarterectomy. A multidisciplinary consensus statement from the ad hoc Committee, American Heart Association. Review. Stroke 26: 188–201
12. Randomised trial of endarterectomy for recently symptomatic carotid stenosis: final results of the MRC European Carotid Surgery Trial (ECST) (1998) Lancet 351: 1379–1387
13. Rothwell PM, Warlow CP (1999) Prediction of benefit from carotid endarterectomy in individual patients: a risk-modelling study. European Carotid Surgery Trialists' Collaborative Group. Lancet 353: 2105–2110

Correspondence: Alain Barth, Department of Neurosurgery, University Hospital of Bern, 3010 Bern, Switzerland. e-mail: alain.barth@insel.ch

Acta Neurochir (2005) [Suppl] 94: 133–136
© Springer-Verlag 2005
Printed in Austria

Surgical treatment for bilateral carotid arterial stenosis

T. Tsukahara, T. Hatano, E. Ogino, T. Aoyama, T. Nakakuki, and **M. Murakami**

Department of Neurosurgery and Clinical Research Center, National Hospital Organization, Kyoto Medical Center, Kyoto, Japan

Summary

Carotid endarterectomy (CEA) is a beneficial procedure for patients with high-grade carotid stenosis. However, patients with bilateral carotid stenosis have a higher surgical risk during CEA. Since the introduction of carotid stenting (CAS) may decrease some of the surgical complications of CEA, a combined treatment using CEA and CAS may be favorable for patients with bilateral carotid stenosis. We analyzed the safety and efficacy of this treatment strategy. Eighteen patients with bilateral carotid stenosis were treated from January 2000. Bilateral CEA was performed on the first two patients, CAS then CEA of contra-lateral symptomatic side in 13 patients, and bilateral CAS in three patients. There were no perioperative neurological complications or strokes during the follow-up period (mean 17 months). The combined treatment of CAS and CEA was a safe and effective strategy for bilateral carotid stenosis.

Keywords: Carotid endarterectomy (CEA), carotid artery stenting (CAS), bilateral carotid stenosis.

Introduction

The North American Symptomatic Carotid Endarterectomy Trial (NASCET) demonstrated the highly beneficial effect of endarterectomy (CEA) in patients with high-grade carotid stenosis [1]. NASCET also demonstrated that a contra-lateral carotid lesion increases the perioperative risk of stroke associated with a severely stenosed ipsilateral carotid artery, although the long-term outcome of patients who had undergone CEA was considerably better than that for medically treated patients [2]. Since hemodynamic stroke of the contra-lateral cerebral hemisphere during cross clamping of the carotid arteries and lower cranial nerve palsy are major surgical complications of CEA, introduction of carotid artery angioplasty and placement of stent (CAS) may be a safer treatment. This study examined the results of our combined CAS and CEA therapy for patients with bilateral carotid stenosis.

Clinical material and methods

Patient population

Between January 2000 and December 2003, we surgically treated 219 patients with carotid stenosis. Surgical treatment (CEA or CAS) was used for 1) angiographical severe stenosis (60% to 99% stenosis), 2) echographical severe stenosis (75% to 99% stenosis) and 3) symptomatic stenosis with intra-luminal ulceration. CEA and CAS were performed for 145 and 111 lesions, respectively.

Eighteen patients (8.2%; 16 male, mean age 71.1 years, range 56–80) had bilateral carotid stenosis. For the bilateral stenoses, we treated the symptomatic side first; except when high hemodynamic risk was anticipated during CEA for the contra-lateral symptomatic side; CAS was then performed first. Bilateral CEA were performed in the first 2 cases, CAS before CEA in 13 cases, and bilateral CAS in 3 cases.

CEA was performed under general anesthesia with the intra-operative monitors of INVOS (SaO2), EEG, and SEP. Intra-operative carotid arterial shunt was not used during cross clamping.

CAS was performed under local anesthesia. Pre-dilatation was performed after distal protection was inserted in the internal carotid artery, then a stent (Smart®) was placed. A balloon occlusion test (BOT) of contra-lateral ICA was then performed for selective cases.

Representative cases and results

Case 1

A 76-year-old man with a history of hypertension and hyperlipidemia developed left amaurosis fugax and was referred to our hospital. His angiography revealed bilateral internal carotid artery stenosis (Fig. 1A, B). Stenting was performed for the right internal carotid artery stenosis. The angiography immediately after stenting showed sufficient dilatation of the lesion (Fig. 1C). Ten days later, CEA was performed for symptomatic left internal carotid artery stenosis. The CT angiography after CEA showed excellent dilata-

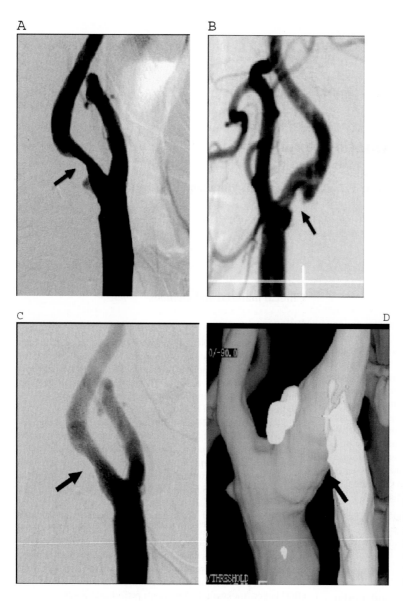

Fig. 1. (A) Right carotid angiogram showing asymptomatic stenosis of internal carotid artery. (Arrow). (B) Left carotid angiogram showing symptomatic severe stenosis of left internal carotid artery. (Arrow). (C) Angiogram taken immediately after stenting shows sufficient dilatation of the lesion. (Arrow). (D) A CT angiography after CEA shows excellent dilatation of the lesion

tion of the lesion (Figure 1D). No complications occurred during either of these procedures. A follow-up angiogram six months after stenting showed no restenosis. There were no ischemic symptoms during the follow-up period.

Case 2

A 69-year-old man with a history of unstable angina pectoris, hypertension, and hyperlipidemia developed repetitive transient left hemiparesis. His MRI showed multiple cerebral infarction. His angiography revealed right internal and left common carotid artery stenosis (Fig. 2A, B). Stenting was performed for the symptomatic right internal carotid artery stenosis. One

week later, stenting was performed for asymptomatic left internal carotid artery stenosis. The angiography after stenting showed sufficient dilatation of the lesions (Fig. 2C, D). There was no periprocedural complication.

Surgical results

Vascular dilatation

Stenosis of the carotid arteries was relieved in all cases after CEA or CAS. Mean stenotic rates of the carotid arteries were 82% in CEA cases and 65% in CAS cases preoperatively. They were 0% after CEA and 6% after CAS, respectively.

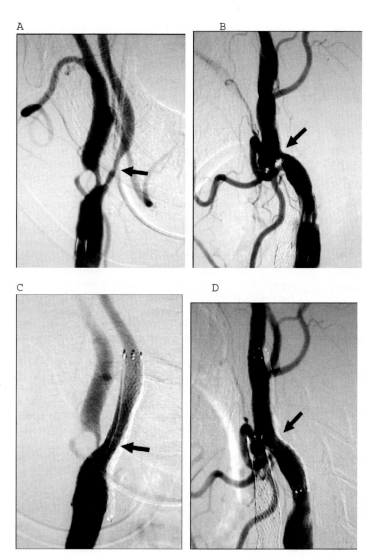

Fig. 2. (A) Right carotid angiogram showing symptomatic stenosis of internal carotid artery. (Arrow). (B) Left carotid angiogram showing asymptomatic stenosis of internal carotid artery. (Arrow). (C) Angiogram taken immediately after stenting shows sufficient dilatation of the lesion. (Arrow). (D) Angiogram taken immediately after stenting shows sufficient dilatation of the lesion. (Arrow)

Character of the plaques of CEA cases

Symptomatic plaques in 13 cases showed intraluminal thrombi in 4, ulceration in 9, intraplaque hemorrhage in 4, and calcification in 3. Asymptomatic plaques in 4 cases showed one ulceration and one calcification.

Surgical complications

There were no neurological deteriorations after treatments, although diffusion weighted brain MRI showed asymptomatic small ischemic lesions in three of nine cases after CAS and none after CEA.

Palsy of lower cranial nerves was not apparent in any of the treated cases.

Follow-up

Mean follow-up period of the surgically treated cases was 16 months. Follow-up angiography was performed in all cases at least six months after treatment. No re-stenosis or recurrent stroke occurred during the follow-up period (mean 16 months).

Discussion

Although CEA is highly beneficial in patients with high-grade carotid stenosis, surgical indication for bilateral carotid stenosis is still controversial [1, 2, 4]. When considering a treatment procedure for bilateral carotid stenosis, the risk of hemodynamic stroke on the contralateral side during surgery should be taken into account. To avoid this risk, it is sometimes necessary to treat the asymptomatic lesion on the other side. The treatment order of bilateral lesions is another important factor to be considered.

Since the introduction of CAS, treatment options for carotid stenosis have changed. CEA is an establish method, and its beneficial effect has been confirmed by randomized studies. However, CEA represents a high risk for patients with contra-lateral ICA lesion, distal ICA lesion, higher level lesion, and other medical risk factors [6]. On the other hand, CAS is a newly developed method, and its beneficial effects are not as established as CEA. However, CAS may be performed for such lesions with less risk. Safety of carotid percutaneous intervention has been improved by the introduction of carotid stenting with self-expandable stents and distal embolization blocking system.

CAS has been routinely performed in clinical practice, especially in Japan. Since many Japanese patients with carotid stenosis have higher cervical lesions compared with European patients, special attention is needed to avoid complications like lower cranial nerve palsy in Japanese patients [7]. The timing of contra-lateral CEA is also of concern when both carotid arteries are involved. Before the introduction of CAS, bilateral CEA was performed at varying surgical intervals. Many surgeons considered a delay of several weeks appropriate in preventing complications such as neurological deficits, nerve injuries, and vocal cord paralysis and its resultant respiratory failure [5, 6]. CAS offers a great advantage in avoiding this life threatening complication.

Although CAS is a less-invasive surgical method, it may be a high risk treatment for soft plaque, eccentric or tortuous lesion, and narrow residual lumen with massive carotid plaque. Consequently, CEA should be chosen for patients with these lesions.

Therefore, combined therapy using CAS and CEA is benefical for patients with bilateral carotid stenoses.

References

1. Ferguson GG, Eliasziw M, Barr HWK, Clagett GP, Barnes RW, Wallace MC, Taylor DW, Haynes RB, Finan JW, Hachinski VC, Barnett HJM, for the North American Symptomatic Carotid Endarterectomy Trial (NASCET) Collaborators (1999) The North American symptomatic carotid endarterectomy trial surgical results in 1415 patients. Stroke: 1751–1758
2. Gasecki AP, Eliasziw M, Ferguson GG, Hachinski V, Barnett HJM, for the North American Symptomatic Carotid Endarterectomy Trial (NASCET) Group (1995) Long-term prognosis and effect of endarterectomy in patients with symptomatic severe carotid stenosis and contralateral carotid stenosis or occlusion: results from NASCET. J Neurosurg 83: 778–782
3. Kiesz RS, Rozek MM, Bouknight D (2001) Bilateral carotid stenting combined with three-vessel percutaneous coronary intervention in single setting. Catheterization and Cardiovascular Interventions 52: 100–104
4. McCarthy WJ, Wang R, Pearce WH, Flinn WR, Yao JST (1993) Carotid endarterectomy with an occluded contralateral carotid artery. Am J Surg 166: 168–172
5. Rodriguez-Lopez JA, Diethrich EB, Olsen DM (2001) Postoperative morbidity of closely staged bilateral carotid endarterectomies: an intersurgical interval of 4 days or less. Annals Vascular Surg 15(4): 457–464
6. Sundt TM, Sandok BA, Whisnant JP (1975) Carotid endarterectomy complications and preoperative assessment of risk. Mayo Clinic Proceedings 50: 301–330
7. Tsukahara T, Akiyama Y, Nomura M, Hashimoto N (1997) Carotid endarterectomy (CEA); standard techniques and ways to avoid complications. Jpn J Neurosurg (Tokyo) 6: 731–736

Correspondence: Tetsuya Tsukahara, Department of Neurosurgery, National Hospital Organization, Kyoto Medical Center, 1-1 Mukaihata-cho, Fushimi-ku, Kyoto, 612-8555, Japan. e-mail: ttsukaha@kyotolan.hosp.go.jp

Acta Neurochir (2005) [Suppl] 94: 137–141
© Springer-Verlag 2005
Printed in Austria

Stenting for vertebrobasilar artery stenosis

T. Hatano, T. Tsukahara, E. Ogino, T. Aoyama, T. Nakakuki, and **M. Murakami**

Department of Neurosurgery and Clinical Research Center, National Hospital Organization, Kyoto Medical Center, Kyoto, Japan

Summary

We report our experience with stenting for symptomatic vertebro-basilar artery stenosis. One hundred and sixteen patients with verte-brobasilar artery stenosis (101 vertebral ostial stenosis, 15 intra-cranial vertebrobasilar artery stenosis) were treated with stenting. Indication criteria of treatment were 1) symptomatic lesion, 2) angiographical stenosis more than 60%. Under local anesthesia, pre-dilatation was first performed, then stents were placed to the le-sion. Successful dilatation was obtained in 115 cases. The stenosis rate reduced to 2% post-stenting in ostial lesions and 16% in intra-cranial lesions. Transient neurological complications developed in 2 patients. Follow-up angiographies more than 6 months after stenting were performed in 94 patients with ostial lesions and all patients with intracranial lesions. Of these, 8 patients (9.5%) with ostial lesions and 4 patients (27%) with intracranial lesions developed restenosis. All patients with restenosis were treated successfully with PTA (percuta-neous transluminal angioplasty). During the follow-up period, 3 pa-tients developed recurrence of VBI (vertebro-basilar insufficiency) symptoms due to restenosis. One patient developed brain stem in-farction due to in-stent occlusion 8 months after stenting.

Conclusion. Stenting for vertebrobasilar artery stenoses is feasible and safe. Prevention of restenosis, especially in intracranial arteries, is the next problem to be solved.

Keywords: Stent; vertebrobasilar artery stenosis.

Introduction

In the treatment of vertebrobasilar artery insuffi-ciency, medical therapy had been the mainstay of treatment because of the high morbidity rate associ-ated with surgical treatment [1, 7, 12]. Recently, percu-taneous transluminal angioplasty (PTA) has evolved to a viable treatment of these lesions. PTA, however, sometimes induces wall dissection and elastic recoil, which results in insufficient dilatation, or, on rare occa-sions, abrupt closure. Furthermore, the restenosis rate after PTA is high [3, 6, 10, 14]. Using stents may re-solve these problems. We investigated the feasibility, safety and outcome of stenting for vertebrobasilar artery stenosis.

Stenting for vertebral artery ostial stenosis

Patients and methods

A total of 101 patients with symptomatic vertebral artery ostial stenoses were treated with stenting in our hospital between October 1997 and April 2004. These patients consisted of 85 males and 16 females with a mean age of 71.5 years (range 46–84 years). Indica-tions for stenting were clinically symptomatic patients having over 60% angiographical stenoses.

Procedure

Aspirin and ticlopidine were administered for at least one week before treatment and one month after treatment. In all but one case, the endovascular tech-nique was performed via a transfemoral approach under local anesthesia. After placement of femoral artery access sheaths (8F-25 cm or 6F-90 cm), heparin was administered. During the procedure, the patient's activated clotting time was adjusted to greater than 250 seconds. A guiding catheter (90–100 cm in length, 8F in diameter) or an ultra-long sheath (90 cm in length, 6F in diameter) with a coaxial catheter (125 cm in length, 6F in diameter) and a guidewire was guided to the subclavian artery just proximal to the ostium of the vertebral artery. Firstly the lesion was dilated with an undersized semicompliant balloon. After predilatation, we evaluated the characteristics of the plaque and the normal size of the vessels using in-travascular ultrasound (IVUS). Then, an appropriate stent was applied to the lesion. Balloon-expandable type stents were used in all cases. After careful posi-tioning, the stent was deployed. Figure 1 illustrates what we consider to be the best position for stents. Re-

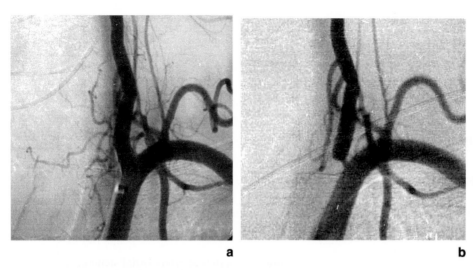

Fig. 1. (a) Anteroposterior left subclavian angiogram demonstrating left vertebral artery ostial stenosis. (b) Angiography after stenting showed excellent dilatation of the lesion

cently, we moderately over-dilated stents, ranging from 0.3 mm to 1 mm. Follow-up angiography was performed six months after stenting. Restenosis was defined as greater than 50% stenosis.

Results

Successful dilatation, defined as less than 30% residual stenosis, was obtained in 100 of 101 cases (99%). The stenosis rate, which was 81% pre-stenting, reduced to 2% post-stenting. The angiograms just after stenting did not show any wall dissections of lesions or any distal occlusions of major intracranial branches. Transient neurological complications occurred in 2 patients (hemiparesis, visual acuity disturbance). No patients experienced permanent neurological complications. Follow-up angiographies more than 6 months after stenting were performed in 94 patients. Of these, 8 patients developed restenosis (9.5%). All patients with restenosis were treated successfully with PTA. As for clinical symptoms, 58% of total patients improved 30 days after stenting. During the follow-up period, two patients developed recurrence of transient VBI symptoms due to restenosis. No patients developed any strokes in the posterior circulation.

Representative case

A 71-year-old man with a history of hypertension and angina developed vertigo and hemiataxia and consulted our hospital. MRI showed a left cerebellar infarction and angiography showed right vertebral artery occlusion and left vertebral artery ostial stenosis (Fig. 1 a). Ten days after admission, we performed stenting for left vertebral artery stenosis. A guiding catheter was positioned in the left subclavian artery. After predilatation, a Palmaz stent (1 cm in length) was applied to the lesion. Angiography after stenting showed excellent dilatation of the lesion (Fig. 1 b). A follow-up angiogram 6 months after stenting showed no restenosis. The patient's symptoms almost disappeared 3 months after stenting.

Stenting for intracranial vertebrobasilar artery stenosis

Patients and methods

Twelve patients with intracranial vertebral artery stenosis and 3 patients with basilar artery stenosis were treated with stenting. These patients included 12 males and 3 females, with a mean age of 68.2 years (53–79 years). Indication for endovascular treatment of intracranial arterial lesions was clinically symptomatic patients with over 60% angiographical stenoses. In the treatment of intracranial artery stenosis, PTA was firstly performed in all patients. Stenting was performed only in cases with insufficient dilatation, dissection or restenosis after PTA.

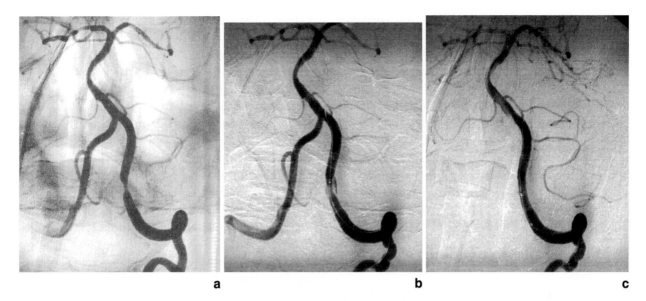

Fig. 2. (a) Anteroposterior left VA angiogram demonstrating stenosis of the left intracranial vertebral artery. (b) Angiography after PTA showed wall dissection (arrow). (c) After stenting, the lesion was sufficiently dilated

Procedure

Stenting methods for these lesions were basically the same as those for ostial lesions. Percutaneous access was achieved via a femoral artery, where a 6F or 8F sheath was introduced. A 6F guiding catheter was advanced up to the level of the second cervical vertebra. Using a load-mapping technique, a 0.014 inch wire was advanced to the second portion of one of the posterior cerebral arteries. PTA was performed with a 2.0–3.0 × 9.0 mm coronary balloon. The stents we used in intracranial lesions were flexible and had a low profile (S670, S660 stent). Stents were expanded to a diameter slightly less than the diameter of the lumen of the normal distal artery. Angiographical follow-up was performed 1 month, 3 months and 6 months after stenting.

Results

Technical success rate was 100% and complication rate was 0%. The stenosis rate, which was 84% pre-stenting, reduced to 16% post-stenting. Four patients (27%) developed restenosis. All patients with restenosis were treated with PTA successfully. In all, 80% of patients were clinically improved 30 days after stenting. Two patients developed transient episodes of VBI due to restenosis within six months of stenting. One patient developed in-stent occlusion 8 months after stenting and 2 months after the 2nd PTA for restenosis. This patient suffered a major stroke.

Representative case

A 78 year-old male with a history of hypertension and diabetes mellitus presented with dizziness and ataxia. MRI imaging revealed a small area of infarction within the left cerebellar hemisphere. His angiography revealed left vertebral artery stenosis (Fig. 2 a). Endovascular treatment was performed 3 weeks after onset. A 6F guiding catheter was positioned at the left vertebral artery. The lesion was crossed with a 0.014-inch wire. PTA was performed with an undersized semicompliant balloon (2.5 mm × 9 mm). Angiography just after PTA showed wall dissection (Fig. 2 b). Stenting was performed using an S660 stent with a nominal diameter of 2.5 mm and a length of 9 mm. The stent-deployment balloon was inflated to a pressure of 10 atm (unconstrained diameter of 2.5 mm). After stenting, the lesion was sufficiently dilated without complications (Fig. 2 c). Follow-up angiography 6 months after stenting revealed no restenosis.

Discussion

Transient ischemic attacks of posterior circulation are associated with a 22% to 35% risk of stroke in five years, and infarction of the vertebrobasilar artery carries a serious prognosis [2, 5, 16]. Although open surgery, such as carotid-vertebral transposition, endarterectomy and bypass surgery, have been performed for obstructive lesions of vertebrobasilar arteries, they are technically demanding and fraught with complications [12]. Medical treatment such as anticoagulation and antiplatelet aggregation therapy does not consistently benefit patients [24]. PTA for vertebrobasilar artery stenosis was introduced in the early 1980s as an alternative to surgery by Sundt *et al.* [13]. Its usefulness has been limited by immediate complications including elastic recoil, wall dissection and vessel rupture [3, 6, 10, 14]. These limitations have fueled interest in treating these lesions by using stents. Theoretically, stenting improves acute and long-term patency and reduces the risk of acute closure from dissection by trapping plaque material between the stent and arterial wall.

Stenting for vertebral artery ostial stenosis

The vertebral artery origin is easily accessible with an endovascular technique, so PTA has become the treatment of choice for these lesions since the 1980s [3, 6]. The usefulness of PTA has been limited by some factors. Arterio-ostial stenoses involving vertebral artery ostial lesions are more elastic than non-arterio-ostial lesions. Therefore, these lesions are resistant to PTA. The use of larger balloons in an attempt to overcome recoil often results in dissection. The difficulty in achieving an adequate dilatation of the vertebral artery origin with PTA only and the potentially high restenosis rate have encouraged the use of stents at this site. In our series, lesions were accessible to stents in all cases. Successful dilatation was obtained in all patients except the initial case. Since 2001, we have performed moderate over-dilatation of stents without any complications. Between 1997 and 2000, the restenosis rate after stenting was 12%. Since 2001, restenosis rate has been reduced to 4.5%. Moderate over-dilatation of stents can be effective in preventing restenosis at this site. The low restenosis rate and low complication rate of stenting for ostial lesions may justify performing primary stenting for vertebral artery ostial stenosis.

Stenting for intracranial vertebrobasilar artery

The tortuous nature of atherosclerotic intracranial vertebrobasilar arteries has limited the use of stents in this area. Although stent devices are less flexible and trackable than PTA balloon catheters, the advent of new-generation, flexible stents has enabled reliable and atraumatic access to intracranial arteries [4, 8, 9, 11]. In our series, technical success was achieved in all

patients. The mean stenosis rate was reduced to 16% after stenting in our patients, whereas other reported series had greater than 40% mean stenosis after balloon angioplasty [10]. Although this residual stenosis rate after stenting was smaller than that of PTA for intracranial arteries, it was greater than that of the ostial lesions in our patients. Intracranial arteries are delicate and thin-walled vessels, with a greater risk for rupture, which can result in lethal bleeding [10]. Therefore, we only under-dilate in these arteries, the relative under-dilatation can prevent procedural complications, such as subarachnoid hemorrhage. Indeed, the complication rate was 0% in our patients. This result was better than that of reported series after PTA or stenting [4, 8–11]. On the other hand, the restenosis rate after stenting for intracranial lesions was high, accounting for 27% of total patients. We speculated that reasons were due to the small diameter of intracranial arteries and under-dilatation of stents. Prevention of restenosis in the intracranial artery is the next problem to be solved. Using self-expandable stents or drug-eluting stents may be an answer to this problem.

References

1. Ausman JI, Shrontz CE, Pearce JE, Diaz FG, Crecelius JL (1985) Vertebrobasilar insufficiency. A review. Arch Neurol 42: 803–808
2. Cartlidge NE, Whisnant JP, Elveback LR (1977) Carotid and vertebral-basilar transient cerebral ischemic attacks. A community study, Ronchester, Minnesota. Mayo Clin Proc 52: 117–120
3. Courtheoux P, Tournade A, Theron J, Henriet JP, Maiza D, Derlon JM, Pelouze G, Evrard C (1985) Transcutaneous angioplasty of vertebral artery atheromatous ostial stricture. Neuroradiology 27: 259–264
4. Gomez CR, Misra VK, Liu MW, Wadlington VR, Terry JB, Tulyapronchote R, Campbell MS (2000) Elective stenting of symptomatic basilar artery stenosis. Stroke 31: 95–99
5. Heyman A, Wilkinson WE, Hurwitz BJ, Haynes CS, Utley CM (1984) Clinical and epidemiologic aspects of vertebrobasilar and nonfocal cerebral ischemia. In: Bergler R, Bauer RB (eds) Vertebrobasilar arterial occlusion disease. Medical and surgical management. Raven Press, New York pp 27–36
6. Higashida RT, Tsai FY, Halbach VV, Dowd CF, Smith T, Fraser K, Hieshima GB (1993) Transluminal angioplasty for atherosclerotic disease of vertebral and basilar arteries. J Neurosurg 78: 192–198
7. Hopkins LN, Martin NA, Hadley MN, Spetzler RF, Budny J, Carter LP (1984) Vertebrobasilar insufficiency. Part 2. Microsurgical treatment of intracranial vertebrobasilar disease. Review. J Neurosurg 66: 662–674
8. Levy EI, Horowitz MB, Koebbe CJ, Jungreis CC, Pride GL, Dutton K, Purdy PD (2001) Transluminal stent-assisted angioplasty of the intracranial vertebrobasilar system for medically refractory, posterior circulation ischemia: early results. Neurosurgery 48: 1215–1223

9. Levy EI, Hanel RA, Boulos AS, Bendok BR, Kim SH, Gibbons KJ, Qureshi AI, Guterman LR, Hopkins LN (2003) Comparison of periprocedure complications resulting from direct stent placement compared with those due to conventional and staged stent placement in the basilar artery. J Neurosurg 99: 653–660

10. Marks MP, Marcellus M, Norbash AM, Steinberg GK, Tong D, Albers GW (1999) Outcome of angioplasty for atherosclerotic intracranial stenosis. Stroke 30: 1065–1069

11. Rasmussen PA, Perl J, Barr JD, Markarian GZ, Katzan I, Sila C, Krieger D, Furlan AJ, Masaryk TJ (2000) Stent-assisted angioplasty of intracranial vertebrobasilar atherosclerosis: an initial experience. J Neurosurg 92: 771–778

12. Spetzler RF, Hadley MN, Martin NA, Hopkins LN, Carter LP, Budny J (1987) Vertebrobasilar insufficiency. Part 1: Microsurgical treatment of extracranial vertebrobasilar disease. J Neurosurg 66: 648–661

13. Sundt TM Jr, Smith HC, Campbell JK, Vlietstra RE, Cucchiara RF, Stanson AW (1980) Transluminal angioplasty for basilar artery stenosis. Mayo Clin Proc 55: 673–680

14. Terada T, Higashida RT, Halbach VV, Dowd CF, Nakai E, Yokote H, Itakura T, Hieshima GB (1996) Transluminal angioplasty for atherosclerotic disease of the distal vertebral and basilar arteries. J Neurol Neurosurg Psychiatry 60: 337–381

15. Prognosis of patients with symptomatic vertebral or basilar artery stenosis. The Warfarin-Aspirin Symptomatic Intracranial Disease (WASID) Study Group (1999) Stroke 29: 1389–1392

16. Whisnant JP, Cartlidge NE, Elveback LR (1978) Carotid and vertebral-basilar transient ischemic attacks: effects of anticoagrants, hypertension, and cardiac disorders on survival and stroke occurrence – a population study. Ann Neurol 3: 107–115

Correspondence: Taketo Hatano, 1-1 Mukaihata-cho, Fukakusa, Fushimi-ku, Kyoto City, Kyoto-fu, Japan. e-mail: taketo@sc4.so-net.ne.jp

Acta Neurochir (2005) [Suppl] 94: 143–148
© Springer-Verlag 2005
Printed in Austria

Extracranial-intracranial bypass
The ELANA technique: high flow revascularization of the brain

H. J. Streefkerk, J. P. Bremmer, and **C. A. Tulleken**

Department of Neurosurgery, ELANA Research Group, Brain Division, Rudolf Magnus Institute, University Medical Center, Utrecht, The Netherlands

Summary

High flow revascularization of the brain is hampered by the fact that temporary occusion of a major cerebral artery is necessary to create the distal anastomosis, which may result in brain ischemia. The excimer laser-assisted non-occlusive anastomosis (ELANA) technique circumvents this problem. In this paper we elucidate the development of a non-occlusive way to make anastomoses to the major cerebral arteries.

Keywords: ELANA technique; cerebral revascularization; vascular anastomosis; non-occlusive anastomosis; EC/IC bypass; IC/IC bypass.

Introduction

The idea to increase the amount of blood flow to the ischemic brain, bypassing any stenoses or occlusions, seems so simple. However, it is still difficult to define which group of patients, who are at risk for a major stroke, will benefit from Extracranial-to-Intracranial (EC/IC) bypass surgery. EC/IC Bypass surgery was developed to improve the cerebral blood flow (CBF) in patients with complete carotid occlusion or ICA stenosis not amenable to extracranial endarterectomy. The International randomized EC/IC Bypass Study showed that the conventional EC/IC bypass, in which the superficial temporal artery (STA) is connected to a cortical branch of the middle cerebral artery (MCA), does not prevent the occurrence of stroke or transient ischemic attacks (TIAs) in patients with symptomatic atherosclerotic lesions of the MCA and/or internal carotid artery (ICA) compared to a non-surgical treated group [1, 2]. The most important critique on the study concerned the evaluation of patients before exclusion or inclusion and randomization in the study [4]. Apart from the clinical criteria, the only additional examination consisted of bilateral carotid angiography. It is therefore not surprising that a new EC/IC bypass trial has been launched in which patients are examined with more advanced techniques to measure the CBF and the oxygen extraction of the brain [3]. Normaly, changes in cerebral perfusion pressure (CPP) have little effect on the CBF due to the autoregulation capacity of the brain. If the CPP decreases the cerebral blood volume (CBV) increases because of the autoregulated vasodilation, thus preserving adequate CBF. Autoregulation fails when the capacity for vasodilation has been exceeded and CBF begins to decline. At that stage, the brain still has the capacity to extract more oxygen increased oxygen extraction fraction (OEF) when oxygen supply has decreased due to diminished CBF. Sufficient augmentation of the blood supply should increase the CBF and decrease the OEF.

However, the conventional STA-MCA bypass only has a limited capacity to increase the blood flow to the brain due to the relatively small size of both donor an recipient bloodvessel. It is possible to create a bypass with a higher capacity by choosing a larger donor vessel, like the more proximal segments of the STA or the external carotid artery (ECA), and/or to interpose a large venous graft between donor and recipient vessel. One of the advantages to use a cortical branch of the MCA as recipient vessel, is that these branches usually have many collaterals. Therefore, it is quite safe to temporarily occlude such a branch in order to create the distal anastomosis of the bypass, using the conventional anastomosis technique originally described by Carrel [5], and improved by Yasargil for use in EC/IC bypass procedures [22, 23]. Even if there are no collaterals, the occlusion of a cortical branch creates temporary ischemia in only a very small part of the brain which may not be clinically relevant. To make a very

high capacity bypass to the brain, a larger (more proximal) recipient artery should be chosen [7]. However,
these vessels do not have many collaterals, so occlusion will create temporary ischemia in a rather large
portion of the brain. Patients at risk for cerebral ischemia usually use their collaterals already at maximum,
diminishing even further the window of time during
which the surgeon may create a conventional anastomosis. Also, the risk of hyperperfusion after the cre-
ation of the bypass increases when choosing a more
proximal recipient vessel. So, in order to safely create
high flow bypasses to the brain and thus increase the
CBF, it is necessary to choose a large donor vessel
(i.e. the ECA), to use an interposing vein graft, and to
connect that graft to a proximal cerebral artery in a
non-occlusive way. In this paper we want to elaborate
on the techniques with which we have tried to create
such a bypass.

In 1902, Carrel described the principles for creating vascular anastomoses, which have hardly changed
during the last century [5]. The recipient artery is temporarily occluded with two clamps. Between them, an
opening is cut into the wall. The end of the donor vessel is connected to the recipient vessel with the endothelial layers of both vessels closely approximated. Still
the backbone of modern vascular surgery, Carrel's
technique has been highly successful. However, its inherent flaw is the temporary occlusion of the recipient
vessel. A critically ischemic area may become infarcted
during the procedure. As the brain is extremely dependent on a continuous blood supply, Carrel's techniques
are almost impossible to use on cerebral arteries. It is
therefore surprising that no attempts have been made
to develop a non-occlusive anastomosis technique,
apart from the animal experiments by Eck and Yahr
[6, 21].

Materials and methods

Twenty-five years ago we started animal experiments in order to
make high-flow revascularization procedures of the brain a safe and
effective procedure. First, the end of the donor vessel is connected to
the recipient artery using sutures, which pass through the wall of the
recipient artery superficially, and fully through the wall of the donor
vessel. Subsequently, a cutting device, which is introduced into the
donor vessel, is used to make a hole in the wall of the recipient artery,
leaving part of the adventitial and medial layers of the recipient
artery exposed to the blood stream. This is contrary to Carrel's adage
that close approximation of the endothelial layers is an absolute pre-
requisite for a successful anastomosis, which may explain why so few
surgeons followed this line of thinking. Exposure of the other layers
of the blood vessel to the blood stream would lead to thrombus formation and occlusion.

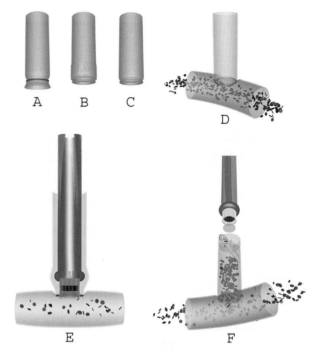

Fig. 1. The ELANA technique. (A) A platinum ring is placed over
the end of the donor vessel. (B) The end of the donor vessel is then
everted over the platinum ring. (C) The donor vessel is fixated to
the platinum ring with several sutures, after which the excessive end
of the everted part is cut of. (D) The donor vessel is then attached to
the recipient vessel using sutures which pass the platinum ring, completely pass the wall of the donor vessel, and only superficially pene-
trate the wall of the recipient vessel. (E) The ELANA catheter is
introduced into the open end of the donor vessel, so that the tip
touches the wall of the recipient vessel inside the platinum ring. Vacuum suction is aplied, ensuring a firm fixation of the laser fibers to
the vessel wall. When the laser is activated, a full-thickness portion
(flap) of the wall of the recipient artery is cut out. (F) Due to the
continued vacuum suction, the flap is recovered when the catheter is
withdrawn from the now functional anastomosis

In many animal experiments we showed that non-occlusive anastomoses will remain patent, thanks to 2 technical innovations [14, 17,
18, 20]. The first was the use of the Excimer laser (Fig. 2E) to cut a
full-thickness disc of recipient artery wall at the anastomosis site.
The laser catheter consists of two concentric circles of 60 micron fibres arranged around the periphery of a thin-walled catheter with an
internal diameter of 2.0 mm. A small metal grid is mounted 0.5 mm
from the tip. The catheter is introduced into the donor vessel, so that
the tip touches the wall of the recipient artery (Fig. 1E). Vacuum is
then induced within the lumen of the catheter, causing a firm fixation
of the wall to the grid and the laser fibres. When the laser is activated
a full-thickness disc of recipient artery wall is cut out, creating a functional anastomosis. The second innovation is the application of a
platinum ring with a diameter of 2.8 mm, which is attached onto the
end of the donor vessel (Fig. 1A, B, C). The donor vessel is then
connected to the recipient vessel (Fig. 1D), using sutures around the
platinum ring, which fully pass through the wall of the donor and
superficially pass the wall of the recipient artery. The effect of the
platinum ring is fourfold: 1) It flattens the wall inside the ring, which
facilitates the penetration of the laser tip over its full circumference;

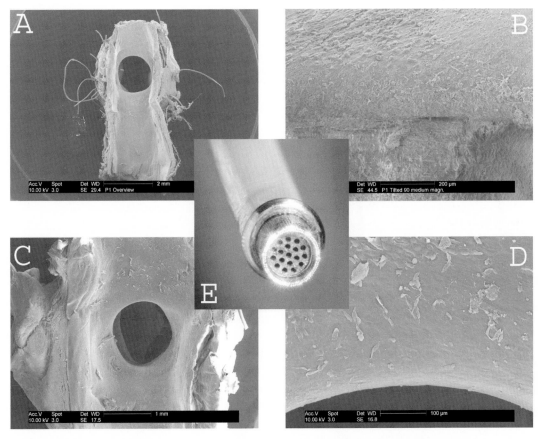

Fig. 2. Scanning electron microscopic *(SEM)* images of 2 anastomoses (A, B, C, D) and an image of the ELANA catheter tip (E). In (A), the inside of the posterior cerebral artery is shown at the site of the anastomosis with the bypass, three weeks after its construction (see text). The bypass is coming towards the camera, and its lumen is clearly visible. A high magnification image of the edge of the vessel wall (B), which has been ablated by the excimer laser (E) shows a smooth surface with re-endothelialization. Similar images of an anastomosis with the intracranial internal carotid artery (C and D) were taken more than 5 years after its construction (see text). The laser edge is very well re-endothelialized in the high magnification image (D)

2) The ring dictates the shape of the anastomosis, which is always round with a diameter of 2.8 mm; 3) It guides the tip to the correct position; 4) The ring prevents the tip from further entering the lumen after penetration of the wall, because it stops the catheter at a circular protuberance, 1.5 mm from the tip.

Results

During the last seven years the excimer laser-assisted non-occlusive anastomosis (ELANA) technique, has been applied in 170 patients with giant intracranial aneurysms, skull base tumours, or progressive brain ischemia [12, 13, 15, 16, 19]. The long term patency was 90% with an average flow in the bypass of 150 ml/min. In one patient with a giant aneurysm of the basilar artery we used the ELANA technique twice to create a connection between the internal carotid artery and the posterior cerebral artery. He died three weeks after the operation because of re-

spiratory failure. Angiography showed that the bypass was patent and at autopsy both anastomoses appeared fully endothelialised, which was later confirmed by scanning electron microscopic evaluation (Fig. 2A, with a high magnification in 2B). Another patient, in whom we ligated the internal carotid artery after the construction of a bypass because of a skull base tumour, died 5 years later because of tumour recurrence. The ELANA anastomosis was removed at autopsy for scanning electron microscopy (Fig. 2C, with high magnification in 2D). The anastomosis site was well endothelialised and the rim of recipient artery wall with the adventitial and medial layers had disappeared.

Our group has published on the clinical results of the ELANA technique in a small series of 15 patients with a high risk of recurrent stroke with promising results [8, 10]. We offer an ELANA EC/IC bypass procedure

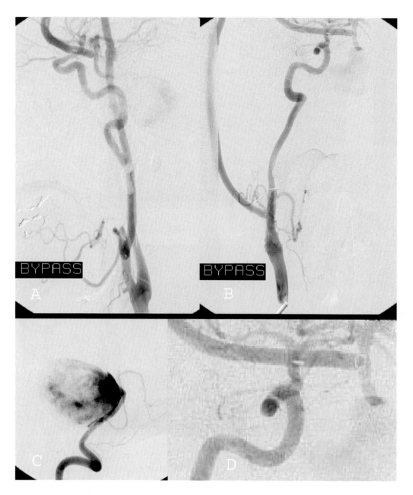

Fig. 3. Pre- and postoperative angiograms of the BA aneurysm and the bypass. In (C) the giant aneurysm is shown. The ECA-BA bypass is shown from a lateral view in (A), and from a frontal view in (B). A closeup of the distal anastomosis to the BA is shown in (D). Note the small platinum ring which has been attached to the distal BA

only to those patients who have ongoing symptoms of cerebral ischemia, after unilateral or bilateral ICA occlusion has been observed, despite antithrombotic treatment and endarterectomy of a contralateral ICA stenosis or ipsilateral ECA, and in whom the symptoms are likely to be of haemodynamic origin. An exception has been made for a patient who presented with repeated episodes of vertebrobasilar ischemia because of vertebral artery occlusion and stenosis. An ICA-posterior cerebral artery segment P1 bypass procedure was performed, effectively creating a new posterior communicating artery [15]. All patients had a proven hypoperfusion of the brain. In this very carefully selected group of patients we have been able to create EC/IC and IC/IC bypasses to all proximal cerebral arteries of the brain, depending on the location and extend of the occlusive vascular lesions. Several times we could not proceed with the ELANA tech-

nique because of severe athereosclerosis of the ICA, the proximal MCA, or the proximal ACA. We then created a conventional EC/IC bypass to a nonsclerotic cortical branch of the MCA, because using a sclerotic recipient vessel may lead to rupture of the anastomosis.

So, it is possible to consider every cerebral artery as a recipient artery for bypass surgery. Recently, we treated a patient with a giant VA-BA aneurysm (Fig. 3c), which was increasing in size during the last months. The last two months our patient could not continue his work as a policeman, and suffered from progressive brainstem deficits with dysarthria, swallow problems, vertigo and ultimately a tetraparesis. He obviously had a bad prognosis, and we expected that his life-expectancy would be very short. Clinically, our patient did not tolerate bilateral VA occlusion, in order to reverse the flow in the BA and thus preventing the aneurysm from growing. Therefore, a "jump" bypass was considered between the intracranial ICA and the PCA, like the bypass made in the afore-mentioned patient. We also considered making an ECA-PCA bypass. Both bypasses should than supply sufficient bloodflow to the posterior circulation, while ligation of both VAs would reverse the flow in the aneurysm. We started by occluding the left VA using two endovascular balloons. Our patient tolerated this without problems. We then operated him. Using a pterional approach, we found that the BA-bifurcation was located quite high, and the BA, distally of the aneurysm, looked very healthy and accessible. Of course, creating a conventional anastomosis to the BA was out of the question. In the literature we could find only one case under deep hypothermic circulatory arrest during which a conventional anastomosis to the BA was made [11]. The ELANA technique allowed us to attach a venous graft to the BA through the small opening formed by the ICA, the A1 and the optic nerve, without occuding the BA. A nice flap of BA wall was retracted and this anastomosis was used to create an ECA-BA bypass, through which a flow of 55 ml/min was observed. This flow was observed with the right VA still open. We then ligated also this VA and the flow through the bypass increased to 95 ml/min. Due to the reversed flow in the aneurysm, there was now a high chance that a thrombus will create within the aneurysm, which hopefully would not occlude the BA itself. BA occlusion, however, was not likely to occur because of the continued flow to the PCAs, SCAs and AICAs. Angiography showed that the bypass supplied the posterior circulation (Fig. 3A, B, D), and our patient was improving and started to talk and move his limbs. After the operation his condition stabilized. There were signs of improvement. Two weeks later, MRA and CTA scans showed progression of thrombus formation within the aneurysm. However, there was also some progression of the neurological deficits. Four weeks later, the patient suffered a fatal subarachnoidal haemorrhage, which probably originated from the remnant of the aneurysm.

Discussion

The ELANA technique is an additional tool in the neurosurgical armamentarium. It can be used to attach blood vessels to otherwise inaccessible cerebral vessels, creating high flows. Whether to use this technique in patients endangered for stroke is still undefined. We have selected only those patients who have suffered multiple TIAs or minor stroke due to ICA occlusions inaccessible for endarterectomy, and who have a proven hypoperfusion of the brain. The results of the new EC/IC bypass trial might show that even more patients will improve when treated with revascularization techniques.

Various techniques to apply the platinum ring onto the recipient vessel are under investigation. The latest developments in our laboratory concentrate on the possibility of making a facilitated sutureless ELANA. The first results of animal experiments on rabbits using this method look very promising.

Acknowledgments

We want to thank all members of the ELANA Researchgroup Utrecht for their continued support both in the experimental animal laboratory as well as in the theatre. Next to the authors, the ELANA Researchgroup Utrecht consists of Mansvelt Beck HJ, Verdaasdonk RM, van der Zwan A, Verweij B and Münker M.

References

1. Failure of extracranial-intracranial arterial bypass to reduce the risk of ischemic stroke. Results of an international randomized trial. The EC/IC Bypass Study Group (1985). N Engl J Med 313: 1191–1200
2. The International Cooperative Study of Extracranial/Intracranial Arterial Anastomosis (EC/IC Bypass Study) methodology and entry characteristics. The EC/IC Bypass Study group (1985). Stroke 16: 397–406
3. Adams HP Jr, Powers WJ, Grubb RL Jr, Clarke WR, Woolson RF (2001) Preview of a new trial of extracranial-to-intracranial arterial anastomosis: the carotid occlusion surgery study. Neurosurg Clin N Am 12: 613–618
4. Ausman JI, Diaz FG (1986) Critique of the extracranial-intracranial bypass study. Surg Neurol 26: 218–221
5. Carrel A (1902) La technique opératoire des anastomoses vasculaires et de la transplantation des vicères. Lyon Med 98: 859–864
6. Eck NV (1877) On the question of ligature of the portal vein. Voen Med Zh 130: 1–22
7. Hillen B, Hoogstraten HW, Post L (1986) A mathematical model of the flow in the circle of Willis. J Biomech 19: 187–194
8. Klijn CJ, Kappelle LJ, van der Grond J, van Gijn J, Tulleken CA (1998) A new type of extracranial/intracranial bypass for recurrent haemodynamic transient ischaemic attacks. Cerebrovasc Dis 8: 184–187
9. Klijn CJ, Kappelle LJ, van der Zwan A, van der Gijn J, Tulleken CA (2002) Excimer laser-assisted high-flow extracranial/intracranial bypass in patients with symptomatic carotid artery occlusion at high risk of recurrent cerebral ischemia: safety and long-term outcome. Stroke 33: 2451–2458
10. Klijn CJ, van Gijn J (2003) Extracranial to intracranial bypass. (Review). Adv Neurol 92: 329–333
11. Sekhar LN, Chandler JP, Alyono D (1998) Saphenous vein graft reconstruction of an unclippable giant basilar artery aneurysm performed with the patient under deep hypothermic circulatory arrest: technical case report. Neurosurgery 42: 667–673

12. Streefkerk HJ, van der Zwan A, Verdaasdonk RM, Beck HJ, Tulleken CA (2003) Cerebral revascularization. (Review). Adv Tech Stand Neurosurg 28: 145–225

13. Streefkerk HJ, Wolfs JF, Sorteberg W, Sorteberg AG, Tulleken CA (2004) The ELANA technique: Constructing a high flow bypass using a non-occlusive anastomosis on the ICA and a conventional anastomosis on the SCA in the treatment of a fusiform giant basilar trunk aneurysm. Acta Neurochir (Wien) 146: 1009–1019

14. Tulleken CA, Schilte GF, Berendsen W, van Dieren A (1988) New type of end-to-side anastomosis for small arteries: a technical and scanning electron microscopic study in rats. Neurosurgery 22: 604–608

15. Tulleken CA, Streefkerk HJ, van der Zwan A (2002) Construction of a new posterior communicating artery in a patient with poor posterior fossa circulation: technical case report. Neurosurgery 50: 415–420

16. Tulleken CA, van der Zwan A, Verdaasdonk RM, Mansvelt Beck RJ, Moreira Pereira Ramos L, Kappelle LJ (1999) High-flow excimer laser-assisted extra-intracranial and intra-intracranial bypass. Operative Techniques Neurosurg 2: 142–148

17. Tulleken CA, van Dieren A, Verdaasdonk RM, Berendsen W (1992) End-to-side anastomosis of small vessels using an Nd:YAG laser with a hemispherical contact probe. Technical note. J Neurosurg 76: 546–549

18. Tulleken CA, Verdaasdonk RM (1995) First clinical experience with excimer assisted high flow bypass surgery of the brain. Acta Neurochir (Wien) 134: 66–70

19. van der Zwan A, Tulleken CA, Hillen B (2001) Flow quantification of the non-occlusive excimer laser-assisted EC-IC bypass. Acta Neurochir (Wien) 143: 647–654

20. Wolfs JF, van den Ham LF, ter Laak MP, van der Zwan A, Tulleken CA (2000) Scanning electron microscopic evaluation of nonocclusive excimer laser-assisted anastomosis in rabbits. Acta Neurochir (Wien) 142: 1399–1407

21. Yahr WZ, Strully KJ, Hurwitt ES (1964) Non-occlusive small arterial anastomosis with a neodymium laser. Surg Forum 15: 224–226

22. Yasargil MG (1967) Experimental small vessel surgery in the dog including patching and grafting of cerebral vessels and the formation of functional extra-intracranial shunts. In: Donaghy RM, Yasargil MG (eds) Micro-vascular surgery. Thieme, Stuttgart and Mosby, St. Louis, pp 87–126

23. Yasargil MG (1969) Microsurgery applied to neurosurgery. Thieme, Stuttgart New York London

Correspondence: Henk Johan Streefkerk, Department of Neurosurgery, HP. Nr. G03.124, University Medical Center Utrecht, Heidelberglaan 100, 3584 CX, Utrecht, The Netherlands. e-mail: H.J.N.Streefkerk@ELANA-online.org

Acta Neurochir (2005) [Suppl] 94: 149–152
© Springer-Verlag 2005
Printed in Austria

Moyamoya angiopathy in Europe

N. Khan and **Y. Yonekawa**

Department of Neurosurgery, University Hospital Zurich, Zurich, Switzerland

Summary

Over the past 6 years we at the Neurosurgery Department in Zürich have had the opportunity to manage increasing numbers of patients, especially children, with Moyamoya angiopathy. With increasing awareness of presence of this angiopathy in Europe the number of referrals from all across Europe is constantly on the increase. We have also been able to readdress the presence of the entity of Moyamoya angiopathy i.e. both the Moyamoya disease and the Moyamoya syndrome in the European population. Thorough presurgical workup is mandatory for evaluation of surgical candidates for the type of effective revascularisation procedure and therefore for their successful management. Apart from scrutinizing the routine yet indispensable presenting symptomatology with clinical examination of the patients, our preoperative diagnostic workup mainly consists of a 6 vessel cerebral angiography, cerebral perfusion studies with HMPAO-SPECT and $H_2^{15}O$-PET examinations and transcranial Doppler. Longterm follow-up of these patients is indispensable and of great interest to us in terms of etiology and progression of the disease process as well as the choice of effective revascularisation procedure especially in our European population.

Keywords: Moyamoya; angiopathy; syndrome; extracranial-intracranial EC-IC bypass; anastomosis; indirect revascularisation.

Introduction

Moyamoya disease or as officially termed in Japan as the spontaneous occlusion of the circle of Willis was first described in 1955 by Takeuchi and Shimizu [13]. Their first case described in the literature demonstrated a unique and typical angiographic presentation consisting of a bilateral stenosis of the intracranial ICA beginning at the terminal portion of the ICA with formation of an abnormal vascular network of collaterals in the basal ganglia resembling "a puff of smoke drifting in the air" and hence the coining of the name Moyamoya, which in Japanese means so. This disease entity has long been believed to exist in prevelance in Japan and south east Asian countries [1, 14]. Our own present experience, as described in this report, shows an increase in the number of cases detected

all across Europe, as is observed with the progressive increase in the number of patients referred to us for surgical management from several European centres. The combination of the Moyamoya disease i.e. the presence of the positive angiographical findings as mentioned above, in combination with other rare congenital or acquired systemic diseases is termed the Moyamoya syndrome (Table 1) [15–17]. For simplification we have coined the term referred to as the "Moyamoya angiopathy" including both the Moyamoya disease and the Moyamoya syndrome form of presentation. We present our pre- and postoperative

Table 1. *Summarises the different congenital and systemic diseases accompanying the Moyamoya angiopathy and hence classification into the Moyamoya syndrome*

Systemic and congenital diseases in Moyamoya Syndrome

Pts.	Age in years	
1	17	Grange Syndrome
2	13	Compound Haemoglobinopathy
3	4	G6PD Dehydrogenase deficiency
4	5	Protein S deficiency
5	10	Trisomy 21
6	17	Neurofibromatosis type 1
7	12	Neurofibromatosis type 1
8	11	Trisomy 21
9	6	operated for PDA, pupillary sphincter dysplasia
10	4	operated for PDA, pupillary sphincter dysplasia
11	5	Neurofibromatosis type 1
12	5	Morning glory optic disc anomaly
13	11	Factor V deficiency, compensated cardiac valvular defect
14	7	Neurofibromatosis type 1
15	25	Haemolytic anaemia
16	42	Neurofibromatosis type 1, inicidental aneurysms, pituitary adenoma

PDA Patent ductus arteriosus.

management experience in this European patient population.

Materials and methods

Fourty two patients were diagnosed and managed with the diagnosis of Moyamoya angiopathy from 1997 to 2003 at the neurosurgical Department of the University Hospital in Zürich. These patients were referred from all across Europe as well as were from within Switzerland. Majority of them were of European-caucasian origin, two patients were of Asian and 1 of Arabic parentage. Preoperative evaluation was carried out with clinical examination, 6 vessel cerebral angiography, hemodynamic studies of HMPAO-SPECT and/or $H_2^{15}O$-PET and transcranial Doppler. Depending on the extent of angiopathy on the 6 vessel cerebral angiography and the territorial hemodynamic perfusion deficits in the region of middle cerebral MCA, anterior cerebral ACA and posterior cerebral artery PCA, a combination of direct and indirect revascularisation was undertaken. Postoperative follow-up ranged from 3 months to 2 years.

Results

Preoperative examinations

There were 29 children (average age 8 years) and 13 adults (average age 38 years). Moyamoya disease was seen in 26 of the patients (11 adults vs 15 children) and Moyamoya syndrome in 16 patients (2 adults vs 14 children). The major disease syndromes presenting in combination with the moyamoya angiopathy and hence termed the Moyamoya syndrome are presented in Table 1. Preoperative clinical symptomatolgy consisted of repeated TIAs in 32 patients, focal epileptic seizures in 7, cognitive deficits in 9 and simple headache on a daily basis in 5. Focal ischemic/infarct changes were seen on preoperative CT/MRI in all but 3 patients. These were mainly seen in the child Moyamoya group. Only 2 of the adult patients presented with an initial presentation of hemorrhage in the basal ganglia region. Typical angiographic changes of bilateral carotid stenosis/occlusion with basal moyamoya collateral formation was seen in 37 patients. In one case unilateral ICA stenosis was seen and in another 2 cases a unilateral ICA stenosis was accompanied with contralateral ACA and MCA stenosis with bilateral Moyamoya collaterals. Two patients with Moyamoya syndrome presented with atypical angiographical changes of bilateral ICA stenosis at the level of ICA bifurcation with additional cholidoectatic dilatation of the ICA in the petrosal part and absence of typical Moyamoya collaterals. In seven patients the posterior circulation PCA was also affected angiographically.

Table 2. *Surgical revascularisation: direct and indirect revascularisation procedures*

Direct Bypass
STA-MCA n = 42, 36 bilateral (Angular A., Prerolandic A., Posterior parietal A., Posterior temporal A.) Posterior auricular artery and Occipital artery used in 2 and 1 case respectively where STA was not suitable
STA-ACA n = 17, 2 bilateral (Middle internal frontal A.)
STA-PCA n = 1
Indirect Revascularisation
Frontal durasyangiosis n = 32
Fronatal durasynangiosis with dura-periost n = 12
Frontal arteriosynangiosis n = 4
Arteriosynangiosis with Occipital artery n = 3
Occipital durasynangiosis n = 1

Preoperative hemodynamic studies with SPECT and PET were performed in all patients. The perfusion reserve deficits after a Diamox challenge in the respective arterial territorial distribution of the middle (MCA), anterior (ACA), and the posterior (PCA) cerebral arteries was taken as the main parameter in the surgical decision making process of the number and location of the revacularisation procedures to be performed (Table 2).

Bilateral classical superficial temporal artery to branch of middle cerebral artery (STA-MCA) bypass was performed in all patients. In 36 patients this was performed bilaterally. The parietal branch of the STA was anastomosed end to side with either the angular, prerolandic, rolandic, posterior parietal or temporal branches of the MCA. Occipital artery (OA) was used in one case instead of the STA and in 2 cases the posterior auricular artery was the donor vessel due to the small calibre of the STA. Additional STA-ACA anastomosis was performed in 17 patients using the middle internal frontal branch of the ACA. OA-PCA direct anastomosis was performed in the sitting position in only one case. In cases where the donor vessel was not available or of too small a calibre or length indirect anastomosis using the durasynangiosis or arteriosynangiosis technique was performed in the frontal (32 patients) and occipital regions (4 patients).

Postoperative follow-up:

Was performed at 3 months postoperatively in all patients. Additional follow-up has been carried out to upto 2 years (mean follow up range 3 months to 2 years). Four patients await follow-up. Twenty eight of the 38 patients had a good outcome (no further TIAs, stroke or seizures, no headaches, improvement in cognitive functions in 5/9 patients), fair outcome was seen

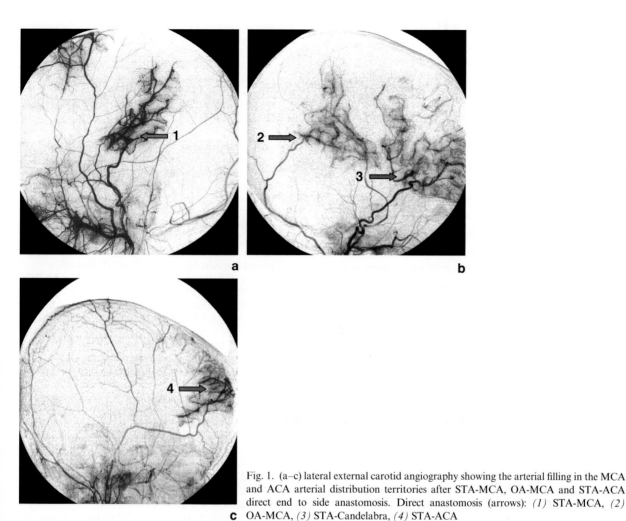

Fig. 1. (a–c) lateral external carotid angiography showing the arterial filling in the MCA and ACA arterial distribution territories after STA-MCA, OA-MCA and STA-ACA direct end to side anastomosis. Direct anastomosis (arrows): *(1)* STA-MCA, *(2)* OA-MCA, *(3)* STA-Candelabra, *(4)* STA-ACA

in 8/38 patients (fewer TIAs, less headache episodes, improvement of speech function, repeat hemorrhage in one adult patient). Acute postoperative clinical worsening was seen in one patient with contralateral ischemia and in another patient with contralateral MCA territorial infarct with massive cerebral edema resulting in death in this patient. Postoperative angiographies performed at 3 months demonstrated functional and effective direct anastomosis, as seen with arterial filling in the distribution territories of the respective cortical arteries (STA-MCA, STA-ACA) as seen in Fig. 1. The noticeable effect of indirect durasynangiosis and arteriosynangiosis was not always seen at 3 months hence demonstrating the immediate effect and usefulness of a direct anastomosis compared to the indirect method of revascularisation. Improvement of cerebral perfusion reserves on postoperative diamox challenge $H_2^{15}O$-PET examinations was seen in 68%

of the patients with unchanged perfusion reserves in the rest of the patients. No worsening of perfusion reserves, nor any steal phenomenon were observed.

Discussion

Over the past few years we have developed a systematic presurgical workup protocol for patients with Moyamoya angiopathy at our neurosurgery Department of the University hospital in Zürich directing us in the planning of the optimal surgical procedure for each individual patient. In recent literature on Moyamoya angiopathy the direct and indirect methods of revascularisation have been extensively reported and compared with each other [2–12]. In our present experience the direct EC-IC bypass cerebral revascularisation procedure is and remains the gold standard in the management of Moyamoya angiopathy in children and adults. Also multiple, direct EC-IC bypass procedures are advocated and performed when possible. The choice of the number of bypasses to be performed depends greatly on the preoperative angiographical staging and most importantly on the cerebral hemodynamic reserve capacities measures with $H_2^{15}O$-PET examinations. When a direct bypass is technically not possible (unavailability of or too small donor or cortical vessel calibre) indirect revascularisation procedures like durasynangiosis, arteriosynangiosis are performed. The cerebral perfusion status in the frontal region needs special attention. Since Moyamoya in children younger than 5 years with repeated frontal ischemia can be devastating in terms of mental and cognitive development, prevention of severe mental retardation therefore justifies early surgical intervention in the frontal region. The role of direct surgical revascularisation of the anterior circulation is therefore to be further developed and customarised [7, 12].

Conclusion

Our present experience provides evidence for the need of early detection of the Moyamoya angiopathy, especially in children, and the usefulness of multiple direct microanastomosis for effective revascularisation in the affected ACA, MCA and PCA regions of interest. This supports the revival of the long forgotten direct extracranial – intracranial EC-IC bypass procedure and hence the importance and indispensable role of microsurgery per se and the need for its continuing use in further training in neurosurgery.

References

1. Fukui M (1997) Current state of study on moyamoya disease in Japan. Review. Surg Neurol 47: 138–143
2. Golby AJ, Marks MP, Thompson RC, Steinberg GK (1999) Direct and combined revascularization in pediatric moyamoya disease. Neurosurgery 45: 50–60
3. Houkin K, Kamiyama H, Takahashi A, Kuroda S, Abe H (1997) Combined revascularization surgery for childhood moyamoya disease: STA-MCA and encephalo-duro-arterio-myo-synangiosis. Childs Nerv Syst 13: 24–29
4. Houkin K, Kuroda S, Ishikawa T, Abe H (2000) Neovascularization (angiogenesis) after revascularization in moyamoya disease. Which technique is most useful for moyamoya disease? Acta Neurochir (Wien) 142: 269–276
5. Houkin K, Kuroda S, Nakayama N (2001) Cerebral revascularization for moyamoya disease in children. Neurosurg Clin N Am 12: 575–584
6. Ikezaki K (2000) Rational approach to treatment of moyamoya disease in childhood. Review. J Child Neurol 15: 350–356
7. Iwama T, Hashimoto N, Tsukahara T, Miyake H (1997) Superficial temporal artery to anterior cerebral artery direct anastomosis in patients with moyamoya disease. Clin Neurol Neurosurg [Suppl] 2 99: 134–136
8. Khan N, Schuknecht B, Boltshauser E, Capone A, Buck A, Imhof HG, Yonekawa Y (2003) Moyamoya disease and Moyamoya syndrome: experience in Europe; choice of revascularisation procedures. Acta Neurochir (Wien) 145: 1061–1071
9. Matsushima T, Fujiwara S, Nagata S, Fujii K, Fukui M, Kitamura K, Hasuo K (1989) Surgical treatment for paediatric patients with moyamoya disease by indirect revascularization procedures (EDAS, EMS, EMAS). Acta Neurochir (Wien) 98: 135–140
10. Matsushima T, Inoue T, Ikezaki K, Imamura T (1998) Multiple indirect procedure for the surgical treatment of children with moyamoya disease. A comparison with single indirect anastomosis with direct anastomosis. Neurosurg Focus 5: 1–5
11. Scott RM (1995) Surgical treatment of moyamoya syndrome in children. Pediatr Neurosurg 22: 39–48
12. Suzuki Y, Negoro M, Shibuya M, Yoshida J, Negoro T, Watanabe K (1997) Surgical treatment for pediatric moyamoya disease: Use of the superficial temporal artery for both areas supplied by the anterior and middle cerebral arteries. Neurosurgery 40: 324–330
13. Takeuchi K, Shimizu K (1957) Hypoplasia of the bilateral internal carotid arteries. Brain and Nerve 9: 37–43
14. Yonekawa Y, Goto Y, Ogata N (1992) Moyamoya disease: Diagnosis, treatment and recent achievement. Part IV. Specific medical disease and stroke. In: Barnett HJ, Mohr JP, Stein BM, Yatsu FM (eds) Stroke: pathophysiology, diagnosis, management. Livingstone, New York, pp 721–747
15. Yonekawa Y, Handa H, Okuno T (1988) Moyamoya disease diagnosis, treatment and recent achievement. Stroke 1: 805–829
16. Yonekawa Y, Khan N (2003) Moyamoya disease. Review. Adv Neurol 92: 113–118
17. Yonekawa Y, Taub E (1999) Moyamoya disease: Status 1998 Neurologist 5: 13–23

Correspondence: Nadia Khan, Neurochirurgische Universitätsklinik Zurich, Frauenklinikstrasse 10, 8091 Zurich, Switzerland. e-mail: nadia.khan@usz.ch

Acta Neurochir (2005) [Suppl] 94: 153–157
© Springer-Verlag 2005
Printed in Austria

Cerebral revascularization model in a swine

M. Reinert[1], **C. Brekenfeld**[2], **P. Taussky**[1], **R. Andres**[1], **A. Barth**[1], and **R. W. Seiler**[1]

[1] Department of Neurosurgery, University Hospital of Bern, Bern, Switzerland
[2] Department of Neuroradiology, University Hospital of Bern, Bern, Switzerland

Summary

The purpose of this study was to analyze the suitability of the cerebral vasculature of the pig regarding a revascularization procedure.

In two 60 kg pigs the femoral artery was exposed and canulated for selective angiography and interventional procedures. After the angiography, the pigs were brought to the animal OR for craniotomy and analysis of the intracranial cerebral arteries and the surgical exposure of the carotid arteries under the microscope.

Angiography demonstrated the presence of a true internal-, external carotid artery and vertebral arteries. Both the vertebral and internal carotid arteries are feeding a rete mirabilis both at the cranial base and the cranio-cervical junction. At these sites further advancement of the angiography catheter was not possible. Out of these rete mirabilis, an intracranial carotid artery and an intracranial vertebral artery were formed, respectively. The intracranial cerebral vessels were of the dimension of 1 mm and less. The extracranial portion of the internal carotid artery was 2.5 mm of diameter.

From these findings, we conclude that a direct cerebral revascularization procedure of the intracranial vessels is not possible in the swine. However, a global revascularization procedure on the extracranial portion of the internal carotid artery is thus feasible, both using a low- and high-flow anastamosis technique.

Keywords: Cerebral revascularization; model; pig; angiography; anatomy.

Introduction

Cerebral revascularization is being performed in patients with moyamoya disease by using a direct extracranial-intracranial (EC-IC) anastomosis technique [7]. Further cerebral revascularization is indicated in patients suffering of large blood vessels anomalies such as aneurysms or carotid occlusion [6, 10]. In these patients a direct high-flow anastomosis technique may be necessary by using a technique without any temporary occlusion. The development of new diagnostic techniques such as the $^{15}O_2$ extraction method in the positron emission tomography (PET) has led to the analysis of patients having a hemodynamic compromise. Patients with clinical symptomatic carotid occlusion and increased hemispheric oxygen extraction fraction (OEF) > 1.130 may benefit of a surgical revascularization procedure [1, 2, 9]. In ongoing multicenter studies in Japan (Japanese Carotid Atherosclerosis Study: JCST) [2] and the United States (carotid occlusion surgery study: COSS) [2] [4] patients are being recruited. The recent reports of the interim analysis in both studies are in favour for the combined surgically and medically treated group [8].

The possibility of measuring the OEF prior and after a revascularization procedure has led to the idea of comparing two surgical procedures, such as a standard EC-IC bypass and an excimer laser assisted non-occlusive anastomosis (ELANA)-technique, which is basically an immediate high-flow anastomosis without any temporary occlusion [5]. An appropriate animal model is thus necessary. The literature of the cerebral vasculature of the pig was however not conclusive on the exact anatomy and blood flow territory of the internal carotid artery [3] and the role of the rete mirabilis at the cranial base.

Prior to starting any PET and revascularization study, the exact anatomical situation and possible operative and interventional approaches need to be defined.

Materials and methods

Two 60 kg pigs were sedated with atropine, xylazine and ketamine. An intravenous line was placed in the ear. Anesthesia was initiated with thiopentone and the animals were then intubated and ventilated. Anesthesia was maintained with fentanyl and thiopentone. The femoral artery was surgically exposed and canulated with a 6 french catheter sheath for selective angiography and interventional procedures. Thereafter, the animals were transported to the angiography-suite (CAS500, Toshiba Ltd. Japan, Matrix 1024 × 1024, biplanar).

The following procedures were performed in Pig 1

Selective angiography of the truncus bicaroticus, common carotid, right internal and external artery, left internal and external carotid artery was performed. Thereafter, both vertebral arteries were selectively canulated. The animal was then transported to the animal operating theatre. A right sided craniectomy to the skull base was performed. The dura was opened and the brain was exposed. From the cranial base, the intracranial portion of the internal carotid artery, following the rete mirabilis, was exposed and followed to the first bifurcation.

The following procedures were performed in Pig 2

After selective angiography with a microcatheter, the left internal carotid artery was occluded with coils up to the rete mirabilis. Thereafter a left external carotid angiogram was performed, followed by canulation of the right internal carotid artery and occlusion with coils. The occlusion was documented and collaterals from the external carotid artery were assessed by a control angiogram of the common carotid artery. Next, the vertebral artery was catheterized and a vertebrobasilar angiogram was performed. The animal was then brought to the animal operating theatre. On both sides the common carotid, internal and external carotid arteries were exposed. Finally, the arteries were excised including the intravascular coils.

Intraoperativ images were performed using a digital camera (Sony DSC-T1 and Nikon Coolpix 990). The images were processed using Corel Draw® (Corel-Draw 9.0, Ottawa, Canada).

Results

The pig has a truncus bicaroticus which splits into a left and right common carotid artery. The common carotid artery divides into an internal and external carotid artery. The internal carotid arteries supply the major part of the brain except the brain stem and the cerebellum. The extracranial portion of the internal carotid artery ends in a rete mirabilis, which is a sort of vascular sponge out of which forms the intracranial portion of the internal carotid artery.

The intracranial portion of the internal carotid artery then divides into the caudal communicating artery and the end-segment of the internal carotid artery. The first branch leaving the internal carotid artery is the caudal communicating artery. The internal carotid artery then turns rostrally to give off several smaller middle cerebral arteries. From this point, the artery is called rostral cerebral artery (Figs. 1 and 2).

The extracranial vertebral artery also ends in a caudal rete mirabilis just at the cranio-caudal junction before entering the dura. This caudal rete mirabilis is, however, not as prominent as the rostral one. Out of this caudal rete mirabilis results an intracranial vertebral artery which then gives rise to the basilar artery together with the contralateral vertebral artery (Fig. 1d).

Selective angiography of the extracranial portion of the internal carotid artery showed "primitive" arteries between the internal carotid arteries and the basilar artery (Fig. 1b).

Angiographic dimensions of the extracranial and intracranial vessels

The extracranial internal carotid artery measured 2.5 mm in diameter at the bifurcation. Before entering the rete mirabilis the internal carotid artery measured 2 mm. The internal carotid artery following the rete mirabilis was of the dimension of 1 mm in diameter (Fig. 1b). The diameter of the rostral artery and the caudal communicating artery was of 0.5 mm and 0.4 mm respectively. The intracranial vertebral artery and basilar artery diameters were below 1 mm.

Coil occlusion of the internal carotid arteries

After occlusion of the left internal carotid artery with coils, a strong collateralization via the rete mirabilis from the right side was seen (Fig. 1c). After occlusion of both internal carotid arteries, the vertebral angiography showed a fine contrast filling in the anterior circulation via the caudal communicating artery. The external carotid angiogram showed that it is not involved in the perfusion of the brain except with a tiny contrast filling over an ethmoidal anastomosis. The ophthalmic artery splits off from the external carotid artery. Selective injection of the vertebral artery after occlusion of both internal carotid arteries leads to a contrast filling of the caudal communicating arteries

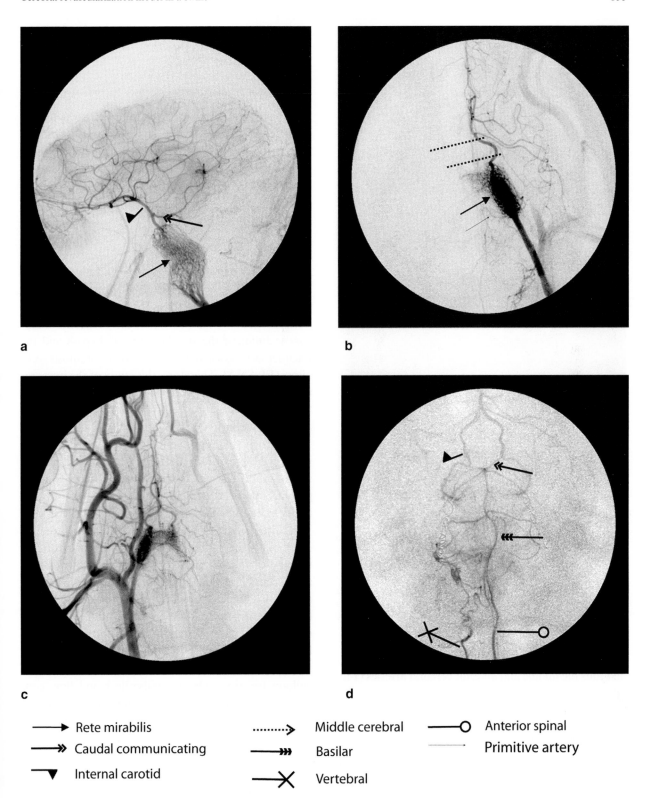

Fig. 1. (a) Lateral left internal carotid angiogram showing the rete mirabilis, the caudal communicating artery and the intracranial carotid artery. (b) Anterior-posterior left internal carotid artery angiogram showing the primitive artery, the rete mirabilis and the middle cerebral artery branches. (c) Anterior-posterior right common carotid angiogram after coiling of the left internal carotid artery: showing the cross-flow over the rete mirabilis. (d) Anterior-posterior right vertebral angiogram after coiling of both internal carotid arteries: showing the right vertebral artery, the anterior spinal artery, the basilar artery, the caudal communicating artery and the internal carotid artery

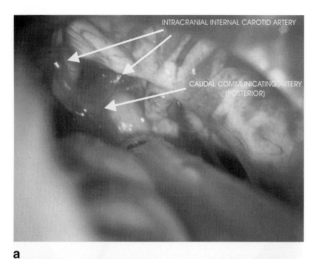

a

b

Fig. 2. (a) Intraoperative view of the internal carotid splitting into the caudal communicating artery and the end-segment of the internal carotid artery. (b) Operative exposure of the common carotid, internal and external carotid arteries. This exposure is suitable for performing a high flow anastomosis, using for example the excimer laser assisted high-flow anastomosis technique. The schematic bypass is shown in green. In this exposure, the occlusion of the carotid artery is induced by coiling of the vessel lumen

and thus the middle and anterior cerebral arteries (Fig. 1d).

Intraoperative situs

Rightsided craniectomy

The craniectomy or craniotomy is a laborious bony work, to finally reach the dura. After opening of the dura under the operating microscope and retraction of the brain, the intracranial carotid artery was demonstrated, as well as its branches. These vessels were

extremely fine, with a diameter of 1 mm for the intracranial carotid artery (Fig. 2a).

Preparation of the carotid arteries

The preparation of the carotid arteries was technically achieved without any complications. The common carotid artery was 3.2 mm in diameter, depending of manipulation and thus vasospasm. The internal carotid artery at the bifurcation site was 2.5 mm in diameter (Fig. 2b).

Discussion

The purpose of this study was to find out if a swine model is suitable for a cerebral revascularization procedure. The specific aim was to assess the swine as a possible model to test the difference between two bypass techniques: the standard EC-IC bypass and the Excimer laser assisted non-occlusive anastamosis technique (ELANA). Therefore, this study of the intracranial blood vessel situation and dimensions was performed as the situation could not be clarified from the accessible literature.

Four new findings were observed in this study, which were previously not expressly stated. First, the rete mirabilis can not be passed by a selective angiographic microcatheter. Second, the external carotid artery does not participate in the cerebral perfusion. The third finding is that the intracranial anatomical situation is such that a microvascular anastomosis technique is at the limit of the technically possible, and certainly not suitable for an ELANA-Bypass procedure. The fourth finding is the difference of the diameters of the internal carotid artery prior to and after the rete mirabilis, eventhough there were no other vessels leaving the rete mirabilis. We hypothesize that this may only be possible if the rete mirabilis has a sort of balloon function, where a pulsatile blood flow converges into a more continuous blood flow. A higher flow rate could also be possible but is less probable to our view since the blood pressure decrease over the rete mirabilis must be considerable.

An experimental revascularization procedure can, however, still be considered in the swine, by performing a bypass on the extracranial portion of the internal carotid artery. By doing this we could test the difference in OEF using a low-flow versus a high-flow bypass technique. The practicability of this new setup will be tested in another series of pigs.

References

1. Derdeyn CP, Videen TO, Grubb RL Jr, Powers WJ (2001) Comparison of PET oxygen extraction fraction methods for the prediction of stroke risk. J Nucl Med 42: 1195–1197
2. Endo S, Kuwayama N, Hirashima Y (2004) Japan carotid atherosclerosis study: JCAS. Neurol Med Chir (Tokyo) 44: 215–217
3. Getty R (1975) The anatomy of the domestic animal, 5th edn. Saunders, Philadelphia London Toronto, pp 1309–1320
4. Grubb RL, Powers WJ, Derdeyn CP, Adams HP, Clarke WR (2003) The carotid occlusion surgery study. Neurosurg Focus 14: Article 9
5. Kappelle LJ, Klijn CJ, Tulleken CA (2002) Management of patients with symptomatic carotid artery occlusion. Clin Exp Hypertens 24: 631–637
6. Kato Y, Sano H, Imizu S, Yoneda M, Viral M, Nagata J, Kanno T (2003) Surgical strategies for treatment of giant or large intracranial aneurysms: our experience with 139 cases. Minim Invasive Neurosurg 46: 339–343
7. Khan N, Schuknecht B, Boltshauser E, Capone A, Buck A, Imhof HG, Yonekawa Y (2003) Moyamoya disease and moyamoya syndrome: experience in Europe; choice of revascularisation procedures. Acta Neurochir (Wien) 145: 1061–1071
8. Kuwayama N (2004) 2nd Swiss Japanese Joint Conference on Cerebral Stroke. University Hospital Zurich
9. Neff KW, Horn P, Dinter D, Vajkoczy P, Schmiedek P, Duber C (2004) Extracranial-intracranial arterial bypass surgery improves total brain blood supply in selected symptomatic patients with unilateral internal carotid artery occlusion and insufficient collateralization. Neuroradiology (print)
10. Nussbaum ES, Mendez A, Camarata P, Sebring L (2003) Surgical management of fusiform aneurysms of the peripheral posteroinferior cerebellar artery. Neurosurgery 53: 831–835

Correspondence: Michael Reinert, Klinik für Neurochirurgie, Inselspital Bern, Universität Bern, 3010 Bern, Switzerland. e-mail: michael.reinert@neurochirurgie-bern.ch

Acta Neurochir (2005) [Suppl] 94: 159–163
© Springer-Verlag 2005
Printed in Austria

Prediction of cerebral blood flow restoration after extracranial-intracranial bypass surgery using superficial temporal artery duplex ultrasonography (STDU)

T. Inoue[1] and **S. Fujimoto**[2]

[1] Department of Neurosurgery, Cerebrovascular Center and Clinical Research Institute, National Hospital Organization Kyushu Medical Center, Fukuoka, Japan
[2] Cerebrovascular Disease, Cerebrovascular Center and Clinical Research Institute, National Hospital Organization Kyushu Medical Center, Fukuoka, Japan

Summary

We investigated the availability of superficial temporal artery (STA) duplex ultrasonography (STDU) for evaluating the improvement of cerebral hemodynamics after extracranial-intracranial (EC-IC) bypass. This study included 56 consecutive patients who underwent EC-IC bypass for occlusive disease of their cerebral arteries. STA duplex ultrasonography (STDU) was performed to measure the flow velocity, pulsatility index, and diameter of ipsilateral STA before and 14 days after EC-IC bypass. Regional cerebral blood flow (rCBF) and acetazolamide (ACZ) reactivity of ipsilateral MCA territory were evaluated by quantitative single photon emission computed tomography. The mean flow velocities of ipsilateral STA were significantly higher ($p < 0.0001$) and PI value was significantly lower ($p < 0.0001$) 14 days after EC-IC bypass than before. The diameter of ipsilateral STA was also larger 14 days after EC-IC bypass than before ($p < 0.0001$). STA mean flow velocity was significantly correlated with the rCBF 14 days after EC-IC bypass ($R = 0.55$, $p < 0.0001$). The post-surgical STA mean flow velocity cut-off value over 58.2 cm/sec yielded the highest diagnostic accuracy (sensitivity, 75%; specificity, 74%) for excellent rCBF value (≥ 40 ml/100 g/min) after EC-IC bypass. The ipsilateral STA mean blood flow velocity is a highly sensitive parameter for predicting rCBF in the ipsilateral MCA territory after EC-IC bypass.

Keywords: EC-IC bypass; duplex ultrasonography; cerebral blood flow.

Introduction

Extracranial-intracranial (EC-IC) bypass surgery is a well known method to increase the regional cerebral blood flow (rCBF) and to improve the cerebral hemodynamic failure [7]. The randomized trial on strictly selected patients with severe cerebral hemodynamic failure has just been finalised in Japan (Japan EC-IC bypass Trial: JET study). In the interim report of JET study (JET Study Group, personal communication),

EC-IC bypass was effective in reducing major stroke or death for 2 years after surgery for patients with severe hemispheric hemodynamic failure due to cerebral artery occlusive disease [4].

After an EC-IC bypass procedure, patients should be required to undergo postoperative evaluation whether cerebral hemodynamics have improved. Since single photon emission computed tomography (SPECT) and positron emission tomography (PET) for the measurement of cerebral hemodynamics are expensive, complicated, and time consuming, they may not be appropriate modalities to use repeatedly after EC-IC bypass.

Arakawa *et al.* [1] reported for the first time the availability of STA flow velocity measured by duplex ultrasonography for evaluating the extent of the collateral flow through STA-MCA anastomosis. They indicated that the end diastolic flow velocity ratio of the operated STA to the contralateral STA is a highly sensitive parameter for prediction of the angiogram-documented bypass flow in patients who underwent this procedure unilaterally. Encouraged by their results, in the present study we aimed to investigate the availability of STA duplex ultrasonography (STDU) for evaluating the improvement of cerebral hemodynamics after EC-IC bypass.

Subjects and methods

Patients

Fifty six consecutive patients who underwent EC-IC bypass procedure for cerebral artery occlusive diseases in our Cerebrovascular

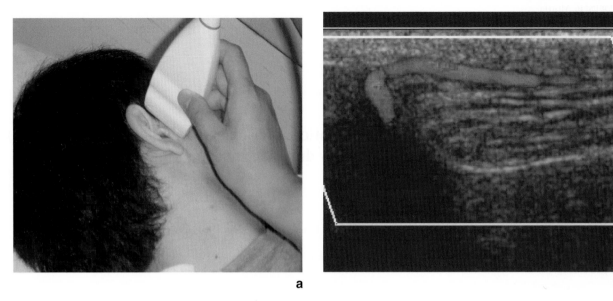

                                                                                                                              a   b

Fig. 1. STDU study. The transducer was placed in the temporal region before the external opening of the acoustic canal (a) and STA was displayed on the B-mode image with color Doppler (b)

Center from June 2001 to January 2004 were prospectively included in the present study. All patients gave informed consent to undergo cerebral angiography and EC-IC bypass procedure. In accordance with the entry criteria of the JET study, we adopted the following criteria as indication for EC-IC bypass: a) symptomatic internal carotid artery (ICA)/MCA stenosis of $\geq 70\%$ in diameter or occlusion; b) fair activities of daily life corresponding to modified Rankin Scale of 2 or less; c) small or no brain infarction on magnetic resonance imaging (MRI); and d) rCBF of the ipsilateral MCA less than 32 ml/100 g/min (corresponding to 80% of normal value) and acetazolamide (ACZ) reactivity less than 10% in quantitative SPECT study with ACZ challenge. Patients with a marginally greater rCBF and ACZ reactivity than the criterion were included in the present study only when they were diagnosed as having a moyamoya disease. The degree of carotid stenosis was assessed using cerebral digital subtraction angiography (DSA) with the method documented in the North American Symptomatic Carotid Endarterectomy Trial (NASCET) study [5]. All patients underwent DSA, MRI, and STDU before and 14 days after EC-IC bypass.

STDU

The Philips (USA) HDI-5000 with the 12-to-5 MHz linear array transducer was used. For the examinations of STA, each patient was examined in a supine position with his head turned away from the side to be scanned. The transducer was placed in the temporal region before the external opening of the acoustic canal and STA was displayed on the B-mode image with color Doppler (Fig. 1). The diameter of bilateral STA was measured. On the longitudinal scans, the sample volume was set within the STA at the point proximal to its bifurcation. The incident angle between the STA and the Doppler beam was kept at 60 degrees or less. Range-gated pulsed Doppler ultrasound was used to measure the blood flow velocity of the STA. Absolute values of peak-systolic (PSV), end-diastolic (EDV), and mean flow velocity (MFV) of bilateral STA were mea-

sured using the maximum frequency envelope. The pulsatility index (PI) for the individual arteries was calculated with the following formula: $PI = (PSV - EDV)/MFV$.

SPECT

The SPECT apparatus was the PRISM 2000X (two-head SPECT system, Picker, USA), and N-isopropil-p-[^{123}I]-iodoamphetamine (^{123}I-IMP) was used as the tracer. An elliptical region of interest (ROI), more than 16 cm^2 in size, was located in the cortical area in the MCA territory of each side. Areas of infarct, if present, were carefully excluded from the ROI. The resting rCBF values were measured quantitatively using the ARG method before and 14 days after CEA [2]. The rCBF values were also measured after the ACZ challenge test. Vasodilatory capacity (ACZ reactivity) was expressed using the following equation: ACZ reactivity = (post-ACZ CBF − resting rCBF)/resting rCBF. The rCBF after surgery was classified into 3 groups: excellent rCBF group (Group A; rCBF of the ipsilateral MCA was 40 ml/100 g/min or more); fair rCBF group (Group B; rCBF was 32 ml/100 g/min or more and less than 40 ml/100 g/min); and low rCBF group (Group C; rCBF was less than 32 ml/100 g/min).

Data analysis

Changes in parameters of both STDU and SPECT were observed, and the relationships between the parameters were investigated. The correlation between changes in rCBF of the MCA territory and the STA flow velocity was also evaluated. In univariate analysis, the chi-square test, paired t-test, and two-way repeated-measured ANOVA were used. Post hoc analysis was done using Scheffe's multiple comparison test. Linear-regression analysis and the Pearson Correlation Coefficient were used to evaluate the correlation between changes in rCBF of the MCA territory and the STA flow velocity. A p value < 0.05 was considered to be significant.

Table 1. *The parameters of STDU and SPECT before and after STA-MCA anastomosis*

		Before surgery	After surgery	p
STDU (STA)				
– Flow velocity	cm/sec			
Peak systolic		65.0 ± 20.6	89.6 ± 20.5	<0.0001
End diastolic		14.8 ± 5.4	39.8 ± 14.1	<0.0001
Mean		28.0 ± 8.9	56.8 ± 17.7	<0.0001
– PI		1.85 ± 0.53	0.93 ± 0.27	<0.0001
– Diameter	mm	1.56 ± 0.24	2.25 ± 0.40	<0.0001
SPECT (MCA terrotory)				
– rCBF	ml/100 g/min	29.7 ± 5.1	37.0 ± 7.4	<0.0001
– ACZ reactivity		0.04 ± 0.16	0.26 ± 0.21	<0.0001

Results

Patient demographics

Thirty six men and 20 women aged 57.1 ± 12.5 (mean ± SD) years were included. All of their cerebral artery occlusive diseases were symptomatic. Forty-four patients had brain infarction and 12 had transient ischemic attacks or transient monocular blindness.

Complications were not observed during any of the STA-MCA anastomosis procedures. New neurological symptoms did not occur in any patient during 14 days after surgery.

Angiographical and MRI findings

In the pre-surgical cerebral angiography, the vascular lesions were classified as follows: ICA occlusion in 30 (origin, 17; distal portion, 13), distal ICA stenosis in 9, MCA occlusion in 11, and MCA stenosis in 6. There were 14 patients with moyamoya disease. There were no extensive collateral pathways such as supplying blood flow to the entire MCA territory. In the cerebral angiography 14 days after EC-IC bypass, anastomosed bypass flow was patent in all patients.

The pre-surgical MRI studies revealed symptomatic or asymptomatic ischemic lesions in the ipsilateral ICA territory to the EC-IC bypass in 44 patients. There were not any new ischemic or hemorrhagic lesions on the MRI studies 14 days after EC-IC bypass.

STDU and SPECT findings

The peak-systolic, end-diastolic, and mean flow velocities of the ipsilateral STA were significantly higher (p < 0.0001 in each) and PI value was significantly lower (p < 0.0001) 14 days after EC-IC bypass than

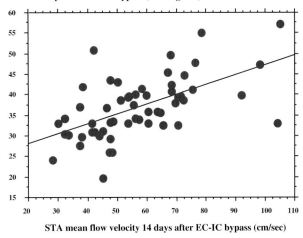

rCBF 14 days after EC-IC bypass (ml/100g/min)

STA mean flow velocity 14 days after EC-IC bypass (cm/sec)

Fig. 2. The post-surgical STA mean flow velocity according to the rCBF grade. The post-surgical rCBF grade of the MCA territory had significant association with the STA mean flow velocity (p < 0.001)

before (Table 1). The diameter of the ipsilateral STA was also larger 14 days after EC-IC bypass than before (p < 0.0001, Table 1). The rCBF and ACZ reactivity of the ipsilateral MCA territory were significantly higher 14 days after EC-IC bypass than before (p < 0.0001 and p < 0.0001, respectively, Table 1).

All 3 parameters of STA flow velocity were significantly correlated with the rCBF (p < 0.0001 in each). Among the 3 parameters, the mean flow velocity had the strongest correlation with the rCBF (R = 0.55, p < 0.0001, Fig. 2). The STA diameter did not have correlation with the rCBF. The ACZ reactivity was not correlated with any parameters of STDU.

The pre-surgical STA mean flow velocity or diameter did not differ among the 3 groups according to the post-surgical rCBF grade. The post-surgical STA mean flow velocity in Group C (42.9 ± 10.5 cm/

STA mean flow velocity 14 days after EC-IC bypass (cm/sec)

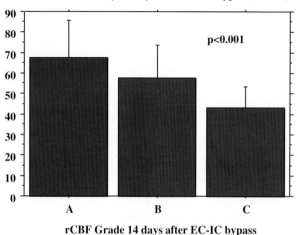

Fig. 3. Correlation between STA mean flow velocity and rCBF in the MCA territory 2 weeks after STA-MCA anastomosis

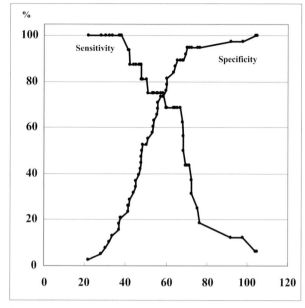

STA mean flow velocity 14 days after EC-IC bypass (cm/sec)

Fig. 4. Diagnostic accuracy of STA mean flow velocity for detection of excellent rCBF in the ipsilateral MCA territory after STA-MCA anastomosis

sec) was significantly lower than that in Group A (66.7 ± 21.2 cm/sec, p < 0.001) or Group B (58.1 ± 15.7 cm/sec, p < 0.05) (Fig. 3). On the other hand, the post-surgical diameter of the STA had no significant association with the post-surgical rCBF grade of the MCA territory. There was no significant difference as to changes in the ACZ reactivity among the 3 rCBF Groups.

Diagnostic accuracy of STA mean flow velocity for predicting rCBF of the MCA territory

With regard to the sensitivity-specificity curve analysis, the post-surgical STA mean flow velocity cut-off value over 58.2 cm/sec yielded the highest diagnostic accuracy (sensitivity; 75%, specificity; 74%) for favorable rCBF value (≥40 ml/100 g/min) after STA-MCA anastomosis (Fig. 4).

Discussions

This is the first report using STDU to assess changes in STA flow velocity and diameter before and after EC-IC bypass and to correlate these data with parameters obtained by SPECT.

In the present study, remarkable changes in the STA flow velocity, PI value, and diameter were observed and these could reflect the patency and effectiveness of the bypass flow. The PI value was well known as reflecting the vascular resistance. Commonly, the PI value in the external carotid artery (ECA) system was higher than that in the ICA system. A remarkable post-surgical decrease in PI value could mean that the ipsilateral STA flow became to be ICA pattern from ECA pattern. STA is a superficial artery, and is easily detectable by STDU. Moreover, STDU is noninvasive, repeatable, and available at bed side or outpatient clinic without any contraindications in comparison with SPECT, MRI, or DSA. Using STDU, we can easily and serially confirm the patency and changes in bypass flow via STA after EC-IC bypass.

The STA mean flow velocity was significantly correlated with the rCBF of the MCA territory after EC-IC bypass. Moreover, the post-surgical rCBF grade of the MCA territory had significant association with the STA mean flow velocity. In the present study, only the patients with severe cerebral hemodynamic failure were included according to the pre-surgical SPECT studies. The development in blood flow via STA-MCA anastomosis would have an association with pre-surgical cerebral hemodynamics. Previous studies revealed the relationships between an abundant blood flow via the anastomosed bypass and the pre-surgical reduced vasodilatory capacity [3, 6]. In our patients, both rCBF and ACZ reactivity of the ipsilateral MCA territory significantly increased after EC-IC bypass. However, the post-surgical cerebral angiography revealed no development in the natural intracranial collateral pathway such as leptomeningeal anastomosis or anterior and posterior communicating arteries. In patients with severe hemodynamic failure due to poor collateral pathway, an improvement in the cerebral hemodynamics could depend on the blood flow via STA-MCA anastomosis.

STA diameter had no significant correlation with the rCBF of the ipsilateral MCA territory. According to the post-surgical rCBF grade, there was no significant difference in STA diameter. In the process of the development in bypass flow via STA after EC-IC bypass, there might be a limitation in the post-surgical dilation of STA and the further increase in the STA blood flow might depend on an increase in the STA flow velocity.

Arakawa *et al.* [1] have reported that the end diastolic flow velocity ratio of the operated STA to the contralateral one is a highly sensitive parameter for evaluating the extent of the bypass flow in patients who underwent EC-IC bypass unilaterally. Combining our method with theirs, we can easily predict the post-surgical rCBF grade as well as the extent of the collateral flow through STA-MCA anastomosis instead of SPECT and cerebral angiography. In conclusion, STDU is a method available for evaluating cerebral hemodynamics in patients who undergo EC-IC bypass.

References

1. Arakawa S, Kamouchi M, Okada Y, Kishikawa K, Omae T, Inoue T, Ibayashi S, Fujishima M (2003) Ultrasonographically predicting the extent of collateral flow through superficial temporal artery-to-middle cerebral artery anastomosis. AJNR Am J Neuroradiol 24: 886–891
2. Iida H, Itoh H, Nakazawa M, Hatazawa J, Nishimura H, Onishi Y, Uemura K (1994) Quantitative mapping of regional cerebral blood flow using iodine-123-IMP and SPECT. J Nucl Med 35: 2019–2030
3. Iwama T, Hashimoto N, Takagi Y, Tsukahara T, Hayashida K (1997) Predictability of extracranial/intracranial bypass function: a retrospective study of patients with occlusive cerebrovascular disease. Neurosurgery 40: 53–60
4. JET Study Group. Japanese EC-IC trial (JET study): study design and interim analysis (in Japanese). (2002) Surg Cereb Stroke. (Jpn) 30: 97–100
5. North American Symptomatic Carotid Endarterectomy Trial Collaborators (1991). Beneficial effect of carotid endarterectomy in symptomatic patients with high-grade carotid stenosis. N Engl J Med 325: 445–453
6. Yamashita T, Kashiwagi S, Nakano S, Takasago T, Abiko S, Shiroyama Y, Hayashi M, Ito H (1991) The effect of EC-IC bypass surgery on resting cerebral blood flow and cerebrovascular reserve capacity studied with stable XE-CT and acetazolamide test. Neuroradiology 33: 217–222
7. Yasargil MG (1960) Diagnosis and indications for operations in cerebrovascular disease. Chapter 4B. In: Yasargil MG (ed) Microsurgery. Applied to neurosurgery. Thieme, Stuttgart New York London, pp 95–119

Correspondence: Tooru Inoue, Department of Neurosurgery and Clinical Research Institute, National Hospital Organization Kyushu Medical Center, 1-8-1 Jigyohama, Chuo-ku, Fukuoka 810-8563, Japan. e-mail: fujimoto@qmed.hosp.go.jp

Venous system

Acta Neurochir (2005) [Suppl] 94: 167–175
© Springer-Verlag 2005
Printed in Austria

Neurosurgery and the intracranial venous system

M. Sindou[1], **J. Auque**[2], and **E. Jouanneau**[1]

[1] Department of Neurosurgery, Hopital Neurologique, University of Lyon, Lyon, France
[2] Department of Neurosurgery, Centre Hospitalo-Universitaire, University of Nancy, Nancy, France

Summary

Neurosurgery and the intracranial venous system

1) Numerous of the so-called «unpredictable» post-operative complications are likely to be related to the lack of prevention or non-recognition of venous problems, especially damages to the dangerous venous structures, namely: the major dural sinuses, the deep cerebral veins and some of the dominant superficial veins like the vein of Labbé.
2) Tumors invading the major dural sinuses (superior sagittal sinus, torcular, transverse sinus) – especially meningiomas – leave the surgeon confronted with a dilemma: leave the fragment invading the sinus and have a higher risk of recurrence, or attempt at total removal with or without venous reconstruction and expose the patient to a potentially greater operative danger. Such situations have been encountered in 106 patients over the last 25 years. For decision-making, meningiomas were classified into six types according to the degree of sinus invasion. Type 1: meningioma attached to outer surface of the sinus wall; Type II: one lateral recess invaded; Type III: one lateral wall invaded; Type IV: one lateral wall and the roof of the sinus both invaded; Types V and VI: sinus totally occluded, one wall being free of tumor in type V.

In brief, our surgical policy was the following: *Type I*: excision of outer layer and coagulation of dural attachment; *Type II*: removal of intraluminal fragment through the recess, then repair of the dural defect by resuturing recess. *Type III*: resection of sinus wall and repair with patch (fascia temporalis). *Type IV*: resection of both invaded walls and reconstruction of the two resected walls with patch. *Type V*: this type can be recognized from type VI only by direct surgical exploration of the sinus lumen. Opposite wall to the tumor side is free of tumor, it is possible to reconstruct the two resected walls with patch. *Type VI*: removal of involved portion of sinus and restoration with venous bypass.
3) As 20% of the patients presenting with manifestations of intracranial hypertension due to occlusion of posterior third of the superior sagittal sinus, torcular, predominant lateral sinus or internal jugular vein(s) develop severe intracranial hypertension, venous revascularisation by sino-jugular bypass – implanted proximally to the occlusion and directed to the jugular venous system (external or internal jugular vein) – can be a solution.

Keywords: Cerebral veins; dural sinuses; intracranial venous system; parasagittal meningiomas; vascular microsurgery; venous occlusion; venous reconstruction.

Introduction

No doubt that numbers of harmful events after intracranial surgery are related to iatrogenic venous damages. They manifest as locally-developed oedema, regional or diffuse brain swelling – some being fatal because of uncontrollable intracranial hypertension – and/or hemorrhagic infarcts, sometimes devastating and erroneously attributed to so-called default in hemostasis.

Ignoring the cerebral venous system during surgery would entail disastrous consequences; therefore good knowledge of venous anatomy and physiology is of prime importance [5, 13, 26, 30, 39]. A complete and detailed pre-operative setting including venous angio-MR, and if necessary DSA with late venous phases, helps to determine optimal surgical strategy. A sustained effort during surgery to respect the venous system, especially the so-called "dangerous veins", is an obligation for the surgeon.

Radical removal of tumors invading the major dural sinuses implicates to preserve and/or repair the venous circulation. Also, restoration of the venous flow may contribute to the cure of neurological diseases due to impairment in venous circulation.

Preservation of the «dangerous» venous structures

Injury or acute occlusion of important intracranial venous structures during surgery might provoke brain swelling and/or venous hemorrhagic infarcts, that could lead to vital or at least severe functional disturbances.

The dural sinuses

The major dural sinuses carry a considerable amount of blood; foremost the superior sagittal sinus (SSS). Its anterior third receives the prefrontal afferent veins; its posterior radiological landmark is around the coronal suture. It is generally admitted that its sacrifice is well tolerated. Actually, severe mental disorders, personality changes, loss of recent memory with a general slowing of thought processes and activity, or even akinetic mutism, may occur if sacrificed and/or if frontal veins are compromised. The midthird receives the numerous and voluminous cortical veins of the central group. Interruption of this portion entails high risks of (bilateral) hemiplegia and akinesia. The posterior third, as well as the torcular Herophili which receives the straight sinus, drains a considerable amount of blood. Interruption would inevitably provokes potentially fatal intracranial hypertension.

The lateral sinuses (LS) ensure a symetric drainage in only 20% of the cases; in the extreme, one LS may drain the SSS in totality (most often the right one) and the other the straight sinus.

The transverse sinus (TS) may be atretic on one side, the remaining sigmoid sinus draining the inferior cerebral veins (i.e. the Labbé system). The sigmoid sinus (SS) drains the posterior fossa. It receives the superior and the inferior petrosal sinuses and also (unconstant) veins coming from the lateral aspect of pons and medulla. SS has frequent anastomoses with the cutaneous venous network through the mastoid emissary vein. When the sigmoid segment of the lateral sinus is atretic, the transverse sinus with its affluents drains toward the opposite side.

All these anatomical configurations (see details in reference 2) have surgical implications and must be taken into account before considering interrupting sinus.

The superficial veins

Any of the superficial veins of a certain calibre has presumably a functional role. However, as shown by experience, some of them are more "dangerous" to sacrifice than others. The superficial veins belong to three "systems": the midline afferents to the SSS, the inferior cerebral afferents to the TS and the superficial sylvian afferents to the cavernous sinus. These three systems are strongly interconnected, but in very variable ways from one individual case to another. The main anastomotic veins are the Trolard, the Labbé and the great superficial sylvian, all of them bearing important surgical implications.

Midline afferent veins enter into the SSS. They are met during interhemispheric approaches [22]. 70% of parasagittal venous drainage is evident within the sector two cm posterior to the coronal suture; it corresponds to the central group. Sacrifice of the midline central group is risky. The sacrifice of the other midline veins, unless they are of large calibre, does not appear so hazardous. The vein of Trolard, or superior anastomotic vein, links the superficial sylvian system to the SSS. It usually penetrates the SSS in the post-central region.

Inferior cerebral veins are cortical bridging veins that channel into the basal sinuses and/or into the deep venous system. They are met in the skull base approaches. Juxta-basal veins may be sacrificed only if they are small and do not contribute predominantly to the system of Labbé. The vein of Labbé, or inferior anastomotic vein, creates an anastomosis between the superficial sylvian vein and the TS before its junction with the SS. Necessity of the respect of Labbé, especially in the dominant hemisphere, is mandatory to avoid posterior hemispheric infarction.

The superficial sylvian vein is formed by anastomosis of the temporo-sylvian veins; these veins are connected with the midline veins upward and the juxta-basal temporal veins downward. It enters predominantly the cavernous sinus, either directly or through the sphenoparietal sinus. Many variations are possible. Sacrificing the superficial sylvian vein is risky when it is of large calibre and poorly anastomosed.

Skull base approaches must be prepared taking into account the anatomical organization of the superficial venous system (see details and literature quotations in reference 5) (Fig. 1).

The deep veins of the brain

The deep veins of the brain are the ones which drain toward the deep venous confluent of Galen. The denomination of venous confluent is appropriate since – in addition to the two internal cerebral veins – the Galenic system receives the two basilar veins of Rosenthal, and also veins from the corpus callosum, the cerebellum (mainly the vermian precentral vein) and the occipital cortex. A good knowledge of the deep veins is important for surgery in the lateral ventricles

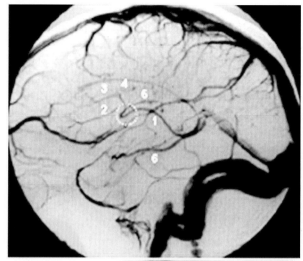

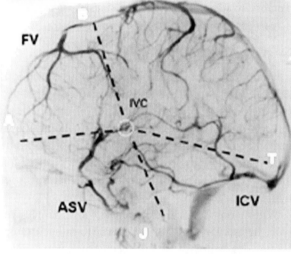

Fig. 1. *Top: Deep cerebral veins (V) and landmark of the interventricular venous confluent (IVC)*: DSA by carotid injection, venous phase, lateral view. The interventricular venous confluent (dotted circle) is formed by confluence of the septal V *(2)*, caudate V *(3, 4)*, and thalamo-striate V *(5)*. Confluence gives rise to the internal cerebral vein *(1)*. On lateral view, this confluent has an almost – constant situation and corresponds to the interventricular foramen of Monro. This point may contribute a useful anatomical – imaging reference. [NB: basilar vein *(6)*; confluence of internal cerebral veins and basilar veins gives Galen Vein. *Bottom: Superficial veins involved in (supratentorial) skull base approaches*: Three groups of veins can be distinguished: the middle afferent frontal V, the inferior cerebral V (i.e. the Labbé system) and the sylvian V. These three groups can be delimited by three "triangles". (1) The triangle corresponding to the frontal group of veins *(FV)* is delimited by the three following landmarks: interventricular venous confluent *(IVC)*, bregma *(B)* and the anterior limit of anterior cranial fossa *(A)*. (2) The triangle corresponding to the inferior group *(ICV)* is delimited by: IVC, Torcular *(T)* and Jugular foramen *(J)*. (3) The triangle corresponding to the anterior sylvian group *(ASV)* is delimited by: IVC, A and J landmarks. Skull base approaches must be designed so that the proeminent venous drainage(s) be respected

and of course in the third ventricle and pineal region [4, 6, 38]. There is a general agreement that the sacrifice of the vein of Galen or of one of its main tributaries should be considered as a high risk, although animal experiments and a few reported clinical observations showed otherwise.

The thalamostriate vein represents an important anatomic landmark when accessing the third ventricle through the lateral ventricle by the interthalamotrigonal approach. It drains the deep white matter of the hemisphere, the internal capsule and the caudate nucleus. This vein has to be sometimes sacrified in this approach. Consequences vary depending on the authors: from little or none to venous infarction of basal ganglia. Because consequences can be severe, sacrificing the thalamostriate vein is justified only if widening the exposure of the third ventricle is absolutely necessary [11].

Veins of the posterior fossa

It is important to consider venous anatomy when dealing with posterior fossa surgery [20, 28]. The sitting position entails the risk of air embolism from sinus and/or vein opening. The cerebellum is exposed to swelling or infarction in case of venous interruption.

Most experts in posterior fossa surgery, especially those who favor infratentorial supracerebellar approaches, estimate that the sacrifice of the precentral vermian vein in order to approach the pineal region is without danger.

The classical statement that the superior petrosal vein can be interrupted without danger needs to be reconsidered. As a matter of fact, swelling of the cerebellar hemisphere after sacrificing a voluminous petrosal vein is not unfrequently observed.

Avoidance of venous occlusions during surgery

The role played by venous occlusions occurring during surgery in post-operative hemorrhagic infarcts is undeniable [3, 19]. Approaches to treat "difficult" lesions suggest that the association of venous sacrifice(s) to brain retraction entails significantly higher risk of brain damage than retraction alone. It has been experimentally shown that parenchymal retraction of one hour duration, in opposition to retraction combined to venous sacrifice, produces a subcortical infarct in 13% and 60% of animals, respectively [15, 16].

Retraction of the brain provokes a local congestion

by compressing the cortical venous network, reduction in venous flow by stretching the bridging veins, and thrombosis of veins if compression of the retractor or a cotonoïd is prolonged. Excessive brain retraction can be avoided by specially designed approaches obeying two principles: the one of minimally invasive opening and the one of bone removal associated with craniotomy at the base of the skull. The key-hole approaches protect from important retraction and consequently avulsing veins.

Bone removal associated to craniotomies for skull base approaches, by increasing the field-view angle and the working-cone [1, 35], makes brain retraction unnecessary. Extended approaches as fronto-basal, orbital, zygomatic, orbito-zygomatic, at the level of the roof of the external auditory meatus, transpetrosal or extreme lateral of the foramen magnum, have become classical (see literature review in reference 24). Limited opening of the dura-mater to the minimum required is the most effective mean to avoid excessive retraction by the self-retractor.

In the eventuality of necessary prolonged retraction, releasing the retractor from time to time decreases damaging phenomena. Removing the blade approximately five minutes every fifteen minutes is considered beneficial.

It may happen that a bridging vein acts as a limitation. To be preserved, the vein has to be dissected free from arachnoid and cortex at a length of 10 to 20 mm [37]. It also may happen that a big vein inside a fissure or a sulcus performs as an obstacle. Because interruption would entail the risk to provoke "a cascade" of intraluminal coagulation of the neighbouring pial veins, it is justified to attempt its preservation. If conservation seems difficult, before deciding sacrifice a gentle temporary clamping for a few minutes with a microforceps or a small temporary clip may be useful to test the absence of consecutive regional congestion.

When an important vein has been ruptured, its reconstruction may be considered. For this purpose, the silicone tubing technique has been developed. "A silicone tube that is most suitable to the size of the vein origin is selected and inserted into the distal segment of the vein and fixed with a 10-0 monofilament nylon circumferential tie. The other end of the silicone tube is then inserted into the proximal end of the vein and tied" [23].

Frequent is the circumstance in which a (punctiform) wound is made in a vein wall during dissection. Rather than to coagulate the vein, hemostasis can be attempted by simply wrapping the wall with a small piece of Surgicel. If this is not sufficient, obliteration of the wound can be made by a very localized microcoagulation with a sharp bipolar forceps or by placing a single suture with a 10-0 nylon thread. But in all cases, whatever the technique used, quality of hemostasis has to be checked by jugular compression at the neck or with local patency test using two forceps, as classical in microvascular surgery.

Finally, it must be stressed that respect of the venous system results from a constant belief of the importance of preserving veins and a sustained effort to do it during the whole operation.

Tumors invading the major dural sinuses

Surgery

Tumors invading the major dural sinuses (superior sagittal sinus, torcular, transverse sinuses) specially meningiomas – leave the surgeon confronted with a difficult dilemma: leave the fragment invading the sinus and have a higher risk of recurrence, or attempt a total removal (with or without venous reconstruction) and expose the patient to potentially greater operative danger.

Within our surgical experience with 106 patients over the last 25 years, our policy was to rather attempt a total removal with venous reconstruction whenever it could be considered as "reasonable" [29, 31]. For decision-making, meningiomas were classified into six types according to the degree of sinus invasion [29, 30, 34]. Type 1: meningioma attached to outer surface of the sinus wall; Type II: lateral recess invaded; Type III: one lateral wall invaded; Type IV: one entire lateral wall and the roof of the sinus both invaded; Types V and VI: sinus totally occluded, one wall being free of tumor in type V (Fig. 2).

Based of this classification, surgery was attempted according the following scheme [29, 30, 34]. Type I: excision of the outer layer, leaving a clean inner layer with coagulation of the dural attachment; Type II: removal of the intraluminal fragment through the recess, then repair of the recess defect by resuturing the wound or by closing it with a (narrow) patch, or – provided it is not stenotic-sealing of the opening with a (tangentially positioned) aneurysm clip; Type III: resection of the invaded sinus wall and repair with patch (fascia temporalis); Type IV: resection of both invaded wall

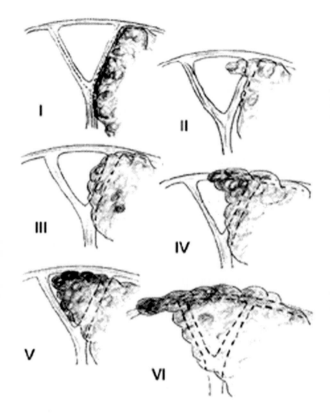

Fig. 2. Classification of meningiomas according to the degree of dural venous sinus involvement. *Type I*: meningioma attached to outer surface of the sinus wall; *Type II*: lateral recess invaded; *Type III*: one lateral wall invaded; *Type IV*: one entire lateral wall and the roof of the sinus both invaded; *Types V and VI*: sinus totally occluded, one wall being free of tumor in type V. This classification is a simplified one from Krause [17] quoted by Merrem [21] and Bonnal and Brotchi [8]

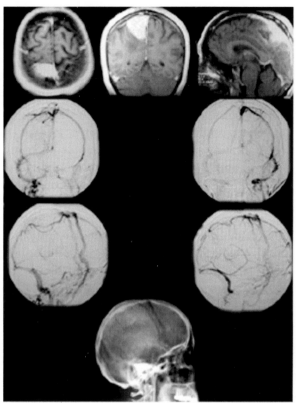

Fig. 3. *Upper row*: Axial, coronal and sagittal sections of T1 weighted MRI, with gadolinium, of a right-sided, midthird, parasagittal meningioma, of type VI. *Middle rows*: Right and left DSA carotid angiograms (AP and lateral views) showing bilateral diploic collateral venous channels draining the anterior part of the (totally occluded) superior sagittal sinus to skull base venous systems. *Lower row*: Plain film of the skull showing the bony aspect of the diploic collateral drainages. Plain X-ray may help to design the bone flap (and also the dural flap) so as to avoid interrupting major venous draining systems

and roof, and reconstruction with patch; Type V: this type can be formally recognized from type VI only by direct surgical exploration of the sinus lumen; as the opposite wall to the tumor side is free of tumor, it is possible to reconstruct the two invaded (and resected) walls with patch, rather than performing a bypass; Type VI: removal of the entire involved portion of sinus and restoration of venous flow with a venous bypass; the site of bypass is on the sagittal sinus for meningiomas involving SSS, between SSS and external jugular vein for meningiomas totally occluding the posterior third and/or the torcular, between TS and the external jugular vein for meningiomas involving the TS.

Surgery is greatly facilitated when the following technical aspects are respected. The semi-sitting (lounging) position allows a good venous return. Risk of air embolism is weak because of the relatively high level of the intracranial venous pressure in these patients. Skin flap and craniotomy should extend across the midline to permit visualization of both sides of the sinus and some 3 cm outside the margins of the occluded sinus. Access should consider cutaneous, pericranial and/or diploic, as well as dural venous pathways, which might be compromised during the approach. Those can be identified on preoperative imaging (venous angio-MRI and DSA with venous phases) (Fig. 3). Then the dura is incised in a circumferential manner around the margin of the tumor insertion on the dura of the convexity, and along the border of the corresponding portion of the superior sagittal sinus. Under the microscope the attatchment of the meningioma to the lateral wall of the sinus and to the neighbouring falx is desinserted by using the cutting effect of the bipolar coagulation forceps. Then an "intracapsular" debulking is carried out so that the meningioma can be dissected from the underlying cortex. Because of frequent discrepancies between images and anatomical lesions, the sinus should be explored through a short incision to disclose any intrasinusal fragment. Temporary control of venous bleeding from the lumen of the sinus, and from afferent veins, can be easily obtained by packing small pledgets of hemostatic material (Surgicel: Johnson and Johnson Medical, Viroflay, France) in the lumen and at the ostia of afferent veins. Balloons or shunts with inflatable balloons should not be used because they do not pass easily through the sinus septa and may disrupt the sinus endothelium. Vascular clamps and aneurysm clips should be avoided because they may injure sinus walls and afferent veins. For venous patching, although the autologous vein would appear as the most suitable material, vein harvesting seems excessive for patching only. The structure of the locally situated dura-mater or fascia temporalis (better than pericranium) are rigid enough to enable blood to flow inside and to use them as patches.

In cases with total invasion of the sinus, bypasses can be indicated to restore venous flow [32]. Bypasses may be performed either prior to removal of the occluded portion (with end-to-side anastomoses) or immediately after its removal (with end-to-end anastomoses). Bypasses must consist of autologous vein (saphenous when a long graft is needed, external jugular vein when only a short graft is necessary) and not of prothesis. (In our series the six cases undergoing a Gore-Tex bypass thrombosed within the first week; five thromboses were asymptomatic, but one was accompanied with a comatous state that was due to acute brain swelling, fortunately, reversible within 10 days. Suture on veins was performed using two hemirunning sutures, with Prolene 8-0 thread [Laboratoire Ethnor, Neuilly/Seine]. To avoid clotting into the reconstructed sinus, heparinotherapy ($2\times$ control) is recommended for at least 21 days and aspirin for the next two months to allow endothelization of the sinus walls.

Patency

Immediate patency essentially depends on the driving pressure within the dural venous system; this was obvious in our observations. Patency two weeks after surgery was studied using DSA in our series. In the 49 patients controlled – of the 52 who had venous reconstruction with patch or bypass-, sinus was patent in 36 cases (that is 73%): 9/9 for lateral recess suturing or patching, 20/23 for wall(s) patching, 7/11 for bypasses with autologous vein, 0/6 (= none) for bypasses with Gore-tex. Absence of long-term patency does not necessarily mean that venous reconstruction was not useful. Progressive occlusion of the venous repair would have given time for compensatory venous pathways to develop. In our series there was no neurological aggravation in those patients with not patent bypass, with the exception of one.

Conclusion

Our surgical experience leads us to advocate – whenever reasonably possible – the total removal of the tumor as the best way of significantly decreasing the recurrence rate of tumour regrowth (3% in our series of 106 patients).

We are also of the opinion that attempting to conserve or restore the venous circulation is preferable. As a matter of fact, the only way to be certain of the absence of wall invasion and of intraluminal tumor fragment, is to explore the wall(s) and open the lumen; this then necessitates reconstructing the sinus. We also think that it is advantageous to restore the venous circulation even if the sinus was occluded preoperatively. As a matter of fact, contrarily to established opinion, the completely occluded portion of the sinus cannot always be resected safely; surgical approach may impair collateral venous pathways. These reconstructions, being time-consuming and technically demanding, are of course only indicated in patients in good general condition.

Attempting radical resection of the tumor followed by venous reconstruction is also favored by other surgical teams [7–10, 12, 14, 25, 27, 36]. Others, although not totally opposed (see references in 34), prefer the conservative method of subtotal resection or staged operation [18]. An intermediate attitude would be to rely on the intra-operative measurement of the sinus pressure, together with consideration of the preoperative angiographic data on the venous circulation, to decide whether or not to reconstruct the venous circulation based on objective hemodynamic values.

But, whatever the procedure chosen may be, decisions should be reevaluated during surgery; one should be ready to stop the operation at any time and to eventually complete it later on, especially in case of imminent brain swelling would threaten.

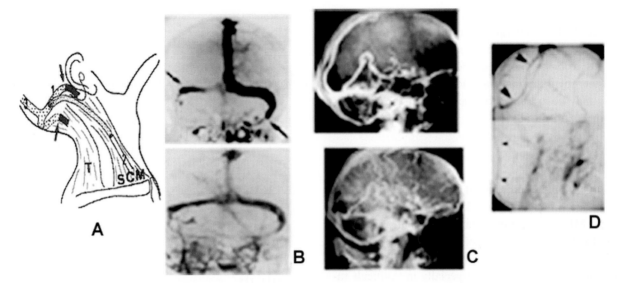

Fig. 4. *Sino-jugular bypasses*: (A) Schematic drawing of a transverse-jugular bypass, between right transverse sinus *(1)* and external jugular vein *(2)*, exposed anteriorly to sterno-cleido-mastoid *(SCM)* and trapezius *(T)* muscles (for – as an example – a bilaterally occluded lateral sinus (small arrows). (B) Post-otitic occlusion of both transverse sinuses in a child. Top: preoperative angiogram (venous phase, AP view) showing occlusion of both transverse sinuses (arrows). Bottom: postoperative angiogram (venous phase, AP view) showing patency of bypass with median saphenous graft (arrowhead). From transverse sinus to external jugular vein, right side. (C) Sino-jugular bypass for intracranial hypertension due to bilateral thrombosis of transverse sinuses, with right dural arterio-venous fistula *(AVF)*. Top: Pre-operative angiogram (lateral view) showing occlusion of the right transverse sinus (arrowhead). The dural AVF is clearly visible with retrograde filling of the sagittal and straight sinuses. Bottom: Post-operative angiogram (lateral view) showing complete removal of AVF and patent sino-jugular bypass (arrowheads). (D) Post-operative control at two weeks by DSA in a patient harbouring a grade VI torcular meningioma, and suffering severe intracranial pressure syndrome. Note the patent sino (sagittal)-jugular (external) bypass performed with a median saphenous vein graft (arrowheads), right side

Surgical restoration of venous flow for intracranial hypertension from venous occlusion

Patients presenting with manifestations of intracranial hypertension due to venous occlusion of posterior third of the superior sagittal sinus, torcular, predominant lateral sinus or internal jugular vein(s), cannot always be controlled efficiently with anti-edema therapy. According to literature estimations, in the order of 20% of cases develop severe intracranial hypertension with progressive loss of vision and/or encephalopathy. In these cases, venous revascularisation by sino-jugular bypass – implanted proximally to the occlusion and directed to the jugular venous system (external or internal jugular vein) – can be the solution [33].

Most frequent causes of "chronic" occlusion of dural sinuses are: 1) fibrosis after infectious thrombophlebitis and/or cruoric thromboses, 2) damage or ligation after trauma or surgery, 3) tumour totally occluding the posterior third of SSS (Intracranial hypertension or encephalopathy can be the revealing mode of a (even small) tumour or a residual fragment left in place occluding the lumen, 4) dural arterio-venous fistulas accompanying sinus thrombosis (restoration of the venous circulation after surgical excision seems to be appropriate because pathogenesis is though to be neo-vascularization after sinus thrombosis).

The rationale for sino-jugular bypass is that it suppresses the cause of intracranial hypertension or makes it reversible. Lumboperitoneal CSF shunting appears to be a simplier technique, but is not without pitfalls and complications. The good clinical long-term results observed in our series of 5 cases of sino-jugular bypasses plead in favour of this procedure as a logical treatment in these circumstances.

The original surgical technique was described in details in 1980 [33] and more recently, briefly, in 2000 [30] (see Fig. 4). Graft (that must be a long graft) has to be harvested from the median saphenous vein. In a eleven patients study (5 personal cases and 6 from the literature), patency rate was 82%; there was no mortality or morbidity. The receiver vein was the internal jugular vein in 5 cases (4 patent), the external jugular vein or a branch in 6 cases (5 patent). These results demonstrate the technical feasibility of restoration of the venous outflow with sino-jugular bypasses achieved with autologous venous grafts. Venous grafts are considered the best material for grafting by almost all the authors involved in experimental as well as in clinical venous reconstruction [32]. Postoperative anticoagulant therapy is an important adjunct for patency. Inocuity may be explained by the fact that the bypass is entirely extra-dural.

Conclusion

Surgery on the Intracranial Venous System requires good neuro-images to work on, not only Venous Angio-MR, as a complement of conventional MRI, but also DSA. As a matter of fact we think that DSA with late venous phases is of prime importance to determine surgical strategy especially in "difficult tumours". For these reasons neurosurgeons must incite neuro-imaging colleagues to be full-partners of neurosurgical management.

References

1. Alaywan M, Sindou M (1990) Fronto-temporal approach with orbito-zygomatic removal. Surgical anatomy. Acta Neurochir (Wien) 104: 79–83
2. Alaywan M, Sindou M (1996) Surgical anatomy of the lateral sinus approaches in the sigmoid region. In: Hakuba A (ed) Surgery of the intracranial venous system. Embryology, anatomy, pathophysiology, neuroradiology, diagnosis, Treatment. First International Workshop on Surgery of the Intracranial Venous System at Osaka September 1994. Springer, Berlin Heidelberg New York Tokyo, pp 63–72
3. Al-Mefty O, Krist AF (1996) The dangerous veins. In: Hakuba A (ed) Surgery of the intracranial venous system. Embryology, anatomy, pathophysiology, neuroradiology, diagnosis, treatment. First International Workshop on Surgery of the Intracranial Venous System at Osaka September 1994. Springer, Berlin Heidelberg New York Tokyo, pp 338–345
4. Apuzzo ML (1977) Surgery of the third ventricle. Williams & Wilkins, Baltimore
5. Auque J (1996) Le sacrifice veineux en neurochirurgie. Evaluation et gestion du risque. Neurochirurgie [Suppl] 1: 32–38
6. Auque J (1996) Microanatomie des veines profondes du cerveau. Neurochirurgie [Suppl] 1: 84–87
7. Bederson JB, Eisenberg MB (1995) Resection and replacement of the superior sagittal sinus for treatment of a parasagittal meningioma: Technical case report. Neurosurgery 37: 1015–1019
8. Bonnal J, Brotchi J (1978) Surgery of the superior sagittal sinus in parasagittal meningiomas. J Neurosurg 48: 935–945
9. Bonnal J, Brotchi J, Stevenaert A, Petrov VT, Mouchette R (1971) Excision of the intrasinusal portion of rolandic parasagittal meningiomas, followed by plastic surgery of the superior longitudinal sinus. Neurochirurgie 17: 341–354
10. Brotchi J, Patay Z, Baleriaux D (1996) Surgery of the superior sagittal sinus and neighbouring veins. In: Hakuba A (ed) Surgery of the intracranial venous system. Embryology, anatomy, pathophysiology, neuroradiology, diagnosis, treatment. First International Workshop on Surgery of the Intracranial Venous

System at Osaka September 1994. Springer, Berlin Heidelberg New York Tokyo, pp 207–219
11. Delandsheer JM, Guyot JF, Jomin M, Scherpereel B, Laine E (1978) Accès au troisième ventricule par voie interthalamotrigonale. Neurochirurgie 24: 419–422
12. Donaghy RM, Wallman LJ, Flanagan MJ, Numoto M (1973) Sagittal sinus repair. Technical note. J Neurosurg 38: 244–248
13. Hakuba A (1996) Surgery of the intracranial venous system. Embryology, anatomy, pathophysiology, neuroradiology, diagnosis, treatment. First International Workshop on Surgery of the Intracranial Venous System at Osaka September 1994. Springer, Berlin Heidelberg New York Tokyo
14. Hakuba A, Huh CW, Tsujikawa S, Nishimura S (1979) Total removal of a parasagittal meningioma of the posterior third of the sagittal sinus and its repair by autogenous vein graft. Case report. J Neurosurg 51: 379–382
15. Kanno T, Kasama A, Shoda M, Yamaguchi C, Kato Y (1989) A pitfall in the interhemispheric translamina terminalis approach for the removal of a craniopharyngioma. Significance of preserving draining veins. Part I. Clinical study. Surg Neurol 32: 111–115
16. Kasama A, Kanno T (1989) A pitfall in the interhemispheric translamina terminalis approach for the removal of a craniopharyngioma. Significance of preserving draining veins. Part II. Experimental study. Surg Neurol 32: 116–120
17. Krause F (1926) Operative Freilegung der Vierhügel, nebst Beobachtungen über Hirndruck und Dekompression. Zentralbl Neurochir 53: 2812–2819
18. Logue V (1975) Parasagittal meningiomas. Adv Tech Stand Neurosurg 2: 171–198
19. Malis LI (1996) Venous involvement in tumor resection. In: Hakuba A (ed) Surgery of the intracranial venous system. Embryology, anatomy, pathophysiology, neuroradiology, diagnosis, treatment. First International Workshop on Surgery of the Intracranial Venous System at Osaka September 1994. Springer, Berlin Heidelberg New York Tokyo pp 281–288
20. Matsushima T, Rhoton AL Jr, de Oliveira E, Peace D (1983) Microsurgical anatomy of the veins of the posterior fossa. J Neurosurg 59: 63–105
21. Merrem G (1970) Die parasagittalen Meningeome. Fedor Krause Gedächtnivorlesung. Acta Neurochir (Wien) 23: 203–216
22. Park J, Hamm IS (2004) Anterior interhemispheric approach for distal anterior cerebral artery aneurysm surgery: Preoperative analysis of the venous anatomy can help to avoid venous infarction. Acta Neurochir (Wien) 146: 973–977
23. Sakaki T, Morimoto T, Takemura K, Miyamoto S, Kyoi K, Utsumi S (1987) Reconstruction of cerebral cortical veins using silicone tubing. Technical note. J Neurosurg 66: 471–473
24. Samii M (1994) Skull base surgery. Anatomy, diagnosis and treatment. 1st International Skull Base Congress Hannover 1992. Karger, Basel
25. Schmid-Elsaesser R, Steiger HJ, Yousry T, Seelos KC, Reulen HJ (1997) Radical resection of meningiomas and arteriousvenous fistulas involving critical dural sinus segments: Experience with intraoperative sinus pressure monitoring and elective sinus reconstruction in 10 patients. Neurosurgery 41: 1005–1018
26. Schmidek HH, Auer LM, Kapp JP (1985) The cerebral venous system. Review. Neurosurgery 17: 663–678
27. Sekhar LN, Tzortzidis FN, Bejjani GK, Schessel DA (1997) Saphenous vein graft bypass of the sigmoid sinus and jugular bulb during the removal of glomus jugular tumors. Report of two cases. J Neurosurg 86: 1036–1041
28. Sindou M (2000) Microvascular decompression for trigeminal neuralgia. Chapter 130. In: Kaye AH, Black P McL (eds) Oper-

ative neurosurgery, vol 2. Churchill-Livingstone, London, pp 1595–1614

29. Sindou M (2001) Meningiomas invading the sagittal or transverse sinuses, resection with venous reconstruction. J Clin Neurosci [Suppl] 1: 8–11

30. Sindou M, Auque J (2000) The intracranial venous system as a neurosurgeon's perspective. Review. Adv Tech Stand Neurosurg 26: 131–216

31. Sindou M, Hallacq P (1996) Microsurgery of the venous system in meningiomas invading the major dural sinuses. In: Hakuba A (ed) Surgery of the intracranial venous system. Embryology, anatomy, pathophysiology, neuroradiology, diagnosis, treatment. First International Workshop on Surgery of the Intracranial Venous System at Osaka September 1994. Springer, Berlin Heidelberg New York Tokyo pp 226–236

32. Sindou M, Mazoyer JF, Fischer G, Pialat J, Fourcade C (1976) Experimental bypass for sagittal sinus repair. Preliminary report. J Neurosurg 44: 325–330

33. Sindou M, Mercier P, Bokor J, Brunon J (1980) Bilateral thrombosis of the transverse sinuses: Microsurgical revascularization with venous bypass. Surg Neurol 13: 215–220

34. Sindou M, Hallacq P (1998) Venous reconstruction in surgery of meningiomas invading the sagittal and transverse sinuses. Skull Base Surgery 8: 57–64

35. Sindou M, Emery E, Acevedo G, Ben-David U (2001) Respective indications for orbital rim, zygomatic arch and orbitozygomatic osteotomies in the surgtical approach to central skull base lesions. Critical, retrospective review in 146 cases. Acta Neurochir (Wien) 143: 967–975

36. Steiger HJ, Reulen HJ, Huber P, Boll J (1989) Radical resection of superior sagittal sinus meningioma with venous interpostion graft and reimplantation of the rolandic veins. Case report. Acta Neurochir (Wien) 100: 108–111

37. Sugita K, Kobayashi S, Yokoo A (1982) Preservation of large bridgings veins during brain retraction. Technical note. J Neurosurg 57: 856–858

38. Yamamoto I, Sato M (1996) Obliteration and its consequences for the deep venous system in surgical approaches to the third ventricle. In: Hakuba A (ed) Surgery of the intracranial venous system. Embryology, anatomy, pathophysiology, neuroradiology, diagnosis, treatment. First International Workshop on Surgery of the Intracranial Venous System at Osaka September 1994. Springer, Berlin Heidelberg New York Tokyo pp 321–329

39. Yasargil MG (1984) Microneurosurgery. Microsurgical anatomy of the basal cisterns and vessels of the brain, diagnostic and studies, vol 1. Thieme, Stuttgart New York

Correspondence: Marc P. Sindou, M.D., D. Sc., Hopital Neurologique P. Wertheimer, Department of Neurosurgery, University of Lyon, 59 Bd Pinel, 69003 Lyon, France. e-mail: marc.sindou@chu-lyon.fr

Acta Neurochir (2005) [Suppl] 94: 177–183
© Springer-Verlag 2005
Printed in Austria

Decompressive craniectomy in severe cerebral venous and dural sinus thrombosis

E. Keller[1], **A. Pangalu**[2], **J. Fandino**[3], **D. Könü**[1], and **Y. Yonekawa**[1]

[1] Department of Neurosurgery, University Hospital Zurich, Zurich, Switzerland
[2] Institute of Neuroradiology, University Hospital Zurich, Zurich, Switzerland
[3] Department of Neurosurgery, University Hospital Bern, Bern, Switzerland

Summary

Objective. To evaluate the outcome of patients with most severe cerebral venous and dural sinus thrombosis (CVT) after decompressive craniectomy. Indications and techniques for decompressive craniectomy and intensive care regimen are discussed.

Methods. Between 2000 and 2004 15 patients with CVT and intracerebral hemorrhage were treated at the Department of Neurosurgery, University Hospital Zurich. Among them, four patients with the most severe illness course were treated with decompressive craniectomy. Indications for decompressive craniectomy were deterioration of level of consciousness with CT signs of space occupying brain edema, venous infarction and congestional bleeding with mass effect, midline shift and obliteration of the basal cisterns.

Results. Among 15 patients with CVT and intraparenchymatous hemorrhage four patients were treated with decompressive craniectomy. Glasgow Coma Scale (GCS) immediately before the operation was in mean 10.2 (range 6 to 13). No patient showed signs of unilateral or bilateral third nerve palsy before surgery. No surgical complications were observed. All four patients who underwent decompressive craniectomy recovered with favourable functional outcome (Glasgow Outcome Scale; GOS 4 and 5). Anticoagulation therapy with heparin was reconvened 12 hours postoperatively with half dosage and 12 hours later with full dosage. No enlargement of existing intraparenchymatous hematoma or other intracranial bleeding complications occurred.

Conclusions. Favorable functional outcome in selected patients with most severe courses of CVT can be achieved after decompressive craniectomy. Postoperative anticoagulation therapy with full dose heparin 24 hours after craniotomy seems to be safe. Precise indications and techniques for combined surgical decompression and thrombectomy deserve to be evaluated in future studies.

Keywords: Cerebral venous and dural sinus thrombosis; venous infarction; congestional bleeding, brain edema; mass effect; intracranial pressure.

Introduction

Cerebral venous and dural sinus thrombosis (CVT) are with an annual incidence of approximately 1.5 to 3 per million adults a rare cause of stroke [28]. Because of early diagnosis and timely medical treatment in recent years morbidity and mortality decreased to 13.5% [30]. In smaller prospective case series papilledema, altered consciousness, coma and intraparenchymatous hemorrhage were suggested to be risk factors for unfavourable outcome [22]. The International Study on Cerebral Vein and Dural Sinus Thrombosis (ISCVT) confirmed that patients with primary CVT (no cancer, no nervous system infection) coma, mental status disorder, hemorrhage on admission CT scan, thrombosis of the deep cerebral venous system, male sex and age > 37 years are at increased risk of bad outcome [30].

The purpose of this report is to evaluate the outcome in a series of patients presenting severe courses of CVT who underwent decompressive craniectomy. A patient with most severe illness course with persistent ICP elevations, treated with decompressive craniectomy, hypothermia and barbiturate coma for 8 weeks is described. Indications for decompressive craniectomy, surgical techniques and timimg to reconvene anticoagulation therapy are discussed.

Materials and methods

Patient population

Between January 2000 and August 2004 15 patients with primary CVT and intraparenchymatous hemorrhage were treated at the Department of Neurosurgery, University Hospital Zurich. Among them, four patients with most severe illness course were treated with decompressive craniectomy. The charts and imaging studies of the 4 surgically treated patients were reviewed. Indications for surgery, surgical technique, perioperative complications, reinstitution of anticoagulation and the outcome were analyzed.

Medical treatment

On admission, all patients were rehydrated with intravenous cristalloids. Antiepileptic treatment with phenytoine or valproate was initiated as early as possible. After surgery, patients initially remained sedated (fentanyl infusion 2–8 ug/kg/h and midazolam 0.1–0.4 mg/kg/h). Subdural catheters (NMT Neuroscience, Frankfurt, Germany) were inserted to provide continuous intracranial pressure (ICP) monitoring. With elevated ICP (>15 mmHg) an emergency CT scan was performed and treatment with osmotherapy, mild hyperventilation and tris-hydroxy-methyl-aminomethane (THAM) buffer was initiated. Patients with intractable ICP-values of 15 mmHg or higher underwent reoperation for extension of bone flap or resection of infarcted tissue. Those patients with persistent high ICP values after the second surgical intervention were eligible for treatment with barbiturate coma combined with mild hypothermia. Medical therapy, barbiturate coma and hypothermia treatment were performed according to a standardized algorithm for treatment of elevated ICP described elsewhere [7]. Barbiturate coma was induced at the same time with induction of hypothermia and was adapted to a burst suppression pattern in continuous EEG-monitoring. Cooling of the patients (target brain temperature 33 °C) was accomplished by using endovascular cooling catheters (Cool Line Catheter and Coolgard System; Alsius Corporation, Irvine, CA, USA) [18].

Decompressive craniectomy

Indications for decompressive craniectomy included progressive neurological deterioration and CT signs of severe space occupying brain edema, venous infarction and congestional bleeding with mass effect, midline shift and obliteration of the basal cisterns with imminent herniation signs. Surgical decompression was defined in terms of an "external decompression" or fronto-temporo-parieto-occipital hemicraniectomy with additional dural patch (duraplasty) to allow adequate brain relaxation or "internal decompression" if resection of infacted cerebral tissue and total clot removal was performed. Replacement of the bone flap was performed within three months after "external decompression" if no signs of edema could be documented. Replacement of the bone flap depended on reduction of edema and was performed within three months after craniectomy. If, the affected brain tissue intraoperative seemed to be completely infarcted, with large space occupying intraparenchymatous hematoma, internal decompression with hematoma evacuation and resection of infarcted tissue was performed. After internal decompression, the bone flap was reinserted during the same operation.

Outcome measurements

Neurological outcome was assessed after three and 12 months in the outpatient clinic by a neurologist using the Glasgow Outcome Scale (GOS) [3]. Those patients who did not show up on control were contacted and asked about their functional status.

Results

Within the last 56 months four of 15 patients with primary CVT and intraparenchymatous bleeding were treated with decompressive craniectomy. Patient and treatment characteristics are given in Table 1. Mean age of the surgically treated patients was

47 ± 13.2 years. As risk factors two patients were using oral contraceptives, in one patient protein S deficiency was identified. Symptoms of CVT, in all cases with headache, occurred between three days and two weeks before admission to our department. Three patients were referred from other hospitals. Diagnoses were confirmed in three patients by intra-arterial digital subtraction angiography and in one patient by CT angiography. Thromboses were localized in two patients in the transverse and sigmoid sinuses, extending into the proximal internal jugular vein, in one patient in the anterior part of the superior sagital sinus and in one patient bilaterally in frontal cortical veins. Glasgow Coma Scale (GCS) immediately before the operation was in mean 10.2 (range 6 to 13). No patient showed signs of unilateral or bilateral third nerve palsy before surgery. In two patients (P2 and P3) craniotomy was performed as an emergency, immediately after the diagnosis was confirmed. In these patients anticoagulation treatment with heparin was started not before surgery, 12 hours after craniotomy with half dosage (9 U/kgBW/hour cont. i.v.) and 24 hours after surgery with full dosage (18 U/kgBW/hour cont. i.v.), adapted to a target thromboplastin time (PTT) of 2 to 2.5 fold. Two patients with secondary deterioration were treated with heparin before surgery, one coming from a foreign hospital, with heparin 10,000 U/24 h cont. i.v., the other with heparin 24,000 U/24 h cont. i.v. All patients were treated with full anticoagulation therapy, initially with heparin, later with phenprocoumon over 6 months. No enlargement of existing intraparenchymatous hematoma or other postoperative intracranial bleeding complications occurred. Two patients (P1 and P4) were treated with external and two patients with internal decompressive surgery. All four patients recovered with good functional outcome (GOS 4 and 5).

In two patients (P2 and P3) intraoperative evaluation showed macroscopically infarcted tissue with intraparenchymatous hemorrhage causing a severe mass effect (Figs. 1 and 2). This two patients were treated primarily with hematoma evacuation and resection of infarcted tissue (internal decompression). In both patients ICP remained below 15 mmHg postoperatively allowing a reduction of the sedation and extubation within three days after surgery. The two patients recovered with good functional outcome, one without deficits (P2), the other one (P3) with slight motoric dysphasia after 8 months. In the other two patients (P1 and P4), intraoperatively, the affected

Table 1. *Patient and treatment characteristics*

Patient date of bleeding	Gender	Age years	Type of thrombosis	Characterization of venous infarction/ hemorrhage	Symptoms	Treatment ICP-monitoring	-Barbiturate coma -Hypothermia	Surgery	VP-shunt	Final outcome
P1 16.4.00	F	39	anterior part of superior sagital sinus	right sided increase of brain volume, right parasagittal congestional bleeding, midline shift, imminent transcingular herniation	headache for 3 days, repeated generalized seizures (GCS 9)	subdural ICP-probe	– –	day 0: Rightsided removal of bone flap + duraplasty day 1: Right sided hematoma evacuation, resection of infarcted tissue	–	GOS 5 no residuals
P2 3.10.03	F	66	frontal cortical veins	bilateral frontal intracerebral hematoma	headache for 2 weeks, decrease of consciousness (GCS 6)	subdural ICP-probe	– –	day 0: Right sided total & left sided subtotal hematoma evacuation	–	GOS 5 no residuals
P3 15.1.04	M	46	left transverse and sigmoid sinus, internal jugular vein	left sided increase of brain volume, congestional temporo-parietal bleeding, midline shift, imminent transcingular herniation	headache for 3 days, rightsided hemiparesis, aphasia, decrease of consciousness (GCS 13)	subdural ICP-probe	– –	day 0: Left sided hematoma evacuation, resection of infarcted tissue	–	GOS 4 slight partial motoric dysphasia
P4 17.6.04	F	37	left transverse and sigmoid sinus, internal jugular vein	left sided increase of brain volume, congestional temporo-parietal bleeding, compression of left sided lateral ventricle, midline shift, imminent transcingular and uncal herniation	headache for 5 days, dysphasia, decrease of consciousness (GCS 13)	subdural ICP-probe ventricular drainage	+ +	day 0: Left sided removal of bone flap + duraplasty day 1: Extension of craniotomy + augmented duraplasty day 28: Ventricular drainage	+	*GOS 4 slight partial motoric dysphasia

M Male; *F* Female; *ICP* Intracranial pressure; *VP* ventriculoperitoneal; *GOS* Glasgow outcome score after one year; *GOS after 8 months.

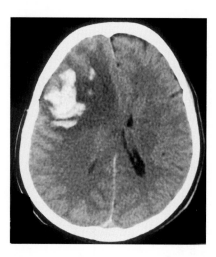

Fig. 1. Patient 1. CT scan, shows right sided frontal mass effect due to intraparenchymal bleeding with midline shift and imminent subfalcine herniation. Day 0 "external decompression" with right hemicraniectomy and duraplasty; day 1 "internal decompression" with right sided hematoma evacuation and resection of infarcted tissue were performed

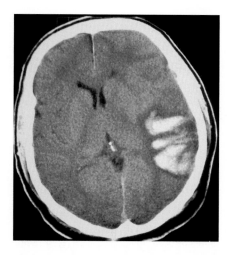

Fig. 3. Patient 3. CT scan, shows a temporo-parietal bleeding with midline shift, compression of the left sided ventricle and subfalcine herniation. Day 0 "internal decompression" with left sided evacuation of the hematoma and resection of infarcted tissue was performed

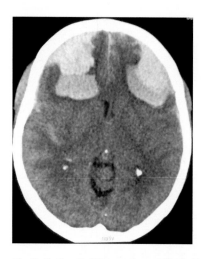

Fig. 2. Patient 2. CT scan, shows bifrontal intraparenchymal hematoma and subarachnoidal bleeding. Day 0 "internal decompression" with right sided total and left sided subtotal hematoma evacuation was performed

brain parenchyma seemed to be only partially infarcted, intraparenchymatous bleeding was more diffuse and hemispheric brain edema was dominant in its space-occupying effect (Figs. 1 and 4). These patients were treated primary with temporo-parieto-occipital craniectomy, removal of a large bone flap and duraplasty (external decompression). In both patients 12 hours after external decompression ICP increased above 15 mmHg. The two patients underwent a second intervention, the first one (P1) with hematoma evacuation and resection of infarcted tissue, the other

one (P4) with an extension of the craniotomy and duraplasty (see below). In P1 sedation could be stopped on day 3, the patient was extubated on day 7. Both patienst recovered without residuals.

P4 showed a most severe illness course over two months. Inspite of immediate treatment with full dose heparin, she deteriorated secondary after 12 hours. This right-handed patient presented with dysphasia, severe left sided brain edema with imminent uncal herniation and diffuse congestional temporo-parietal bleeding in ischemic brain tissue (Fig. 4a and 4b). Therefore, despite extensive brain swelling during craniotomy, only a large bone flap was removed combined with duraplasty without hematoma evacuation and resection of potentially viable tissue. Postoperative CT scan showed massive brain swelling with beginning herniation through the bone defect and still imminent uncal herniation (Fig. 1c). The patient underwent a second intervention for enlargement of the craniectomy and duraplasty (Fig. 1d). Nevertheless, the ICP increased up to 50 mmHg inspite of osmotherapy, THAM and mild hyperventilation. With combined hypothermia and barbiturate coma, the ICP could be controlled and cerebral perfusion pressure (CPP was maintained over 70 mmHg with aggressive fluid replacement and inotropes (noerepinephrine and dobutamine). Barbiturate coma was stopped and the patient had to be rewarmed after 18 days because of severe sepsis syndrome starting from a catheter infection. Intracranial hypertension persisted with ICP

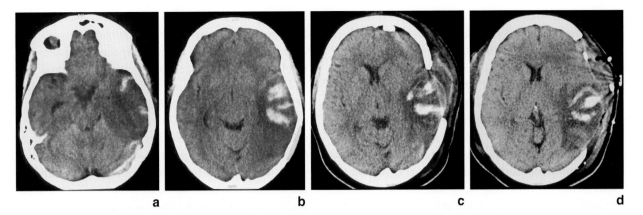

Fig. 4. Patient 4. (a and b) Show mass effect temporo-parietal left sided due to venous congestion and infarction and hemorrhage in the infarcted area. Compression of left sided lateral ventricle, midline shift and uncal herniation. (c) CT scan after first "external decompression". (d) CT scan after second "external decompression" with enlargement of the craniectomy and duraplasty. The compression of the left sided ventricle is diminishing

values between 20 and 30 mmHg. Fundoscopy showed persistent bilateral papilledema. On day 24, the patient was additionally treated with acetazolamide 4 × 250 mg i.v. which was effective in lowering ICP to 15–20 mmHg. On day 28, in CT scans brain swelling was declined and, with a normal size of the ventricular system a ventricular drainage was inserted into the left lateral ventricle. The patient was treated with cerebrospinal fluid (CSF) drainage (150–200 ml/day) and ICP values remained below 15 mmHg. Sedation was stopped after treatment of elevated ICP for 33 days. The patient developed a communicating hydrocephalus and ventriculoperitoneal shunt was inserted. The bone flap was implanted 2 months after surgery. In the 3-month follow-up evaluation of this patient only slight motoric dysphasia was described, otherwise the patient had no neurological deficits.

Discussion

In the largest cohort with 624 CVT patients (ISCVT study) death occurred in 8% and moderate to severe disability in 5.1% [30]. The authors suggested that high-risk patients may benefit from more aggressive therapeutic interventions.

Decompressive surgery for supratentorial arterial ischemic infarctions has been performed for decades [2, 21, 25, 26]. Krayenbühl in 1966 described four patients with CVT and space-occupying local or diffuse brain edema treated with decompressive craniotomy [24]. Three of them recovered with good outcome. In the following years two single case reports and one

case series with three patients treated with decompressive craniectomy were described [4, 6, 8]. All five patients were treated late in deep coma or with signs of diencephalic dysfunction [6] or fixed dilated pupils [4]. In severe middle cerebral artery (MCA) stroke patients, nevertheless, it has been shown that early decompressive craniectomy (before signs of herniation are apparent) improves survival and functional outcome [5, 21].

Indications for decompressive craniectomy in the present series of four patients with CVT were progressive neurological deterioration, together with characteristic CT signs of space occupying mass effect. Risk factors for an unfavourable outcome, identified with the ISCVT study were present in all our patients [30]. All four patients showed intraparenchymatous hemorrhage on admission CT scans, clinical deterioration and were 37 years old or older. GCS before surgery was in mean 10.2 and no patient showed signs of dienencepahlic syndrome or third nerve palsy. With the extended indications our patients were treated early avoiding irreversible brain damage due to herniation. All patients survived with good functional outcome. In previous series, with late decompressive surgery in CVT, three of five patients survived with good functional outcome [4, 6, 8].

In the present series two patients were treated primarily with "internal decompression" (craniectomy with hematoma evacuation and resection of infarcted tissue). In both patients, postoperatively, ICP normalized, sedation could be stopped the first day and the patients could be extubated early. The other two patients were treated with "external decompression" (craniectomy combined with duraplasty). In both of them, pronounced brain edema developed and ICP values increased within the first hours after craniotomy. They both had to be treated with a second surgical decompression. The two patients treated primarily with less invasive external decompression had more prolonged ICU courses. This might be due to bone flaps and dura extension, not being large enough to provide sufficient decompressive effect [11, 20]. On the other hand, with the very early surgical intervention, the affected brain tissue being congested but not yet completely infarcted, external decompression may lead to rapid resolve of venous congestion and reperfusion may attenuate increasing cytotoxic brain edema. In MCA stroke as well as in trauma patients different surgical techniques, decompressive craniectomy with dural augmentation versus internal decompression with removal of infarcted tissue and disimpaction of the uncus are extensively discussed [2, 21, 25, 26]. In this small case series with four patients the benefits of different surgical approaches can not be evaluated. The decision for the surgical technique may depend on the differentiation of viable from non-viable brain. Venous infarcts differ significantly from arterial infarcts in having more edema and less necrosis, explaining a higher potential for recovery [29]. It appears reasonable that, if during surgery it is visible that the affected brain regions are completely infarcted and intraparenchymatous bleeding is localized with extensive mass effect, one prefers primarily haematoma evacuation and resection of infarcted tissue. On the other hand, in patients with only partially infarcted brain parenchyma, diffuse intraparenchymatous bleeding and more prominent effect of space-occupying brain edema the less invasive technique with external decompression is preferred. In particular a little aggressive procedure is the more selected, if the brain region concerned is in a possibly eloquent area as it was with our fourth female patient the case.

As other invasive approaches, small case series with endovascular treatment (balloon angioplasty, rheolytic thrombectomy) or open thrombectomy, combined with thrombolysis (urokinase or tissue plasminogen activator) are described [8–10, 16, 19]. One case report documents the possibility of microsurgical revascularization with a venous bypass [15]. CVT leads to impaired venous outflow, venous congestion, infarction with cytotoxic brain edema and impaired reabsorption of CSF [9, 23]. Intracranial hypertension

develops, worsening these pathogenetic mechanisms. Decompressive surgery may interrupt this vicious circle by diminishing the intracapillary pressure thus resolving venous congestion, improving cerebral perfusion and allowing time for cortical collateral vein drainage [4]. On the other hand, thrombectomy, pharmacologic thrombolysis and venous bypass surgery are causal therapeutical approaches which might be combined with decompressive surgery.

Anticoagulation is the most important therapeutic starting point in medical treatment of CVT even in patients with intraparenchymatous hemorrhage [1, 13, 27]. Heparin restrains the propagation of the clot [12, 29]. Therefore, despite an increased bleeding risk with full dose anticoagulation initiated early after craniotomy [14], in our patients heparin was started 12 hours postoperatively with half dosage (9 U/kg BW/hour cont. i.v.) and 24 hours after surgery with full dosage (18 U/kg BW/hour cont. i.v.), adapted to a target PTT of 2 to 2.5 fold. No enlargement of existing intraparenchymatous hematoma or other intracranial bleeding complications occurred.

With persistent intracranial hypertension after extensive surgical decompression, conventional ICP treatment modalities (osmotherapy, THAM-buffer and mild hyperventilation) may be insufficient. In patients with extensive brain edema the insert of a ventricle probe for CSF drainage is often not possible by the compression of the side ventricles. In these most severe cases, treatment with barbiturate coma and/or mild hypothermia with ICP lowering and neuroprotective properties [18] are to be considered.

Patients with persistent papilledema and intracranial hypertension inspite of decreased brain edema, normal ventricles on neuroimaging and normal CSF composition fullfill the criteria of pseudotumor cerebri [17]. In these patients visual loss may be insidious and ventriculoperitoneal shunting may be performed.

In conclusion: Favourable funtional outcome in selected patients with most severe courses of CVT can be achieved by early decompressive craniectomy. Indications for early surgery are progressive deterioration instead of adequate anticoagulation therapy, with CT signs of mass effect by space occupying brain edema, venous infarction and congestional bleeding, leading to midline shift and/or obliteration of the basal cisterns indicating imminent brain herniation within the next hours or days. Anticoagulation therapy with full dose heparin 24 hours after craniotomy seems to be safe. Results of a larger series would be valuable in supporting our hypothesis that surgery in an early stage of disease may be beneficial and that internal as well as external craniectomy have their place, depending on every individuals clinical and CT findings. In future, techniques for decompressive surgery combined with thrombectomy deserve to be evaluated.

References

1. Bousser MG, Chiras J, Bories J, Castaigne P (1985) Cerebral venous thrombosis – a review of 38 cases. Stroke 16: 199–213
2. Brazis PW (2004) Pseudotumor cerebri. Review. Curr Neurol Neurosci Rep 4: 111–116
3. Chow K, Gobin YP, Saver J, Kidwell C, Dong P, Vinuela F (2000) Endovascular treatment of dural sinus thrombosis with rheolytic thrombectomy and intra-arterial thrombolysis. Stroke 31: 1420–1425
4. Clark K, Nash TM, Hutchison GC (1968) The failure of circumferential craniotomy in acute traumatic cerebral swelling. J Neurosurg 29: 367–371
5. Crassard I, Bousser MG (2004) Cerebral venous thrombosis. Review. J Neuroophthalmol 24: 156–163
6. de Bruijn SF, de Haan RJ, Stam J (2001) Clinical features and prognostic factors of cerebral venous sinus thrombosis in a prospective series of 59 patients. For the Cerebral Venous Sinus Thrombosis Study Group. J Neurol Neurosurg Psychiatry 70: 105–108
7. de Bruijn SF, Stam J (1999) Randomized, placebo-controlled trial of anticoagulant treatment with low-molecular-weight heparin for cerebral sinus thrombosis. Stroke 30: 484–488
8. Einhaupl KM, Villringer A, Meister W, Mehraein S, Garner C, Pellkofer M, Haberl RL, Pfister HW, Schmiedek P (1991) Heparin treatment in sinus venous thrombosis. Lancet 338: 597–600
9. Ekseth K, Bostrom S, Vegfors M (1998) Reversibility of severe sagittal sinus thrombosis with open surgical thrombectomy combined with local infusion of tissue plasminogen activator: technical case report. Neurosurgery 43: 960–965
10. Ferro JM, Canhao P, Stam J, Bousser MG, Barinagarrementeria F, ISCVT Investigators (2004) Prognosis of cerebral vein and dural sinus thrombosis results of the international study on cerebral vein and dural sinus thrombosis (ISCVT). Stroke 35: 664–670
11. Frerichs KU, Deckert M, Kempski O, Schurer L, Einhaupl K, Baethmann A (1994) Cerebral sinus and venous thrombosis in rats induces long-term deficits in brain function and morphology – evidence for a cytotoxic genesis. J Cereb Blood Flow Metab 4: 289–300
12. Gasser S, Khan N, Yonekawa Y, Imhof HG, Keller E (2003) Long-term hypothermia in patients with severe brain edema after poor-grade subarachnoid hemorrhage: feasibility and intensive care complications. J Neurosurg Anesthesiol 15: 240–248
13. Ivamoto HS, Numoto M, Donaghy RM (1974) Surgical decompression for cerebral and cerebellar infacts. Stroke 5: 365–370
14. Jennett B, Snoek J, Bond MR, Brooks N (1981) Disability after severe head injury: observations on the use of the Glasgow Outcome Scale. J Neurol Neurosurg Psychiatry 44: 285–293
15. Keller E, Imhof HG, Gasser S, Terzic A, Yonekawa Y (2003) Endovascular cooling with heat exchange catheters: a new method to induce and maintain hypothermia. Intensive Care Med 29: 939–943
16. Kourtopoulos H, Christie M, Rath B (1994) Open thrombectomy combined with thrombolysis in massive intracranial sinus thrombosis. Acta Neurochir (Wien) 128: 171–173
17. Krayenbuhl HG (1966) Cerebral venous and sinus thrombosis. Clin Neurosurg 14: 1–24
18. Lazio BE, Simard JM (1999) Anticoagulation in neurosurgical patients. Review. Neurosurgery 45: 838–848
19. Persson L, Lilja A (1990) Extensive dural sinus thrombosis treated by surgical removal and local streptokinase infusion. Neurosurgery 26: 117–121
20. Rieke K, Krieger D, Adams HP, Aschoff A, Meyding-Lamade U, Hacke W (1993) Therapeutic strategies in space-occupying cerebellar infarction based on clinical, neuroradiological and neurophysiological data. Cerebrovasc Dis 3: 45–55
21. Rieke K, Schwab S, Krieger D, von Kummer R, Aschoff A, Schuchardt V, Hacke W (1995) Decompressive surgery in space-occupying hemispheric infarction: results of an open, prospective trial. Review. Crit Care Med 23: 1576–1587
22. Robertson SC, Lennarson P, Hasan DM, Traynelis VC (2004) Clinical course and surgical management of massive cerebral infraction. Neurosurgery 55: 55–62
23. Schwab S, Steiner T, Aschoff A, Schwarz S, Steiner HH, Jansen O, Hacke W (1998) Early hemicraniectomy in patients with complete middle cerebral artery infarction. Stroke 29: 1888–1893
24. Sindou M, Mercier P, Bokor J, Brunon J (1980) Bilateral thrombosis of the transverse sinuses: microsurgical revascularization with venous bypass. Surg Neurol 13: 215–220
25. Soleau SW, Schmidt R, Stevens S, Osborn A, MacDonald JD (2003) Extensive experience with dural sinus thrombosis. Neurosurgery 52: 534–544
26. Stam J, de Bruijn SF, deVeber G (2003) Anticoagulation for cerebral sinus thrombosis. Stroke 34: 1054–1055
27. Stam J (2003) Cerebral venous and sinus thrombosis: incidence and causes. Adv Neurol 92: 225–232
28. Stefini R, Latronico N, Cornali C, Rasulo F, Bollati A (1999) Emergent decompressive craniectomy in patients with fixed dilated pupils due cerebral venous and dural sinus thrombosis: report of three cases. Neurosurgery 45: 626–630
29. Weber J, Spring A (2004) Unilaterale dekompressive Kraniektomie bei Thrombose des linken Sinus transversus und sigmoideus. Zentralbl Neurochir 65: 135–140
30. Yonekawa Y, Konu D, Roth P, Keller E (2003) Surgery for acute stroke, chapter 14. In: Bogousslavsky J (ed) Acute stroke treatment, 2nd edn. Dunitz, London New York, pp 209–232

Correspondence: Emanuela Keller, Department of Neurosurgery, University Hospital, Frauenklinikstrasse 10, 8091 Zurich, Switzerland. e-mail: emanuela.keller@usz.ch

Author index

Index of keywords

SpringerNeurosurgery

K. R. H von Wild (ed.)

Re-Engineering of the Damaged Brain and Spinal Cord

Evidence – Based
Neurorehabilitation

In Cooperation with Giorgio A. Brunelli.
2005. XVI, 232 pages. 55 figures.
Hardcover **EUR 120,–**
Reduced price for subscribers to "Acta Neurochirurgica": **EUR 108,–**
(Recommended retail prices)
Net-prices subject to local VAT.
ISBN 3-211-24150-7
Acta Neurochirurgica, Supplement 93

Traumatic Brain Injury (TBI) can lead to loss of skills and to mental cognitive behavioural deficits. Paraplegia after Spinal Cord Injury (SCI) means a life-long sentence of paralysis, sensory loss, dependence and in both, TBI and SCI, waiting for a miracle therapy. Recent advances in functional neurosurgery, neuropros-thesis, robotic devices and cell transplantation have opened up a new era. New drugs and reconstructive surgical concepts are on the horizon. Social reintegra-tion is based on holistic rehabilitation. Psychological treatment can alleviate and strengthen affected life. This book reflects important aspects of physiology and new trans-disciplinary approaches for acute treatment and rehabilitation in neu-rotraumatology by reviewing evidence based concepts as they were discussed among bio and gene-technologists, physicians, neuropsychologists and other therapists at the joint international congress in Brescia 2004.

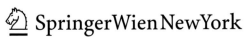 SpringerWienNewYork

P.O. Box 89, Sachsenplatz 4–6, 1201 Vienna, Austria, Fax +43.1.330 24 26, books@springer.at, **springer.at**
Haberstraße 7, 69126 Heidelberg, Germany, Fax +49.6221.345-4229, SDC-bookorder@springer-sbm.com, springeronline.com
P.O. Box 2485, Secaucus, NJ 07096-2485, USA, Fax +1.201.348-4505, orders@springer-ny.com, springeronline.com
Eastern Book Service, 3–13, Hongo 3-chome, Bunkyo-ku, Tokyo 113, Japan, Fax +81.3.38 18 08 64, orders@svt-ebs.co.jp
Prices are subject to change without notice. All errors and omissions excepted.

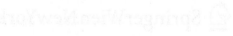

SpringerNeurosurgery

Alberto Alexandre, Albino Bricolo,
Hanno Millesi (eds.)

Advanced Peripheral Nerve Surgery and Minimal Invasive Spinal Surgery

2005. XI, 157 pages.
Hardcover **EUR 98,–**
Reduced price for subscribers to "Acta Neurochirurgica": **EUR 89,–**
(Recommended retail prices)
All prices are net-prices subject to local VAT.
ISBN 3-211-23368-7
Acta Neurochirurgica, Supplement 92

The papers in this volume summarize information about the most recent and effective techniques for treating diffcult functional problems and painful situations by using minimally invasive spinal surgery techniques. Spinal endoscopy both for diagnostic and treatment purposes is presented as well as microsurgical operations for spinal problems, intradiscal techniques for the treatment of disc degenerative pathology, and dynamic stabilization techniques together with an up-to-date review of physiopathology of the diseases. New trends in peripheral nerve surgery are presented. Also the problem of traumatic nerve lesions in different anatomical districts is analyzed with special attention on the theme of thoracic outlet syndrome. The posttraumatic aspects of this disease are discussed both in respect of its causative mechanisms, and its medicolegal aspects.

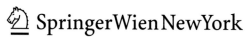 **Springer**Wien NewYork

P.O. Box 89, Sachsenplatz 4–6, 1201 Vienna, Austria, Fax +43.1.330 24 26, books@springer.at, **springer.at**
Haberstraße 7, 69126 Heidelberg, Germany, Fax +49.6221.345-4229, SDC-bookorder@springer-sbm.com, springeronline.com
P.O. Box 2485, Secaucus, NJ 07096-2485, USA, Fax +1.201.348-4505, orders@springer-ny.com, springeronline.com
Eastern Book Service, 3–13, Hongo 3-chome, Bunkyo-ku, Tokyo 113, Japan, Fax +81.3.38 18 08 64, orders@svt-ebs.co.jp
Prices are subject to change without notice. All errors and omissions excepted.

SpringerNeurosurgery

Berndt Wowra, Jörg-Christian Tonn,
Alexander Muacevic (eds.)

Gamma Knife Radiosurgery

European Standards and Perspectives

2005. VII, 111 pages. With partly coloured figures.
Hardcover **EUR 89,–**
Reduced price for subscribers to "Acta Neurochirurgica": **EUR 80,–**
(Recommended retail prices)
Net-prices subject to local VAT.
ISBN 3-211-22870-5
Acta Neurochirurgica, Supplement 91

Gamma knife radiosurgery has grown continually in importance in recent years. However, there was a lack of established clinical and physical quality standards and a good knowledge of the possibilities of radiosurgical treatment for brain lesions. This book fills the gap by giving an overview of the current status of European gamma knife radiosurgery. Leading european experts report on their specialities in this field which is a state-of-the-art summary of the possibilities and results of their current work. The book encompasses all important as well as the more rare indications. All relevant technical and clinical quality standards are addressed. Tailored planning strategies are described for different indications. All professionals who care for patients with neurosurgical disease, such as neurosurgeons, radiosurgeons, radiologists, radiation oncologists and neurologists will find the book highly useful for the management of patients with benign and malignant brain lesions in a multidisciplinary setting.

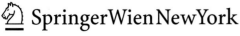 SpringerWien NewYork

P.O. Box 89, Sachsenplatz 4–6, 1201 Vienna, Austria, Fax +43.1.330 24 26, books@springer.at, **springer.at**
Haberstraße 7, 69126 Heidelberg, Germany, Fax +49.6221.345-4229, SDC-bookorder@springer-sbm.com, springeronline.com
P.O. Box 2485, Secaucus, NJ 07096-2485, USA, Fax +1.201.348-4505, orders@springer-ny.com, springeronline.com
Eastern Book Service, 3–13, Hongo 3-chome, Bunkyo-ku, Tokyo 113, Japan, Fax +81.3.38 18 08 64, orders@svt-ebs.co.jp
Prices are subject to change without notice. All errors and omissions excepted.

SpringerNeurosurgery

Berndt Wowra, Jörg-Christian Tonn, Alexander Muacevic (eds.)

Gamma Knife Radiosurgery

SpringerWienNewYork

SpringerNeurosurgery

H.-J. Reulen (ed.)
in collaboration with J. Brennum, Fl. Gjerris,
J. Haase, W. Kanpolat, D. Lang. K. W. Lindsay,
J. Lobo Antunes, D. W. Long, G. Neil Dwyer,
G. Schackert, J. Steers, H. J. Steiger, J. C. Tonn,
T. Trojanowski, P. A. Winkler

Training in Neurosurgery in the Countries of the EU

A Guide to Organize a Training Programme

2004. VIII, 125 pages. 4 figures.
Hardcover **EUR 98,–**
Reduced price for subscribers to "Acta Neurochirurgica": **EUR 89,–**
(Recommended retail prices)
Net-prices subject to local VAT.
ISBN 3-211-21322-8
Acta Neurochirurgica, Supplement 90

Agreed standards and guidelines are the heart and soul of improving the differing training systems and to harmonize neurosurgical training in the European countries. Such standards and guidelines have been laid down in the European Training Charter of the European Union of Medical Specialists and recently novellated.

This book, written by experienced neurosurgeons, offers all those concerned with neurosurgical training – trainers and trainees – practical advice to implement the above mentioned standards and recommendations. It has been written as a manual: "How to do it". It describes the tasks of a chairman (programme director), the tasks of the teaching staff, the organisation of a training curriculum, a rotation plan or a morbidity and mortality conference, the periodic progress evaluation, the course of an external audit and many more important topics. It contains a lot of practical tips, check lists and useful examples.

Well educated young colleagues offer "safe neurosurgery" to our patients.

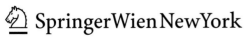 SpringerWienNewYork

P.O. Box 89, Sachsenplatz 4–6, 1201 Vienna, Austria, Fax +43.1.330 24 26, books@springer.at, **springer.at**
Haberstraße 7, 69126 Heidelberg, Germany, Fax +49.6221.345-4229, SDC-bookorder@springer-sbm.com, springeronline.com
P.O. Box 2485, Secaucus, NJ 07096-2485, USA, Fax +1.201.348-4505, orders@springer-ny.com, springeronline.com
Eastern Book Service, 3–13, Hongo 3-chome, Bunkyo-ku, Tokyo 113, Japan, Fax +81.3.38 18 08 64, orders@svt-ebs.co.jp
Prices are subject to change without notice. All errors and omissions excepted.

Springer and the Environment